Essential Medical Facts
Every Clinician Should Know

Robert B. Taylor

Essential Medical Facts Every Clinician Should Know

To Prevent Medical Errors, Pass Board Examinations and Provide Informed Patient Care

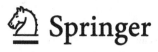 Springer

Robert B. Taylor
Department of Family Medicine
School of Medicine
Oregon Health & Sciences University
3181 SW Sam Jackson Park Road
Portland, Oregon, 97239
USA
taylorr@ohsu.edu

ISBN 978-1-4419-7873-8   e-ISBN 978-1-4419-7874-5
DOI 10.1007/978-1-4419-7874-5
Springer New York Dordrecht Heidelberg London

Printed on acid-free paper

Springer is part of Springer Science+Business Media (www.springer.com)

*To Practicing Clinicians everywhere, who
translate current research into informed and
evidence-based patient care*

*While
Pondering undiff. symptoms and signs,
Help the suffering......;
Reporting progress and....;
Avoiding diagnositic....
And keeping up with essential....*

It might be illusory to imagine that we can learn from the mistakes of others, but the alternative is to make them all ourselves.

Stephens GG. A family doctor's rules for clinical conversations.
J Am Board of Fam Pract 1994; 7(2): 179-181.

Men occasionally stumble across the truth, but most of them pick themselves up and hurry off as if nothing happened.

Winston Churchill. Quoted in: Meyers MA. Happy Accidents.
New York: Arcade Books; 2007. Page 19.

#####

Clinical abilities, mature wisdom and human compassion can all help make us good clinicians.

Knowing essential medical facts can help us avoid mistakes.

Preface

Medical textbooks, continuing education programs and reference sources all provide the knowledge base needed for competent medical practice. This book presents the rest of what you need to know to be an outstanding clinician. *Essential Medical Facts* goes beyond basic teachings, presenting bits of medical knowledge that can help prevent diagnostic blunders and therapeutic missteps. After all, mastery of disease templates and principles of management can make you a good doctor, but that is not enough; you also need your arsenal of discrete medical facts. *Essential Medical Facts* may just allow you to sidestep some of medicine's many hidden landmines, such as the Achilles tendinitis and possible rupture that can occasionally follow use of a quinolone antibiotic.

I have been a medical writer and book editor for more than three decades, much of this time spent compiling huge – think of a volume weighing 10 pounds – clinical reference books, a publication model now becoming an anachronism. Today clinicians hunting for the answers to questions can find more timely information on line, and they can find it faster than searching the index and then the numbered pages of a heavy tome. But medical web sources – both the subscription reference sites and PubMed – often frustrate us when we don't know what question to ask. Enter the "topical book," the book of facts, containing snippets of information that really should be in your memory bank and mine, and that may well be somewhere in the traditional reference sources, but will remain hidden there unless we think to look. The answer to retrieving medical facts is not a book of answers, but a book of prompts. *Essential Medical Facts* is just such a topical book.

Do you need this book? Here is a quiz that can help you decide.

- What types of migraine headache should not be treated with 5-hydroxytriptamine receptor agonists such as sumatriptan (Imitrex)?
- What should you suspect when you find anemia in a long distance runner?
- Can you name an herbal remedy that can decrease the INR (International Normalized Ratio), and thereby reduce the effectiveness of warfarin (Coumadin) anticoagulation?
- Do you know the clue that can help distinguish the neurogenic claudication of spinal stenosis from vascular claudication as a cause of pain in the lower extremities?

- Are you aware of the disease that should be suspected when you find nasal polyps in a child age 12 or younger?
- Which one of the commonly used antiepileptic drugs is associated with an increased risk of impaired cognition in infants at age 3 when there has been in utero exposure?
- Can you describe the clue to early diagnosis of herpes zoster infection of the eye?

If you can't answer most of the seven questions above, don't see the next patient until you have read this book.

Who needs this book? No matter what your area of specialization, you are first and foremost a clinician, a truism with implications in terms of your broad-based knowledge and skills. At some time on our educational journey, each of us chooses a focus of emphasis in medicine, be it surgery, psychiatry, gastroenterology, geriatrics, sports medicine or something else. This book is designed to be a reminder that, however narrow or broad our current scope of practice, all of us need to know medicine's fundamental statistical probabilities and clinical correlations, the evidence-based diagnostic and therapeutic pearls, and the sometimes quirky side effects of drugs we prescribe, even if the information might seem to be outside our personal spheres of expertise.

We need to know about more than just our limited specialty areas because of an awkward reality in medicine: Rare is the patient with one disease, conveniently limited to a single organ or body system. And knowing about your patient's "other" diseases – even if not confined to your favorite organ, system or other area of proficiency – may be vital to success in diagnosis or therapy of your patient's problem.

In the sense that this book is abundantly referenced, the facts presented are evidence-based. I recognize that many of the items presented are the result of a single clinical trial or meta-analysis, or even, in a few cases, the subject of a review article, and may be challenged by conflicting opinion or emerging information. No matter. The statements in this book will, I hope, stick like *Post-It Notes* in your memory, there to alert you just when you might be about to overlook a key clinical finding or make a medication error.

In addition to stating facts and describing the supporting studies, I have added editorial comments in *italics*. These annotations are intended to help clarify the facts reported and as reminders to think further about their implications. Also, because medical books don't need to be dry and boring, in some instances I have included comments to link the stated fact to a favorite clinical aphorism or an event in history. Just for the record, names and circumstances in case histories have been modified to protect confidentiality.

Within the chapters that follow, facts are presented in no special sequence. I have done this for two reasons. First of all, in most chapters I couldn't think of a logical way to order the data. Does a fact about headache logically come before or after a statement about obesity, or is there any reason to discuss one diagnostic pearl before another? Secondly, patients with clinical problems present in random order: If you are seeing a patient with fatigue, the next person may describe backache and the next, a skin rash.

How should you use this "topical" book? Think of it as an exercise in "speed-learning." I recommend that, in contradistinction to the typical medical reference book, you read this book cover to cover. Then, in the clinic or hospital, when you come across a situation that jogs your memory – recall that *Post-It Note* metaphor above – *Essential Medical Facts* can serve as a reference book; find the topic in the index, and then on the book page. You can use the citations provided to check out the source articles on line, which may set the agenda for your own up-to-the-minute literature search. If even a few such searches help avoid serious clinical misadventures, the effort will have been worthwhile.

Thank you for reading this book. If you come across *Essential Medical Facts* that should be included in the future, I would be pleased to receive them by email: taylorr@ohsu.edu

PS. The answers to the seven questions are in the book. You can find each quickly by using the index, or just go ahead and read every chapter.

Portland, OR   Robert B. Taylor

Acknowledgments

Many persons helped with this book, sometimes without even knowing they were doing so. At the top of this list is my family: Anita D. Taylor, MA Ed, an accomplished author, perceptive proofreader and fearless critic; our children Diana and Sharon; and our four grandchildren, Francesca (Frankie), Elizabeth (Masha), Jack, and Anna (Annie). In addition, I want to acknowledge just some of the many physicians who, over the years, have shared their friendship, wisdom, and clinical insights. In no special order, these valued persons are: Doctors Robin Hull, Bob Bomengen, Ray Friedman, Tom Deutsch, John Saultz, Bill Toffler, Scott Fields, Eric Walsh, Rick Deyo, Peter Goodwin, Ben Jones, Joe Scherger, Takashi Yamada, Ryuki Kassai and John Kendall. I offer a special thanks to Coelleda O'Neil, who has helped me with my books for more than two decades. In addition, I gratefully acknowledge the excellent work of my Springer editor, Katharine Cacace.

Contents

Clinical Practice Notice

Everyone involved with the preparation of this book has worked very hard to assure that information presented here is accurate and that it represents accepted clinical practice. These efforts include confirming that drug usage discussed in this text are in accordance with current practice at the time of publication. Nevertheless, therapeutic recommendations and dosage schedules change with reports of ongoing research, updated guideline recommendations, reports of adverse drug reactions, and other new information.

A few drugs mentioned herein have Food and Drug Administration (FDA) clearance for limited use in restricted settings. Some discussions in the book describe novel uses of drugs. It is the responsibility of the clinician to determine the FDA status of any drug selection, drug dosage, or device recommended to patients.

The reader should check the package insert for each drug to determine any change in indications or dosage as well as for any precautions or warnings. This admonition is especially true when the drug considered is new or infrequently used by the clinician.

The use of the information in this book in a specific clinical setting or situation is the professional responsibility of the clinician. The authors, editors, or publisher are not responsible for errors, omissions, adverse effects, or any consequences arising from the use of information in this book, and make no warranty, expressed or implied, with respect to the completeness, timeliness, or accuracy of the book's contents.

Chapter 1
Medical Facts, Errors, and This Book

The education of the doctor which goes on
after he has his degree is, after all,
the most important part of his education.

American surgeon and librarian John Shaw Billings (1838–1939) [1]

This book presents literally hundreds of facts, based on the conclusions of published research reports, meta-analyses and other sources. We clinicians are responsible for knowing the "facts of the day," the current evidence that forms the basis of practice. Although some of these facts can be traced to our professional school education, most have become known after we received our degrees. As an example, most of the drugs we use today – the proton pump inhibitors, the angiotensin converting enzyme (ACE) inhibitors, the statins, the triptans, and more – have been introduced since I received my MD degree, and I have learned about them outside the medical school classroom. Thus for me, and for you, learning about timely and essential facts becomes, in the words of Billings, "the most important part of [our] education."

The following case illustrates the importance of keeping up to date with current facts, both in our own disciplines and in areas that seem outside of our daily scope of practice:

Dr. Kline, a radiologist specializing in mammography in a midwestern city, read with interest the 2008 report by Lambertz et al., telling how "premedication with 4% lidocaine gel significantly reduced discomfort during screening mammography." The authors speculate that the reduced pain of mammography will lessen resistance to future imaging, and hence enhance breast cancer detection [2]. Based on the result of this prospective, double-blinded, placebo-controlled trial, in the fall of 2008, Dr. Kline decided to employ this method in his mammography practice. He followed the described protocol of having a nurse apply 4% lidocaine gel from the clavicles down to the inferior costal margins and laterally to the mid-axillary lines, followed by the application of a plastic wrap.

Dr. Kline's patients generally accepted the lidocaine gel applications well, many commenting on the reduced discomfort with the procedure. Then one morning in December, while beginning her mammography, a 52 year-old patient developed lightheadedness and an irregular heartbeat, followed by a grand mal seizure. She was rushed to the emergency department, subsequently admitted to the hospital. Fortunately, she made a full recovery and was discharged 2 days later.

R.B. Taylor, *Essential Medical Facts Every Clinician Should Know: To Prevent Medical Errors, Pass Board Examinations and Provide Informed Patient Care*, DOI 10.1007/978-1-4419-7874-5_1, © Springer Science+Business Media, LLC 2011

The essential fact that the radiologist probably did not know was this, and I am quoting from the Food and Drug Administration (FDA) web site: "On February 6, 2007, the Food and Drug Administration issued a Public Health Advisory titled: Use of Skin Products Containing Numbing Ingredients for Cosmetic Procedures and Life Threatening Side Effects" [3]. The FDA web site goes on to discuss the risks associated with the application of large amounts of topical anesthetics to the skin, including irregular heartbeat, seizures and death. They describe the instances in which two women, ages 22 and 25, applied topical anesthetics to their legs to reduce the pain of laser hair removal. Following application of the topical anesthetic, they applied plastic wrap to the legs. Both women had seizures, fell into comas, and subsequently died.

There were red flags raised in the cosmetic surgery literature, such as the June, 2008 report by Kaweski describing the use and hazards of topical anesthetic creams in plastic surgery, hazards that included severe toxicity and death [4]. Of course, mammography is not plastic surgery, and the report probably escaped the radiologist's notice.

After his patient's adverse drug reaction, Dr. Kline is likely to have read the January, 2009 Food and Drug Administration public health advisory about the improper use of skin numbing products, a report that took specific note of "a recently published study in *Radiology*." This advisory stated that improper use of skin numbing-products can cause irregular heartbeat, seizures, breathing difficulties, coma and death [5]. By this time all radiologists should have been aware of the potential adverse consequences of the drug – lidocaine – being used.

References

1. Billings JS. Educating the physician. Boston Med Surg. 1894; 131:140.
2. Lambertz CK, Johnson CJ, Montgomery PG, Maxwell JR. Premedication to reduce discomfort during screening mammography. Radiology. 2008; 248(3):765–772.
3. Topical anesthetics. U.S. Food and Drug Administration. Available at: http://www.fda.gov/Drugs/DrugSafety/DrugSafetyPodcasts/ucm079047.htm/. Accessed June 8, 2010.
4. Kaweski S. Plastic Surgery Educational Foundation Technology Assessment Committee. Topical anesthetic creams. Plast Reconstr Surg. 2008; 121(6):2161–2165.
5. Improper use of skin numbing products can be deadly. U.S. Food and Drug Administration. Available at: http://www.fda.gov/ForConsumers/ConsumerUpdates/ucm095147.htm. Accessed August 27, 2009.

Medical Errors Matter

As we begin a book intended to minimize medical errors, I want to pause to consider the scope of the problem. Here are some data: Adverse medical events cause the deaths of up to 100,000 US patients each year, and affect approximately 5–10% of all hospitalized patients [1]. Diagnostic errors for which a correct diagnosis and therapy might have saved the patient's life are detected in up to 5% of autopsies [2]. And by far not all errors involve diagnosis. There are roughly four million emergency medical encounters each year necessitated by adverse drug events. These visits to emergency rooms and clinics cost Americans more than $4 billion [3]. Even physicians and their families are not immune to the epidemic of medical errors. Blendon et al. surveyed 831 practicing physicians, of whom 35% reported errors in their own or a family member's care [4].

Many of these errors are preventable, especially drug-related adverse events which, as Kuehn describes, "may occur as a result of a clinician not applying current knowledge of a drug when prescribing" [3]. Other causes of errors include fatigue, carelessness, inattention, and even mistakes in calculation, which can result in life-threatening "tenfold errors," especially dangerous in children [5]. Nevertheless, even when rushed, fatigued, or distracted, the clinician who is up to date with essential medical facts is less likely to make mistakes.

References

1. West CP. Huschka MM, Novotny PJ, et al. Association of perceived medical errors with resident distress and empathy. JAMA. 2006; 296(9):1071–1078.
2. Newman-Toker DE, Pronovost PJ. Diagnostic errors – the next frontier for patient safety. JAMA. 2009; 301(10):1060.
3. Kuehn BM. FDA initiative aims to reduce medication-related errors. JAMA. 2009; 302(21):2304.
4. Blendon RJ, DesRoches CM, Brodie M, et al. Views of practicing physicians and the public on medical errors. N Engl J Med. 2002; 347(24):1933–1940.
5. Kozer E, Scolnik D, Jarvis AD, Koren G. The effect of detection approaches on the reported incidence of tenfold errors. Drug Saf. 2006; 29(2):169–174.

###

Essential Medical Facts Involve the Full Panorama of Medicine: Epidemiology, Prevention, Diagnosis, Laboratory Testing, Imaging, and Therapy of All Types

Here is a preview of the pages ahead. In Chap. 2, I will describe a five-hospital study leading to the conclusion that antipyretic agents are ineffective in preventing recurrences of febrile seizures. The curious finding that the presence of high levels of serum uric acid in hospitalized patients is an independent predictor of mortality is discussed in Chap. 7. You will read in Chap. 9 about a study that found sublingual vitamin B12 effective therapy for recurrent aphthous stomatitis. Chapter 9 describes the significance of finding a first degree heart block upon electrocardiography. And in Chap. 13, I present some unanticipated findings, such as the report that 1,000 mg of aspirin was similar in effectiveness to 50 or 100 mg of sumatriptan in treating acute migraine.

Some of the study conclusions presented might have immediate clinical value. After all, how far can one go wrong treating recurrent aphthous ulcers with vitamin B12? Others facts, such as the suspicion that leprosy/Hanson disease in the U.S. may be linked to exposure to armadillos just might prove epidemiologically relevant some day. (See Chap. 8.) Or maybe not.

###

This Book Is Written for Clinicians, Those of Us on the Front Lines Actually Seeing Patients

Because this is a clinically oriented book, I made some decisions about how to present the content:

- The section presenting and discussing each fact is short and self-contained, with no need to turn to a later page in the chapter to find the reference citations.
- I have tried to phrase each fact carefully. To do so required using some waffle words, such as "may be associated with," "can be a cause of" or simply "might." After all, much of what is in this book is early knowledge and emerging data, things you should know but that may change over time.
- All the reports of studies described have been truncated, in order to keep this book to a manageable size. Thus what you read in the pages to come are snapshots containing what I believe are the key facts that clinicians need to know. I suggest that you use the cited references to read the full text of papers that seem especially pertinent to your practice.
- I tell the source of many studies: that is, the trial was conducted in Finland or Japan, or at Harvard, the University of California, or the Twin Oaks Institute for Health Awareness. Identifying the location just might have some bearing on the credibility of a published report. And yes, the Twin Oaks Institute is mentioned to make a point about credibility; it does not really exist.
- I have not included all of the statistics included in all the papers. To do so would render many summaries densely unreadable. When you read the phrase "statistically significant," however, you know that the phrase was used by the author(s).
- I have also done my best to avoid, or explain, research jargon and coy phrases, such as "sensitivity analysis" and "noninferiority." At the end of the book is an Appendix: *A Glossary of Statistical Terms*. I hope this glossary will help clarify any questions that arise in regard to research reports described.
- In many cases, I have used quotes taken directly from the published articles. I have done so because many of these papers are quite technical and I want to avoid changing meaning by paraphrasing descriptions of results and conclusions. Each quotation and its source are clearly identified.
- For each of us, some of the facts in this book will be more pertinent than others. There are some, however, that in my opinion as a primary care physician, have the potential to alter what we do the next time a specific situation arises. These items are labeled *practice changers* in the book.

- Finally, readers who know my books are aware that I like to inject some medical history, back-stories and fun into medical writing. An example is the speculation that some deaths in history attributed to poisoning were actually the result of acute appendicitis. (See Chap. 6.) Another example is my favorite Oslerism describing abdominal adhesions as the last refuge of the diagnostically destitute. (Also in Chap. 6.) I tell this to explain the use of quotations, aphorisms, and illustrative cases to help you and me remember our *Essential Medical Facts*.

I think by now you have a clearer picture of what to expect. I will start with an iconoclastic chapter – Challenging Current Medical Misconceptions – looking at some our cherished beliefs through the prism of published evidence. Now, settle in to enjoy and learn.

#####

Chapter 2
Challenging Current Medical Misconceptions

> *It is not hard to learn more.*
> *What is hard is to unlearn when you discover yourself wrong.*
>
> American Scientist Martin H. Fischer
> (1879–1962) [1]

Medicine offers us a treasury of knowledge, and much of `it will be validated over time. But tucked in our reference books and hidden in the seldom-revised PowerPoint slides of our professors and continuing medical education (CME) meeting lecturers are some spurious "facts."

> Charles H., a 56 year old computer store manager, came to his local emergency room, complaining of vague chest discomfort present for about 4 h. Based on an absence of prior history of cardiovascular disease, a normal cardiovascular examination and electrocardiogram (ECG), and a failure to report any pain relief following the administration of sublingual nitroglycerin, the patient was discharged to home with a diagnosis of chest wall pain.
>
> He returned 6 h later with a massive myocardial infarction.

In fact, the absence of known prior heart disease and a normal heart exam and ECG in no way rule out the possibility of a coronary occlusion. The worrisome aspect of this case is the apparent reliance on the patient's response to sublingual nitroglycerine. Over the past few years, several studies have shown that relief of chest pain with nitroglycerine is not a reliable test and does not distinguish between cardiac and non-cardiac chest pain [2–4]. In the study by Steel et al., for example, 260 patients received sublingual nitroglycerine as a diagnostic test for chest pain. They found that nitroglycerin relieved the chest pain in 66% of patients. When used to identify a cardiac origin of chest pain, the diagnostic sensitivity of sublingual nitroglycerine was 72%, and the specificity was 37%. "The positive likelihood ratio for having coronary artery disease if nitroglycerine relieved chest pain was 1.1 (0.96–1.34)" [2]. This is not very good.

Each generation of clinicians builds upon the foundation laid by those who have gone before, but we also often become mired in the murky thinking of our predecessors, reluctant or unable to extricate ourselves. Claudius Galen (129–200 CE), whom Porter calls "the medical colossus of the Roman era," gave us some

R.B. Taylor, *Essential Medical Facts Every Clinician Should Know: To Prevent Medical Errors, Pass Board Examinations and Provide Informed Patient Care*,
DOI 10.1007/978-1-4419-7874-5_2, © Springer Science+Business Media, LLC 2011

misconceptions that endured for a millennium [5]. Galen's errors included teachings that the heart has only two chambers, the liver has five lobes, and hollow nerves carry a "vital spirit" from brain to muscle [6]. A little more recently, eighteenth century Boston physicians advised patients with "griping in the guts" to swallow leaden bullets.

The theory of pernicious pockets of infection around teeth and tonsils causing a host of maladies has been around since the time of Hippocrates. In 1808, American physician-statesman Benjamin Rush advocated removing infected teeth to relieve arthritis. In fact, according to Lambert, writing in 1978 about extracting teeth to improve health, "Almost all physicians between 1910 and 1950 were influenced by the theory, and even now the profession has not entirely escaped its effects, in spite of the fact that modern medical textbooks mention it only to condemn it" [7]. In fact, on a personal note, when I was in medical school ca 1960, I recall one aging community doctor telling how he had greatly helped several arthritis patients by removing all their teeth!

Even more recently, we have used diethylstilbestrol to prevent miscarriage or premature deliveries. We once performed routine episiotomies during childbirth. And we have treated severe hypertension with lumbar sympathectomy, all in the earnest belief that what we were doing was both beneficial and safe. Not too many years ago, the treatment of advanced heart failure routinely included "floating" a Swan–Ganz pulmonary artery catheter [8].

And so we cling tenaciously to some outdated notions, long after they have ceased to be faithful servants. This chapter is about exposing these "plastic pearls." Each of the facts below challenges a cherished clinical misconception.

References

1. Fabing HJ, Marr R, editors: Fischerisms, being a sheaf of sundry and divers utterances culled from the lectures of Martin H. Fischer, professor of Physiology in the University of Cincinnati. Springfield, Illinois: Charles C. Thomas, 1937.
2. Steele R, McNaughton T, McChonahy M, Lam J. Chest pain in emergency department patients: if the pain is relieved by nitroglycerin, is it more likely to be cardiac chest pain? CJEM. 2006; 8(3): 164–169.
3. Henrikson CA, Howell EE, Bush DE. Chest pain relief by nitroglycerin does not predict active coronary artery disease. Ann Intern Med. 2003; 139(12): 979–986.
4. Dierks DB, Boghos E, Guzman H, Amsterdam EA, Kirk JD. Changes in the numeric descriptive scale for pain after sublingual nitroglycerin do not predict cardiac etiology of chest pain. Ann Emerg Med. 2005; 45(6): 581–585.
5. Porter R. The greatest benefit to mankind: a medical history of humanity. New York: Norton, 1997, page 71.
6. Inglis B. A history of medicine. New York: World Publishers, 1965, page 39.
7. Lambert EC. Modern medical mistakes. Bloomington, Indiana: Indiana University Press, 1978, page 27.
8. Shure D. Pulmonary artery catheters – peace at last? N Engl J Med. 2006; 354(21): 2273–2274.

###

Continuous Intrapartum Electronic Fetal Monitoring (EFM) Has Not Been Found to Decrease the Incidence of Fetal Mortality or Cerebral Palsy

EFM is used in 85% of all U.S. deliveries, thus applying what seems reassuring technology to a normal body function – labor and delivery [1]. In fact, continuous EFM brings an increased risk of cesarean delivery and instrument-assisted vaginal births [2, 3]. What it has done is decrease the incidence of neonatal seizures, the only demonstrable benefit [2].

Here is the first of my editorial comments, intended to clarify and sometimes question:

EFM has been part of routine maternity care for the past three decades. It has increased intrapartum anxiety, limited the mobility of laboring mothers, enriched trial lawyers, and led to the presence of unnecessary "C-section" scars on a many an abdominal wall. In the setting of an apparent uncomplicated labor, is it time to discuss the pros and cons of continuous EMF with women, with the realization that the technology is always there if needed at some point in labor?

References

1. Martin JA, Hamilton BE, Sutton PD, Ventura SJ, Menacker F, Munson ML. Births: final data for 2002. Natl Vital Stat Rep. 2003; 52(10): 1–113.
2. Bailey RE. Intrapartum fetal monitoring. Am Fam Phys. 2009; 80(12): 1388–1396.
3. Alfirevic Z, Devane D, Gyte GM. Continuous cardiotocography (CTG) as a form of electronic fetal monitoring (EFM) for fetal assessment during labor. Cochrane Database Syst Rev. 2006; Jul 19(3): CD006066.

###

Visual Assessment Is Not Reliable in Screening Newborns for Significant Hyperbilirubinemia Prior to Discharge from the Nursery

We clinicians like to believe that we are keen observers. To examine this belief, Riskin et al. studied 1,129 neonates, comparing their total serum bilirubin levels with visual estimates by neonatologists (n = 5) and nurses (n = 17) [1]. They found significant variations among estimates by observers. They also found problematic visual estimates in 61.5% of the 109 infants with high-risk total serum bilirubin levels.

The implication here is, of course, that underestimation of high-risk bilirubin levels can lead to poor management. Also, the observers in this study were experienced professionals. Consider that, with early discharges from the mother–baby unit, we rely on the visual estimates of inexperienced parents to detect hyperbilirubinemia once the baby goes home.

Reference

1. Riskin A, Tamir A, Kugelman A, Hemo M, Bader D. Is visual assessment of jaundice reliable as a screening tool to detect significant neonatal hyperbilirubinemia? J Pediatr. 2008; 152(6): 782–787.

Pallor of the Palmar Creases Is Unreliable in Detecting Anemia

This is one of those treasured, but heretofore unexamined, clinical tips that is passed on in lore and texts. I came across it in an on-line book, *Wisdom of the Ageds: Clinical Pearls*, by Ricer, a monograph I actually like a great deal, that consists of a collection of pearls contributed by a number of his colleagues. In this book, however, we find the statement, contributed by one of the *Ageds*: "If the palmar creases are not red when the hand is opened (check with your own), think anemia" [1].

The usefulness of pallor was addressed by three Portland, Oregon internists who made independent assessments of the conjunctiva, face, nails, palms, and palmar creases in 103 patients. Note the distinction between palms and palmar creases. In these various areas in their various patients, the authors concluded that the absence of pallor cannot be counted on to detect anemia, and specifically that neither the nail beds nor palmar creases are of value in assessing the presence or absence of anemia [2].

> On the plus side, they did find that pallor of the conjunctivae, face, and palms together is helpful in confirming the presence of anemia [2].

References

1. Ricer R. Wisdom of the ageds: Clinical pearls. Available at: http://www.familymedicine.uc.edu/ricer/ClinicalPearls.pdf.
2. Nardone DA, Roth KM, Mazur DJ, McAfee JH. Usefulness of physical examination in detecting the presence or absence of anemia. Arch Intern Med. 1990; 150(1): 201–204.

The Levine Sign – Chest Discomfort Described by Placing a Clenched Fist on the Chest – Is Not a Reliable Indicator in Determining the Cause of Chest Pain

In physical examination seminars, students have long been taught to be especially concerned about the chest pain patient who describes the discomfort by placing a clenched fist on the chest. To test the utility of this and other gestures, Marcus et al. conducted a prospective study of 202 patients admitted for chest pain, relating gestures used to troponin levels, functional studies and coronary angiograms.

Of these 202 persons, 11% exhibited the Levine Sign, 35% showed the Palm Sign (placing the palm of the hand on the chest), and 16% used the Arm Sign (touching the left arm).

Four percent showed the Pointing Sign (pointing to the pain site with one finger). None of the sensitivities of the signs exceeded 38%. The Levine Sign and the Arm Sign specificities ranged between 78 and 86%, but their positive predictive values did not exceed 55%. The authors describe these signs as having "poor test characteristics" [1].

One would think that an eponymous physical exam sign – e.g. the Levine Sign – would be bulletproof, but this turns out not to be the case. Actually, the Pointing Sign fared the best of all, with 98% specificity as an indicator of non-ischemic chest discomfort [1].

Reference

1. Marcus GM, Cohen J, Varosy PD. The utility of gestures in patients with chest discomfort. Am J Med. 2007; 120(1): 83–89.

###

Pain Relief Following a GI Cocktail Is Not Limited to Gastrointestinal Disease

Chest pain relieved by a "GI cocktail" (a mixture of viscous lidocaine, liquid antacid and an anticholinergic drug) has traditionally been considered due to gastrointestinal disease, and not myocardial ischemia. I'm sorry to report that some patients with coronary artery disease may report relief after drinking the venerated GI cocktail. Wrenn et al. performed a retrospective review of emergency department patients who had received the GI cocktail, some for abdominal pain and some for chest pain, along with various other drugs. As far as the GI cocktail (and other treatment rendered) was concerned, the authors conclude, "Chest pain patients and abdominal pain patients had a similar frequency of response" [1].

The study, a chart review, was confounded by concomitant administration of narcotics, nitroglycerin, antiemetics, H2-blockers and so forth. Nevertheless, the authors urge that we not put too much faith in the diagnostic value of the response to the GI cocktail.

Reference

1. Wrenn K, Slovis CM., Gongaware J. Using the "GI cocktail:" a descriptive study. Ann Emerg Med. 1995; 26: 687–690.

###

Contrary to Lore, Women with Ovarian Cancer Usually Have Symptoms Which May Be Noted Months Before Diagnosis

Cancer of the ovary is often discovered late in the course of disease. The ovaries can be difficult to palpate on physical examination, there is no practical screening test, and we have always considered the disease to be typically silent until it is far along. However, a case–control study of 212 ovarian cancer patients over age 40 revealed 7 symptoms associated with ovarian cancer: abdominal distension, postmenopausal bleeding, loss of appetite, increased urinary frequency, abdominal pain, rectal bleeding, and abdominal bloating. At least one of these seven symptoms was reported to primary care physicians in 85% of ovarian cancer cases but only by 15% of control patients. The authors further report: "After exclusion of symptoms reported in the 180 days before diagnosis, abdominal distension, urinary frequency, and abdominal pain remained independently associated with a diagnosis of ovarian cancer" [1].

> The symptom with the highest positive predictive value (PPV) was abdominal distension, with a value of 2.5%, meaning that for every 40 women with this symptom, one will have ovarian cancer [1].

Reference

1. Hamilton W, Peters TJ, Bankhead C, Sharp D. Risk of ovarian cancer in women with symptoms in primary care: population based case–control study. BMJ. 2009; 339: b2998.

It Is Safe to Use Opiates to Relieve Abdominal Pain, Even if the Diagnosis Is in Doubt

Many of us have been told that administering narcotics to a patient with acute abdominal pain may make it difficult to determine the diagnosis. In fact, a prospective, randomized, placebo controlled study of 100 consecutive patients with significant abdominal pain who received opiate analgesia or saline indicates that pain relief not only may not interfere with diagnosis, but that the reduction in severity of physical signs may facilitate diagnosis [1].

> The Attard et al. study has been confirmed by a more recent Cochrane Review that concludes: "The review provides some evidence to support the notion that the use of opioid analgesic in patients with acute abdominal pain is helpful in terms of patient comfort and does not retard decisions to treat" [2].
>
> In another study, LoVecchio et al. conducted a randomized, prospective, placebo-controlled trial in which 5 or 10 mg of morphine or placebo were given to 48 patients with abdominal pain. The found statistically significant changes in physical examination findings in both analgesic groups, but not in the placebo group. They go on to note that the changes in physical findings attributed to analgesics did not result in any delay in diagnosis or adverse events [3].

References

1. Attard AR, Corlett MJ, Kidner NJ, Leslie AP, Fraser IA. Safety of early relief for acute abdominal pain. BMJ. 1992; 305: 554–556.
2. Manterola C, Astudillo P, Losada H, Pineda V, Sanhueza A, Vial M. Analgesia in patients with acute abdominal pain. Cochrane Database Syst Rev. 2007; Jul 18(3): CD005660.
3. LoVecchio F, Oster N, Sturmann K, Nelson LS, Flashner S, Finger R. The use of analgesics in patients with acute abdominal pain. J Emerg Med. 1997; 15(6): 775–779.

###

It Seems Safe for Patients with Diverticular Disease to Eat Nuts, Corn and Popcorn, After All

It has long been suggested that persons with diverticular disease should not consume corn, popcorn, nuts and seeds, for fear that some kernel will lodge in a diverticulum, causing inflammation and/or bleeding. In a study of 47,228 adult men enrolled in the Health Professional Follow-up Study from 1986 to 2004, researchers compared food-frequency questionnaires to the incidence of diverticulitis and diverticular bleeding. They found no link between eating corn and diverticulitis, and no association between nut, corn, or popcorn consumption and diverticular bleeding. Most interesting of all to me, the found an inverse relationship between nut and popcorn consumption and the risk of diverticulitis.

> Could it be, then, that eating nuts and popcorn might actually benefit patients with diverticular disease? At least, is it really safe to change our longstanding advice to avoid foods with residual kernels? With diverticulosis present in approximately one third of Americans age 60 and over, the answers to these questions have widespread clinical relevance.

Reference

1. Strate LL, Liu YL, Syngal S, Aldoori WH, Giovannucci E. Nut, corn and popcorn and the incidence of diverticular disease. JAMA. 2008; 300(8): 907–914.

###

Lactic Acidosis May Not Be a Special Risk Associated with Metformin Use, After All

Metformin is a favored oral hypoglycemic medication, and has other helpful attributes as well, several of which are covered in chapters that follow. There has, however, been a cloud over its use – the "well-known" risk of developing lactic acidosis.

Because of this risk metformin has sometimes not been prescribed for patients with cardiovascular or pulmonary disease that might cause hypoxemia, or renal disease that might result in metabolic abnormalities. This concern may change following the report by Salpeter et al., who reviewed pooled data from 347 clinical trials involving metformin and other antidiabetic oral medications. In all, 125,941 subjects were involved. They calculated that the upper limit for the true incidence of lactic acidosis was 4.3 cases per 100,000 years of metformin use, compared with 5.4 cases in patients using other drugs. They conclude: "There is no evidence from prospective comparative trials or from observational cohort studies that metformin is associated with an increased risk of lactic acidosis, or with increased levels of lactate, compared to other anti-hyperglycemic treatments" [1].

> *For as long as I can recall, metformin use has been considered a little risky, especially in older patients or those with cardiopulmonary or renal disease. Who among us wanted to be responsible for causing potentially fatal lactic acidosis, even though none of us seemed able to recall a case? The Cochrane Review cited puts the risk of metformin-induced lactic acidosis as more equivalent to the risk with non-metformin therapies, shedding needed light on what has been a misleading bit of clinical lore.*

Reference

1. Salpeter SR, Greyber E, Pasternak GA, et al. Risk of fatal and nonfatal lactic acidosis with metformin use in type 2 diabetes mellitus. Cochrane Database Syst Rev. 2010; Jan 20(1): CD002967.

Night Pain in Back Pain Patients Might Not Really Be an Ominous Symptom

Night pain, we have been told, is especially worrisome – a red flag. To examine this theory, Harding et al. studied 482 consecutive patients attending a back pain triage clinic. Of these, 213 had night pain, with 90 having pain each night. Among all these night pain patients, no serious pathology was found, leading the authors to challenge the specificity of night pain an indicator of serious disease when the presenting complaint is back pain [1].

> *This study prompted me to wonder: Might the non-specificity of night pain as an indicator of severe pathology in back pain patients extend to other pain syndromes? I search PubMed in vain for studies of night pain in migraine, chest pain, abdominal pain, and pelvic pain. There are clearly some researchable questions here.*

Reference

1. Harding IJ, Davies E, Buchanan E, Fairbank JT. The symptom of night pain in a back pain triage clinic. Spine. 2005; 30(17): 1985–1988.

###

The Prehn Sign Is Not Dependable in Differentiating Between Epididymitis and Testicular Torsion

The Prehn sign describes the maneuver of elevating the contents of a painful scrotum. If the pain is relieved by the maneuver, the diagnosis is likely to be epididymitis; if there is no pain relief, think of testicular torsion as the cause.

Here is what we know about the acutely painful scrotum in boys, adolescents and young men. The most common cause is acute epididymitis. Testicular torsion, a surgical emergency, occurs much less frequently [1]. The diagnosis is suspected clinically and can be confirmed on Doppler study (88% accuracy) or, if the Doppler scan is indeterminate or negative in the face of a worrisome clinical picture, radionuclide scanning (95% accuracy) [2]. What cannot be counted on to make the diagnosis is the Prehn sign, which can often be falsely positive or negative [1, 3].

> The take-home message is this: In young men and boys, the diagnosis of epididymitis should be made with great caution. Although epididymitis is the more likely cause of an acute scrotum, testicular torsion is one of the must-never-miss diagnoses.

References

1. Edelsberg JS, Surh YS. The acute scrotum. Emerg Med Clin North Am. 1988; 6(3): 521–546.
2. Haynes BE, Bessen HA, Haynes VE. The diagnosis of testicular torsion. JAMA. 1983; 249(18): 2522–2527.
3. Petrack EM, Hafeez W. Testicular torsion versus epididymitis: a diagnostic challenge. Pediatr Emerg Care. 1992; 8(6): 347–350.

###

Monofilament Testing Is Not Reliable in the Diagnosis of Peripheral Neuropathy

In a review of previously published studies describing the use of monofilament testing to diagnose peripheral neuropathy, Dros et al. found the method to have sensitivity ranging from 41 to 93% and specificity from 68 to 100%. They concluded: "Despite the frequent use of monofilament testing, little can be said about the test accuracy for detecting neuropathy in feet without visible ulcers" [1].

> Up to half of patients with diabetes mellitus will develop peripheral neuropathy as a complication, and up to half of these persons will lack symptoms. For this reason, an inexpensive and safe diagnostic maneuver to detect the complication is useful. We clinicians have embraced monofilament testing, which is much more elegant that the safety pin – once worn on the lapel of a white coat, and rarely if ever sterilized.
>
> Happily, we not have a better test for detecting peripheral neuropathy, the tuning fork, discussed in Chap. 6.

Reference

1. Dros J, Wewerinke A, Bindels PJ, van Weert HC. Accuracy of monofilament testing to diagnose peripheral neuropathy: a systemic review. Ann Fam Med. 2009; 7(6): 555–558.

Bed Rest Is No Longer the Preferred Treatment for Acute Low Back Strain

A systematic review by Waddell et al. compared the two schools of thought in managing acute low back pain. They identified ten trials of bed rest and eight trials in which patients were advised to remain active. All trials were in a primary care setting. They found that patients advised to continue usual activities, when compared to bed rest patients, reported a faster return to work, fewer recurrent problems, and less chronic disability [1].

> In my early practice years, the 1960s, we admitted acute low back strain patients to the hospital, where they were treated for days with Buck's extension traction. This consisted of taping the lower legs so that, with the patient supine, traction could be applied using a pulley attached to the bed footboard and a cord containing a weight. Named for U.S. surgeon Gordon Buck (1807–1877), the method, to my way of thinking was chiefly a means to enforce bed rest, since it always seemed improbable that the 5 pounds of traction on each leg actually had much effect on the spinal muscles and vertebrae. The way for the patient to escape the contraption and go home was, of course, to report improvement in the back pain.

Reference

1. Waddell G, Feder G, Lewis M. Systematic reviews of bed rest and advice to stay active for acute low back pain. Br J Gen Pract. 1997; 47(423): 647–652.

Spinal Manipulation Is Not Useful in the Treatment of Infant Colic

The domains of chiropractic and allopathy seldom intersect, and so perhaps you did not know that chiropractic manipulation is sometimes recommended for infants with colic. Ernst found three randomized clinical trials studying this method, finding as follows: "The totality of this evidence fails to demonstrate the effectiveness of this treatment" [1].

The method was found unhelpful as therapy for infant colic. But there is another side to the coin. What about the risk of harm? Are there any short- or long-term adverse effects of this intervention?

Reference

1. Ernst E. Chiropractic spinal manipulation for infant colic: a systematic review of randomized clinical trials. Int J Clin Pract. 2009; 63(9): 1351–1353.

It Is Generally Safe to Use Prescription Medications for a Year or Two Following Their Expiration Date

This advice comes from a study done for the U.S. Department of Defense (DoD) by the Food and Drug Administration for 20 years. The purpose of the study to see if money could be saved by extending the shelf life of DoD drugs. Researchers looked at the stability of 122 different drug products. They found: "Based on testing and stability assessment, 88% of the lots were extended for at least 1 year beyond their original expiration date for an average extension of 66 months, but the additional stability period was highly variable" [1].

Medication potency seems to persist past the expiration date. But what about safety of the drug? Might an outdated drug cause some adverse effects? According to The Medical Letter, there are no published reports of toxicity of current drug formulations attributed to use after their expiration date. The historical asterisk here is the incidence of renal tubular damage caused by use of degraded tetracycline in a formula no longer manufactured [2].

I offer a few caveats here. First of all, I suspect that the DoD keeps its drugs in a much better environment – think temperature and humidity control – than most bathroom medicine cabinets. Secondly, an exception to the above expiration date advice is liquid antibiotics, generally prepared when your local pharmacist adds water to a powder, and intended to be fully used or discarded. Finally, if I were taking a drug that is truly vital to my health, and for which dosing is critical, I would pay strict attention to expiration dates.

References

1. Lyon RC, Taylor JS, Porter DA, Prasanna HR, Hussain AS. Stability profiles of drug products extended beyond their labeled expiration dates. J Pharm Sci. 2006; 95(7): 1549–1560.
2. Drugs past their expiration date. Med Lett. 2009; 51(1327–1328): 1–2.

###

Selected Cephalosporins Can Be Used in Patients with a History of Penicillin Allergy

A widely circulated misconception has been the tale that there is a 10% cross-allergy risk between penicillin and all cephalosporins. Not so, according to a recent literature review. It seems that while some cephalosporins – cephalothin, cephalexin, cefadroxil, and cefazolin – have a significant risk of cross-allergy with penicillin, others do not. The safer drugs to use in a setting of a history of penicillin allergy are: cefprozil, cefuroxime, cefpodoxime, ceftazidime, and ceftriaxone [1].

> *Given that there are legions of patients that carry the label "penicillin-allergic," however valid or erroneous this designation might be, knowing that certain cephalosporins can be used in these patients will be helpful in daily practice.*

Reference

1. Pichichero ME. Cephalosporins can be prescribed safely for penicillin-allergic patients. J Fam Pract. 2006; 55(2): 106–107.

###

The Use of Intravenous Drugs Such as Epinephrine in the Setting of Out-of-Hospital Cardiac Arrest Does Not Improve the Odds of Survival to Hospital Discharge

In a study conducted in Norway, researchers randomized 851 adults, mean age 64 years, with non-traumatic out-of-hospital cardiac arrest to receive Advanced Cardiac Life Support Guideline based care with and without access to intravenous (IV) drug access. The use of IV drug access improved adjusted survival to the intensive care unit, but did not differ from no-IV-access in regard to survival to hospital discharge, 1-year survival duration or survival with favorable neurologic outcomes [1].

An earlier study from Sweden examined 10,966 instances of out-of-hospital cardiac arrest and whether or not the patients received epinephrine or were intubated. The researchers found: "Neither in total nor in any subgroup did we find results indicating beneficial effects of any of these two interventions" [2].

> *I am not sure that, in a specific instance of cardiac arrest, there is compelling evidence that IV access and use of epinephrine would be inadvisable, even allowing for the possibility of undesirable epinephrine side effects, such as tachycardia, decreased renal blood flow, and increased myocardial irritability [3]. What the Scandinavian studies do for me, however, is give permission not to use IV pressor agents in instances of out-of-hospital cardiac arrest in which my clinical judgment is that such intervention might be a bad idea.*

References

1. Olasveengen TM, Sunde K, Brunborg C, et al. Intravenous drug administration during out-of-hospital cardiac arrest: a randomized trial. JAMA. 2009; 302(20): 2222–2229.
2. Holmberg M, Holmberg S, Herlitz J. Low chance of survival among patients requiring adrenaline (epinephrine) or intubation after out-of-hospital cardiac arrest in Sweden. Resuscitation. 2002; 54(1): 37–45.
3. Tarazi RC. Sympathomimetic agents in the treatment of shock. Ann Intern Med. 1974; 81(3): 364–371.

###

Patients with Mild or Moderate Depression May Experience Little or No Benefit from the Use of Antidepressant Medication

The default therapy of depression has always been antidepressant medication. If a lower dose brings no relief, we increase the dose. When one drug does not work we try another. In this setting, Fournier et al. wondered about the pharmacologic effect of antidepressant medication relative to pill placebo for patients with less severe depression.

In an analysis of six studies involving 718 patients, researchers found that in the treatment of depression, the response to medication versus placebo differed substantially as a function of baseline severity. That is, the worse the depression, the more useful the antidepressant medication when compared to placebo. Those with less than severe depression often experienced little or no benefit from antidepressant medication compared to placebo [1].

Ghaemi even suggests: "A revival of the concept of neurotic depression would make it possible to identify patients with mild-to-moderate, chronic or episodic dysthymia and anxiety who are unlikely to benefit greatly from antidepressants" [2].

Depression is the common cold of mental illness. We see the disease, whether mild, moderate or severe, in daily practice. After reading this study, I will change my thinking about medication use in depression a little. Perhaps instead of aiming to conquer mild to moderate depression with antidepressants, I will focus a little more on counseling and on relieving symptoms such as sleep disturbances. In patients with mild to moderate depression, I will be less likely to recommend increasing doses of medication when lower doses don't seem to work.

References

1. Fournier JC, DeRubeis RJ, Hollon SD, et al. Antidepressant drug effects and depression severity. JAMA. 2010; 303(1): 47–53.
2. Ghaemi SN. Why antidepressants are not antidepressants: STEP-BD, STAR*D, and the return of neurotic depression. Bipolar Disord. 2008; 10(8): 957–968.

###

Oral Dexamethasone Is Not Helpful in the Treatment of Acute Bronchiolitis in Children

In many settings, corticosteroids are used to treat acute bronchiolitis, a leading cause of morbidity and hospitalization in children. It seems to make sense, after all, that an antiinflammatory medication would reduce airway inflammation in these children. To examine this belief, Cornell et al. conducted a double-blind, randomized trial involving 600 children in 20 emergency departments. These children, experiencing bronchiolitis with wheezing, were treated with a single dose of oral dexamethasone versus placebo. The author of the study reported no significant difference in the rates of hospital admission, the respiratory status after 4 h, and later clinical outcomes [1].

This clinical trial is consistent with the conclusions of a metaanalysis, reported in 2004, involving 1,198 children enrolled in 13 trials. When the outcomes of using systemic glucocorticoids versus placebo in acute viral bronchiolitis were compared, there were no benefits in length of stay or clinical scores [2].

> *This is not to say that systemic glucocorticoids might not be beneficial if the child with bronchiolitis also has chronic lung disease or asthma.*

References

1. Corneli HM, Zorc JJ, Mahajan P, et al. A multicenter, randomized, controlled trial of dexamethasone for bronchiolitis. N Engl J Med. 2007; 357(4): 331–339.
2. Patel H, Platt R, Loranzo JM, Wang EE. Glucocorticoids for acute viral bronchiolitis in infants and young children. Cochrane Database Syst Rev. 2004; (3): CD004878.

###

Short Courses of Steroids Used to Treat Asthma Need Not Be Tapered, and Can Be Simply Stopped

Clinical tradition has long held that when short courses of steroids are used to treat asthma, the drug must eventually be withdrawn by tapering. Several studies have shown this not to be true. Here are two of them:

Clinicians in the United Kingdom studied 35 patients admitted to hospital for asthma, treated with 40 mg of enteric-coated prednisone daily for 10 days, followed by a gradual prednisone taper or by a placebo-tablet taper. There was no significant change in mean peak expiratory flow rate in either group during the 7 days of active or placebo tapering or during the following 10 days [1].

A study conducted in Cleveland, Ohio compared acute asthma patients receiving an 8-day course prednisone (40 mg/day) versus others receiving an 8-day tapered dose of prednisone. The researchers found that the two groups did not differ in the

FEV1 percent predicted, the incidence of relapse, or the incidence of adrenal suppression [2].

Based on these studies and others that I found while reviewing this topic, it seems that we no longer need to taper off our doses when treating acute asthma with short-term prednisone. As a practicing physician, I can state that this simplifies my life a little, as well as the lives of my patients. On a practical basis, writing a prescription for a tapering dose of a drug is always a slight challenge. And then the patient must keep track of drug doses that change each day. Now I wonder if the no-taper-needed method applies to other instances of short-term steroid use, such as severe cases of poison ivy dermatitis.

References

1. O'Driscoll BR, Kalra S, Wilson M, Pickering CA, Carroll KB, Woodcock AA. Double-blind trial of steroid tapering in acute asthma. Lancet. 1993; 341(8841): 324–327.
2. Cydulka RK, Emerman CL. A pilot study of steroid therapy after emergency department treatment of acute asthma: is a taper needed? J Emerg Med. 1998; 16(1): 15–19.

###

Guillain–Barré Syndrome (GBS) Is More Likely to Be Caused by Influenza than by an Influenza Vaccine

Influenza is a more likely antecedent to GBS than influenza vaccination if for no other reason than there are many more instances of influenza infection [1]. Too be sure, GBS is a rare complication of both, and the link with the viral infection is especially difficult to quantify. In this regard, following a study of 405 patients with GBS, Sivadon-Tardy et al. concluded: "Influenza viruses are infrequent triggering agents of GBS but may play a significant role during major influenza epidemics" [1].

It is easier to measure the risks with influenza vaccine. Juurlink et al. describe influenza vaccination as "associated with a small but significantly increased risk for hospitalization for GBS" [2]. Following a study of patients with GBS during the 1992–1993 and 1993–1994 influenza/influenza vaccine seasons, Lasky et al. calculate that influenza carries an "adjusted relative risk of 1.7, [which] suggests slightly more than one additional case of GBS per million persons vaccinated against influenza" [3].

GBS attained some notoriety when the disease afflicted popular actor Andy Griffith in 1983. Also, some medical historians have suggested that the cause of the paralysis suffered by Franklin Delano Roosevelt was not polio, but GBS. The disease came to be associated with influenza vaccine during the swine flu epidemic of 1976. Clinicians should keep in mind that GBS can follow a number of infectious diseases. According to Hahn, the most common antecedent pathogen is Campylobacter jejuni, a frequent cause of gastroenteritis [4].

References

1. Sivadon-Tardy V, Orlikowski D, Porcher R, et al. Guillain–Barré syndrome and virus infection. Clin Infect Dis. 2009; 48(1): 48–56.
2. Juurlilnk DN, Stukel TA, Kwong J, et al. Guillain–Barré syndrome after influenza vaccination in adults: a population-based study. Arch Intern Med. 2006; 166(20): 2217–2221.
3. Lasky, Terracciano GJ, Magder L, et al. The Guillain–Barré syndrome and the 1992–1993 and 1993–1994 influenza vaccines. N Engl J Med. 1998; 339(25): 1797–1802.
4. Hahn AF. Guillain–Barré syndrome. Lancet. 1998; 352(9128): 635–641.

Exposure to Cold May Have Something to Do with Upper Respiratory Infections, After All

Any scientifically grounded physician is likely to state that being exposed to a cold environment – breathing cold air, being "chilled," and so forth – cannot cause a cold. But there is the pesky increase in colds and related respiratory infections that occurs during the winter months. In 2002, Eccles, at the Common Cold Centre in Cardiff, Wales, affirmed, "Present scientific opinion dismisses a cause-and-effect relationship between acute cooling of the body surface and common cold." However, he goes on to propose a hypothesis: "that acute cooling of the body surface causes reflex vasoconstriction in the nose and upper airways, and that this vasoconstrictor response may inhibit respiratory defense and cause the onset of clinical cold symptoms by converting an asymptomatic subclinical viral infection into a symptomatic clinical infection" [1]. Interesting theory.

Then in 2005, Johnson and Eccles, still at the Common Cold Center, studied cold symptoms in patients subjected to acute cooling of the feet. They found, "Acute chilling of the feet causes the onset of common cold symptoms in around 10% of subjects who are chilled" [2].

The latest paper I can find on the topic is by Mourtzoukou and Falagas, in Greece who, following a review of available data, conclude: "Although not all studies agree, most of the available evidence from laboratory and clinical studies suggests that inhaled cold air, cooling of the body surface and cold stress induced by lowering the core body temperature cause pathophysiological responses such as vasoconstriction in the respiratory tract mucosa and suppression of immune responses, which are responsible for increased susceptibility to infections" [3].

> First of all: Yes, there really is a Common Cold Centre at the Cardiff School of Biosciences, Cardiff University. Furthermore, their findings seem to validate my mother's cold weather advice to dress warmly and keep my feet dry.
>
> On a related note, while searching for items that relate to the common cold, I came across a study by Cohen et al., describing the relationship between sleep efficiency and duration and the development of common cold symptoms in 153 healthy adult volunteers. Their conclusion was: "Poorer sleep efficiency and shorter sleep duration in the weeks preceding exposure to a rhinovirus were associated with lower resistance to illness" [4].

References

1. Eccles R. Acute cooling of the body surface and the common cold. Rhinology. 2002; 40: 109–114.
2. Johnson C, Eccles R. Acute cooling of the feet and the onset of common cold symptoms. Fam Pract. 2005; 22(6): 608–613.
3. Mourtzoukou EG, Falagas ME. Exposure to cold and respiratory tract infections. Int J Tuberc Lung Dis. 2007; 11(9): 938–943.
4. Cohen S, Doyle WJ, Alper CM, et al. Sleep habits and susceptibility to the common cold. Arch Intern Med. 2009; 169(1): 62–67.

###

Ginkgo biloba Does Not Prevent Cognitive Decline in Older Adults

The Ginkgo Evaluation of Memory (GEM) study was a randomized, double-blind, placebo controlled trial involving 3,069 community-dwelling persons age 72 and older who took 120 mg of *G. biloba* twice daily or placebo. Participants were followed for a mean of 6.1 years with various tests of neuropsychological function. In the end, compared with placebo, *G. biloba* in the doses used "did not result in less cognitive decline in older adults with normal cognition or with mild cognitive impairment" [1].

> *Somehow, however, I suspect that we will continue to see advertized claims that G. biloba can prevent the cognitive decline of aging and Alzheimer disease.*

Reference

1. Snitz BE, O'Meara ES, Carlson MD, et al. *Ginkgo biloba* for prevention of cognitive decline in older adults: a randomized trial. JAMA. 2009; 302(24): 2662–2670.

###

Antipyretic Agents Do Not Prevent Recurrences of Febrile Seizures

Parents and physicians alike have long endeavored to see that any child with a history of febrile seizures receives an antipyretic medication at the first sniffle, with the intent of preventing a subsequent seizure episode. From Finland comes a study of 231 children who suffered their first febrile seizure. Following acute care, subsequent treatment was with oral ibuprofen, acetaminophen or placebo. The investigators found no significant differences in the recurrence of febrile seizures among the three groups. The temperature was higher in instances of seizure than in those without seizure, and "this phenomenon was independent of the medication given."

The conclusion of the authors was: "Antipyretic agents are ineffective for the prevention of recurrences of febrile seizures and for the lowering of body temperature in patients with a febrile episode that leads to a recurrent febrile seizure" [1].

For me, this study prompts a paradigmatic shift in thinking. As a family physician I am keenly aware that a febrile seizure, especially a first episode, is terrifying to parents, and worrisome to the physician. I recall being called to the homes of frightened parents in the middle of the night. In those settings, after the seizure had run its course, standard therapy was to attack the fever with antipyretics. Now we have a study challenging the utility of antipyretics in preventing recurrences of febrile seizures. But what else do we have? And so thinking may change, but what about practice? I suspect that, in spite of this study, parents and physician will still advocate antipyretics when the child with a history of febrile seizures develops an elevated body temperature, simply because we lack a truly useful method of seizure prevention.

Also, in this study, which focused on preventing febrile seizure recurrence, did you notice that our favorite antipyretics used in children – ibuprofen and acetaminophen – did not seem effective in lowering body temperature?

Reference

1. Strengell T, Uhari M, Tarkka R, et al. Antipyretic agents for preventing recurrences of febrile seizures: randomized controlled trial. Arch Pediatr Adolesc Med. 2009; 163(9): 799–804.

Supplementary Use of Vitamins C and E Does Not Offer Protection Against Heart Disease

The Physicians' Heart Study, active from 1997 to 2007, was a randomized, double-blind, placebo controlled trial of vitamins C and E in regard to major cardiovascular events – nonfatal myocardial infarction, nonfatal stroke, and death due to cardiovascular disease. The subjects were 14,641 male physicians age 50 years and older. At the end of the trial, the investigators concluded that, compared to placebo, neither vitamin had any significant effect on the incidence of cardiovascular events [1].

Will this serve as the definitive study regarding this controversial issue? Perhaps so, at least as far as men are concerned.

Reference

1. Sesso HD, Buring JE, Christen WG, et al. Vitamins E and C in the prevention of cardiovascular disease in men: the Physicians' Health Study II randomized controlled trial. JAMA. 2008; 300(18): 2123–2133.

###

We Do Not Need to Drink Eight Glasses of Water a Day

Common belief holds that we adults should drink eight 8-ounce glasses of water a day (sometimes termed "8 × 8"). Vreeman and Carroll suggest that this misguided notion may have originated with a 1945 recommendation that adults need 2.5 L of water a day. They go on to relate, "An ordinary standard for diverse persons is 1 milliliter for each calorie of food. Most of this quantity is contained in prepared foods." The authors then point out that if the second sentence is ignored and the water content of foods not counted, then one could see how the 8 × 8 instruction could gain traction [1].

Valtin, writing in 2002, holds that rigorous proof for the advice to drink eight 8-ounce glasses of water daily is lacking. He goes on to point out that in some instances – heavy exercise in a hot climate – eight or more 8-ounce glasses of water may be needed daily [2].

Clinicians should keep in mind the rare, but possible, outcomes of heroic water consumption: hyponatremia, water intoxication, or exacerbation of heart failure.

References

1. Vreeman RC, Carroll AE. Medical myths. BMJ. 2007; 335(7633): 1288–1289.
2. Valtin H. "Drink at least eight glasses of water a day." Really? Is there scientific evidence for "8 × 8"? Am J Physiol Regul Integr Comp Physiol. 2002; 283(5): R993–R1004.

Low Dose Vitamin K Does Not Reduce Bleeding in Warfarin Patients with Elevated International Normalized Ratios (INRs)

In a study conducted in 14 anticoagulant clinics, overanticoagulated patients with international normalized ratio values of 4.5 and higher were treated with 1.25 mg of oral vitamin K (n = 347) or placebo (n = 365). Actively bleeding patients were excluded. The conclusion: "Low-dose oral vitamin K did not reduce bleeding in warfarin recipients with INRs of 4.5 to 10.0" [1].

A sidebar to this study is as follows: The day after taking vitamin K or placebo, the former group experienced a 2.8 drop in INR while the latter group had a decrease of 1.4. This means that low-dose vitamin K actually dropped the INR but – and this is a big "but" – did not result in reduced actual bleeding events [1].

Reference

1. Crowther MA, Ageno W, Garcia D, et al. Oral vitamin K versus placebo to correct excessive anticoagulation in patients receiving warfarin: a randomized trial. Ann Intern Med. 2009; 150(5): 293–300.

###

Vitamin B12 Need Not Be Given by Injection

Our classic medical textbooks have assured us that vitamin B12 replacement requires the use of intramuscular (IM) injections, owing to impaired absorption in patients with an intrinsic factor deficiency. A study of 38 newly diagnosed cobalamin deficient patients assigned to receive cyanocobalamin intramuscularly or orally has shown that, at least in the short term, oral administration of high doses of vitamin B12 can provide satisfactory replacement, and in fact may be superior to IM administration [1].

In fact, vitamin B12 is not the only medication previously given chiefly by injection that can safely be administered orally, as I describe next.

Reference

1. Kuzminski AM, Del Giacco EJ, Allen RH, Stabler SP, Lindenbaum J. Effective treatment of cobalamin deficiency with oral cobalamin. Blood. 1998; 92(4): 1191–1198.

Oral Antibiotics Are the Best Outpatient Treatment for Pneumonia

This is the recommendation of the American Thoracic Society and the Infectious Diseases Society of America [1]. Also, a careful literature review by Shatsky also finds no superiority of parenteral therapy over oral therapy for acute sinusitis or for severe urinary tract infections [2].

Getting a "shot" was once considered by many to be the gold standard of therapy, perhaps harking to the early days of penicillin in the 1940s. In fact, at one time, oral penicillin was more expensive than injectable, explaining why, as cruel as is sounds, when I was an intern in a U.S. Public Health Service Hospital in 1961, children with confirmed streptococcal pharyngitis were brought to the hospital daily for 10 days for penicillin injections. This cost-cutting practice was by USPHS/government fiat, a sobering recollection as we anticipate increased federal control over medical care in America.

References

1. Mandell LA, Wunderink RG, Anzuto A, et al. Infectious Diseases Society of America/American Thoracic Society consensus guidelines on the management of community-acquired pneumonia in adults. Clin Infect Dis. 2007; 44(suppl 2): S27–S72.
2. Shatsky M. Evidence for the use of intramuscular injections in outpatient practice. Am Fam Phys. 2009; 79(4): 297–300.

###

Childhood Vaccines Do Not Cause Autism

In 1984, Wakefield et al. published a paper, relating a study of 12 children ages 3–10 referred to a pediatric gastroenterology clinic with a history of normal development followed by loss of acquired skills, including language, together with diarrhea and abdominal pain. In eight of the 12 children the onset of behavioral manifestations followed vaccination against measles, mumps, and rubella [1]. The study did not include a control population.

Then, in 2010, in a stunning development, Lancet, which had published the 1984 paper, retracted the paper, stating: "In particular, the claims in the original paper that the children were 'consecutively referred' and that the investigations were 'approved' by the local ethics committee have been proven to be false" [2].

The Wall Street Journal Health Blog tells a little more of the story. It seems that blood was taken from children at a birthday party, and the families each received a small cash payment. Also, Wakefield received a large research grant from attorneys representing parents of affected children, but did not disclose this funding as a possible conflict of interest [3].

The Lancet retraction comes just 6 months after the "Age of Autism – the Daily Web Newspaper of the Autism Epidemic" honored Dr. Wakefield as the first recipient of its Galileo Award [4]. If the renowned Italian astronomer and mathematician were alive today, I wonder how he would feel about this eponymous recognition.

I present this fact – that childhood vaccines do not cause autism – because, thanks to activist groups and publications such as the one mentioned here, the vaccine-autism myth is likely to persist for a long time to come.

References

1. Wakefield AJ, Murch SH, Anthony A, et al. Ileal-lymphoid-nodular hyperplasia, non-specific colitis, and pervasive developmental disorder in children. The Lancet. 1998; 351(9103): 637–641.
2. The editors of Lancet. Retraction – Ileal-lymphoid-nodular hyperplasia, non-specific colitis, and pervasive developmental disorder in children. Early Online Publication, 2 February 2010. Available at: http://www.thelancet.com/journals/lancet/article/PIIS0140-6736(10)60175-7/fulltext?_eventId=logout/. Accessed February 20, 2010.
3. The end of a paper that linked autism to a vaccine. WSJ (Wall Street Journal) Health Blog. Available at: http://blog.wsj.com/health/2010/02/the-end-of-a-paper-that-linked-autism-to-a-vaccine/.
4. Age of Autism Galileo Award to Doctor Andrew Wakefield. Available at: http://www.ageofautism.com/2009/08/dr-andrew-wakefield-on-dateline-nbc-more-stories-at-age-of-autism/. ccessed February 20, 2010.

#####

Chapter 3
Epidemiologic Realities and Gee-Whiz Facts

When you hear hoofbeats, look for horses, not zebras.

Attributed to Theodore E. Woodward, MD (1914–2005), University of Maryland Hospital, Baltimore, Maryland [1].

Most of us received our professional education in academic medical centers (AMCs), which tend to attract patients with uncommon and difficult-to-manage diseases. In the AMC, learners often encounter advanced systemic lupus erythematosus, Hashimoto thyroiditis, hemochromatosis, and central cord syndrome, and may come to think of these as everyday health problems. Then these learners become licensed health professionals, and most begin seeing ordinary persons with ordinary health problems in community-based settings.

> Jane P., a 20 year college student, visited the student health service in late September with two complaints: For a few days, she had experienced a stuffy nose accompanied by mild general achiness and a low grade fever. Also for a week she had noticed some oval-shaped salmon-colored skin lesions on her chest and back. Concerned about the presentation, the student health physician embarked on a diagnostic mission, determined to connect the complaints and make the diagnosis of Lyme disease, Rocky Mountain spotted fever, or even secondary syphilis. Had the doctor stopped and thought about what occurs most commonly in young women in the fall and spring of the year, he would have made the correct diagnoses, both of them: a viral upper respiratory infection and an unrelated problem of pityriasis rosea.

Nobel Prize nominee Theodore Woodward probably would have advised the student health physician to consider the common diagnoses first, an approach that could have avoided an expensive workup, not to mention the worry experienced by the patient. In the case of the young college student, the common diagnoses were the most benign. In other instances, what is common may also be the most serious, such as lung cancer, methicillin-resistant *Staphylococcus aureus* (MRSA) infection, or sudden infant death syndrome (SIDS). I will come to those shortly, but first let me consider why we should all know some fundamental epidemiologic data, most common causes, and a few other interesting facts.

Sir William Osler (1849–1919) once quipped, "Medicine is a science of uncertainty and an art of probability." Knowing what is probable, what is unlikely and what is truly ridiculous can help make you and me better diagnosticians. I call these

R.B. Taylor, *Essential Medical Facts Every Clinician Should Know: To Prevent Medical Errors, Pass Board Examinations and Provide Informed Patient Care*,
DOI 10.1007/978-1-4419-7874-5_3, © Springer Science+Business Media, LLC 2011

Gee-Whiz Facts. You find them in the introductory paragraphs of research papers and the first few slides of a lecture presentation.

Here is an example: There are almost 30,000 herbal preparations and dietary supplements on the market and half of all American adults take one or more of these herbs or supplements regularly [2]. Knowing this information alerts me to the risk that every other adult patient I see just might be taking an over-the-counter preparation that can interact with medicine I prescribe. (Some of these interactions are described in Chap. 11.)

At this point, I want to stress the importance of epidemiologic facts. Knowing what occurs commonly and what doesn't, what kills people and what is likely to do so, what medicines and herbal remedies your patients are likely to be taking, and what causes some of the problems we face each day can make you a better clinician. These facts also establish the groundwork for the chapters to come on clinical pearls, idiosyncratic drug effects, unexpected clinical findings, and more.

With this introduction, let us look at some Gee-Whiz Facts, beginning with life expectancy, death, disability, drugs and various diseases.

References

1. Woodward TE. Quoted in: Taylor RB. White coat tales: medicine's heroes, heritage, and misadventures. New York: Springer, 2008; page 128.
2. Primary Care Case Reports. 2009;15(6):58.

###

The Overall Life Expectancy at Birth in the United States Is Now 77.7 Years

This figure is based on final data from 2006 [1]. The 77.7 year life expectancy is a big change from the early 1900s, when the average newborn was projected to live about 50 years. Also by comparison, today's death rate is 776 per 100,000 US standard population; in 1908, that ratio was 1,500 per 100,000 persons, with more than one-fourth of all deaths occurring in children under age five [2].

> *I think we can safely state that most of the increase in life expectancy has come through preventive health measures. This includes assuring a safe supply of water and food, immunizations against many communicable diseases, and attention to personal lifestyle choices such exercise, reduced consumption of dietary fats and smoking cessation.*

References

1. National Vital Statistics Reports. 2009;57(14):1.
2. JAMA. 1909;53(19):1567–1568. Reprinted in JAMA 100 Years Ago section in JAMA. 2009;302(17):1915.

###

Heart Disease and Cancer Are the Leading Causes of Death in America

Curiously, the numbers of these two top killers are not far apart. Here, thanks to the National Center for Health Statistics, is the latest tally of leading causes of death in the United States [1]:

Cause		Number of deaths/year 2006
1	Heart disease	631,636
2	Cancer	559,888
3	Stroke	137,119
4	Chronic lower respiratory diseases	124,583
5	Accidents	121,599
6	Diabetes	72,449
7	Alzheimer disease	72,432
8	Influenza and pneumonia	56,326
9	Kidney disease	45,344
10	Septicemia	34,234

The clinical lesson here is that any patient suspected of having heart disease or cancer deserves extra attention to these potentially lethal entities.

Reference

1. Leading causes of death in America. Available at: http://www.cde.gov/nchs/FASTAST/lcod. htm. Accessed January 17, 2010.

The Leading Cause of Death in Young Persons Ages 1–24 Years Is Accidents

And for ages 15–24 years the number two leading cause of death is homicide, a sobering figure as we ponder the literally thousands of years of what-should-have been productive life lost each year [1].

Prevention is always better – and more cost-effective – than cure, and the clinician's most effective intervention may be before the fact and not after injury has occurred. That involves tuning in to risk-taking or self-destructive behavior and counseling the young person, and ideally also the parents.

Reference

1. http://www.nlm.nih.gov/medlineplus/encl/article/001915.htm. Accessed December 9, 2009.

###

In America, the Leading *Actual* Cause of Death – in Contrast to Data Usually Recorded on Death Certificates – Is Smoking

The concept of actual causes of death involves behavior choices that result in lethal diseases. According to Mokdad et al., smoking leads the list with 435,000 deaths, 18% of US deaths [1]. The list was derived by searching a MEDLINE database linking risky behavior and mortality. Here are other items on the list of actual causes of death: poor diet and physical inactivity (400,000), alcohol misuse (85,000), motor vehicle crashes (43,000), incidents involving firearms (29,000), sexual behaviors (20,000), and illicit drug use (17,000).

> *Sharing one or two of these facts with a young patient may just save a life. You might even choose to use an analogy. Think about deaths due to smoking. If you do the math, we lose more than a thousand persons to smoking every day. That is the equivalent of three 747 jetliners crashing each day, killing everyone. Such an image may just make an impact. Of course, you as the physician will never realize that someone's life was saved by giving up cigarettes that day, but that is one of the realities of practicing preventive medicine.*

Reference

1. Mokdad AH, Marks JS, Stroup DF, Gerberding JL. Actual causes of death in the United States, 2000. JAMA. 2004;291:1238–1245.

###

According to One Report, the Fifth Leading Cause of Death in America Is Medical Error

Mokdad et al. compiled their list of actual causes of death by looking at risk behaviors – smoking, alcohol use, and so forth [1]. Such a screen would not capture reports of medical error. Looking at things another way, the Millennium Research Group (MRG), described as the global authority on medical technology market intelligence, analyzed data that suggested that medical errors causes up to 98,000 deaths each year, making clinical errors one of the leading causes of death in the US [2]. That death tally puts errors just ahead of alcohol misuse in the *actual causes* of death sweepstakes. MRG senior analyst David Plow comments, "Generally, medical errors are caused by overcrowded, understaffed clinical areas with complex workflow patterns and incomplete or inefficient communication between clinical areas" [2].

As an example of death due to medical error, Bedell et al. looked at 203 cardiac arrests in a university teaching hospital. Of these, 28 (14%) of arrests followed an iatrogenic complication. Seventeen of these 28 patients died. The most common causes of potentially preventable arrest were medication errors and toxic effects of drugs. The authors concluded that in 18 of the 28 cases, arrest "might have been prevented by stricter attention to the patient's history, findings on physical examination, and laboratory data" [3].

The MRG study seems to have focused on acute care, in which case many errors outside the acute care arena care setting may have been missed, a factor that would only increase the annual total of medical errors. And the Bedell et al. study, from medicine faculty at Harvard Medical School, is a little dated, indicating an opportunity for some investigator to revisit the relationship of medical error and cardiac arrest.

Incidentally, for those who are reading carefully, the 98,000 deaths each year attributed to medical error, if compared to the list of leading causes of death in America presented on page 31, would place medical error in sixth position, not fifth, but we will not quarrel about a single difference in rank between two studies using two different methods. The point is that medical errors are a noteworthy cause of death.

References

1. Mokdad AH, Marks JS, Stroup DF, Gerberding JL. Actual causes of death in the United States, 2000. JAMA. 2004;291:1238–1245.
2. Medical error is the fifth-leading cause of death in the U.S. Available at: http://www. medicalnewstoday.com/articles/75042.php. Accessed January 17, 2010.
3. Bedell SE, Deitz DC, Leeman D, Delbanco TL. Incidence and characteristics of preventable cardiac arrests. JAMA. 1991;65(21):2815–2820.

###

Acute Medication Poisoning Accounts for Nearly Half of All Poisonings Reported in the US

With more than 2.4 million poisonings reported annually, this means that some 1.2 million Americans suffer acute medication poisoning each year [1]. In both adults and children, the most common cause of acute poisoning is analgesics. Most acute poisonings are treated outside a hospital and few are fatal [2].

The tip-off for the family and clinician is often a sudden change in mental status.

References

1. Bronstein AC, Spyker DA, Catilena LR, Green JF, Romack BH, Heard SE. The 2006 annual report of the American Association of Poison Control Center' National Poison Data System. Clin Toxicol. 2007;45(8):815–817.
2. Frithsen IL, Simpson WM Jr. Recognition and management of acute medication poisoning. Am Fam Physician. 2010;81(3):316–323.

###

According to the Morbidity and Mortality Weekly Report (MMWR), the Leading Cause of Disability in US Adults Is Arthritis

According to the report from the CDC (Centers for Disease Control and Prevention), back and spine problems are a close second. Here is the top-ten list, based on 45.1

Condition causing disability	Estimated total persons affected	Percent of persons reporting disability
Arthritis/rheumatism	8,552,000 persons	19.0%
Back/spine problems	7,589,000	16.8
Heart trouble	2,988,000	6.6
Lung/respiratory problem	2,224,000	4.9
Mental or emotional problem	2,203,000	4.9
Diabetes	2,012,000	4.5
Deafness or hearing problem	1,908,000	4.2
Stiffness/deformity of limbs	1,627,000	3.6
Blindness or vision problem	1,460,000	3.2
Stroke	1,076,000	2.4

million persons reporting a disability to the U.S. Census Bureau. The report was released May 1, 2009 and based on 2005 data [1].

I have listed only the top ten causes of disability. If we look lower on the list we find cancer at number 11; cancer tends to kill – or be cured – rather than cause disability. And, a little surprisingly – at least to me – is that senility/dementia/Alzheimer disease is listed number 15, affecting 546,000 persons (1.2% of persons reporting a disability). Is this a meaningful number? Or could there be a reporting bias in the U.S. census, with persons in this category not all being counted?

Also, not all reports agree with the MMWR. The American Heart Association Statistics Committee and Stroke Statistics Subcommittee holds that stroke is the leading cause of disability in the U.S., although that conclusion just might have been influenced by the focus of the group [2].

On a global basis, Sabat hold that dementia is the leading cause of chronic disability, ahead of cerebrovascular and musculoskeletal diseases [3].

References

1. Centers for Disease Control and Prevention (CDC). Prevalence and most common causes of disability among adults – United States, 2005. MMWR Morb Mortal Wkly Rep. 2009;58(16):421–426. Accessed January 17, 2010.
2. Lloyd-Jones D, Adams R. Carnethon M, et al. American Heart Association Statistics Committee and Stroke Statistics Subcommittee. Heart disease and stroke statistics – 2009 update: a report from the American Heart Association Statistics Committee and Stroke Statistics Subcommittee. 2009;119:480–486.
3. Sagat SR. Dementia in developing countries: a tidal wave on the horizon. Lancet. 2009;374(9704):1805–1806.

###

Headache Is the Most Common Pain Condition Resulting in Lost Time from Work

A study of 28,902 working U.S. adults revealed that during a 2-week period, 13% reported time lost from work due to a pain condition. Headache was the most common cause cited (5.4%), followed by back pain (3.2%), arthritis pain (2.0%), and other musculoskeletal pain (2.0%) [1].

In the study cited, headache patients reported a mean loss of 3.5 productive hours/week, while those with back pain or arthritis lost 5.2 h/week [1].

Reference

1. Stewart WF, Ricci JA, Chee E, Morganstein D, Lipton R. Lost time and cost due to common pain conditions in the U.S. workforce. JAMA. 2003;290(18):2443–2454.

If We Look Beyond Skin Cancer, the Most Common Cancer of All, the Next Most Commonly Occurring Malignancy Is Lung Cancer

Here, courtesy of the National Cancer Institute, based on data from the American Cancer Society, is the list of most common cancer types [1]. Of course, breast cancer occurs almost exclusively in women and thus, in spite of a declining incidence, it is still the leading cancer (excluding non-melanoma skin cancer) among US women [2].

Cancer type	Estimated new cases/year
Skin (non-melanoma)	>1,000,000 cases
Lung (including bronchus)	219,440
Breast (female/male)	193,370/1,910
Prostate	192,280
Colorectal	146,970
Bladder	70,980
Melanoma	68,720
Non-Hodgkin lymphoma	65,980
Kidney (renal cell) cancer	49,096
Leukemia (all types)	44,790

The list above shows cancer incidence. Cancer deaths are another story, described next.

References

1. National Cancer Institute. Common cancer types. Available at: http://www.cancer.gov/cancertopics/commoncancers/. Accessed December 10, 2009.
2. Jemal A, Siegel R, Ward I, Hao Y, Xu J, Thun MJ. Cancer statistics, 2009. CA Cancer J Clin. 2009;59(4):225–249.

###

Lung Cancer Is, Far and Away the Leading Cause of Cancer Death in America

As a cause of cancer deaths, colorectal cancer comes in a distant second. Again, courtesy of the National Cancer Institute, here is the Rogue's Gallery of lethal cancers [1].

Cancer type	Estimated deaths/year
Lung (including bronchus)	159,390 deaths
Colorectal	49,920
Breast (female/male)	40,170/440
Pancreatic	35,240
Prostate	27,360
Leukemia (all types)	21,870
Non-Hodgkin lymphoma	19,500
Bladder	14,330
Kidney (renal cell) cancer	11,003
Melanoma	8,650

Just for interest: Pancreatic cancer ranks number four on the list of deaths due to cancer, but did not make the top-ten list of incidence. (It would have been number 11 on an extended list.) The implication is that this cancer, when it occurs, tends to have a grim outlook. On the other end of the spectrum is prostate cancer, a virtual tie with breast cancer as one of the most commonly occurring malignancies, but ranking only fifth as a cause of cancer death.

Reference

1. National Cancer Institute. Common cancer types. Available at: http://www.cancer.gov/cancertopics/commoncancers/. Accessed December 10, 2009.

###

The Most Common Initial Symptom of the Leading US Cancer Killer, Lung Cancer, Is Cough

Lung cancer, the most common cause of cancer death in the United States, has a paltry 15% 5 year survival [1]. Just for the record: Smoking is the major risk factor for lung cancer, and cough is the most common initial symptom [2].

For all these reasons, no wise clinician accepts the patient's self-diagnosis of "smoker's cough" without investigation.

References

1. Collins LG, Haines C, Perkel R, Enck RE. Lung cancer: diagnosis and management. Am Fam Physician. 2007;75(1):56–63.
2. Barro JA, Valladares G, Faria AR. Early diagnosis of lung cancer. Epidemiological variables, clinical variables, staging and treatment. J Bras Pneumol. 2006;32(3):221–227.

Almost One Half of All Persons Report Using a Prescription Drug in the Past Month

And 71% of physician patient visits involve drug therapy, helping facilitate this level of medication consumption. The most frequently prescribed medications were analgesics, antihyperlipemic agents, and antidepressants [1].

We who care for patients might well recall the words of Sir William Osler (1849–1919): "One of the first duties of the physician is to educate the masses not to take medicines."

Reference

1. Centers for Disease Control and Prevention. Therapeutic drug use. Available at: http://www.cdc.gov/nchs/FASTASTS/drugs.htm. Accessed December 10, 2009.

###

According to a Commercial Source, Lipitor (Brand of Atorvastatin) Is the Top of the Proprietary Drug List in Sales

The source is a site titled Drugs.com, which describes itself as "the most popular, comprehensive and up-to-date source of drug information online" [1]. According to this source, here are the top ten prescription drugs, identified by brand name and ranked by sales volume:

1. Lipitor
2. Nexium
3. Plavix
4. Advair Diskus
5. Prevacid
6. Seroquel
7. Singulair
8. Effexor XR
9. OxyContin
10. Actos

The report describes annual sales of more than five billion dollars for Lipitor. Yes, that is billion, with a B. And Americans consumed some two and a half billion dollars worth of OxyContin during the year.

Reference

1. Top 200 drugs for 2008 by sales. Available at: http://www.drugs.com/top200/html. Accessed December 10, 2009.

Americans Spend an Estimated 2.9 Billion Dollars on Over-the-Counter Cold Remedies Each Year

The common cold, aka upper respiratory infection, is the third most common diagnosis in physicians' offices, trailing only hypertension and well-child visits [1]. And at these visits, patients receive some $1.1 billion worth of unneeded antibiotics to treat this ubiquitous viral infection [2].

The various OTC medications may afford patients some small measure of symptomatic relief, and might keep them from inappropriate antibiotic use. But, as we see, cold sufferers often show up in physicians' offices where, unfortunately, on a busy day, it is easier and quicker to hand the patient a prescription than to explain why one is not needed.

References

1. Cherry DK, Woodwell DA, Rechsteiner EA. National Ambulatory Medical Care Survey: 2005 summary. Adv Data. 2007;387;1–39.
2. Fendrick AM, Monto AS, Nightingale B, Sarnes M. The economic burden of respiratory track infection in the United States. Arch Intern Med. 2003;163:487–494.

###

Sudden Infant Death Syndrome Is the Chief Cause of Healthy Infant Deaths

Sudden infant death syndrome is the leading cause of death in healthy US infants, with more than 2,200 deaths each year. Risk factors include a low APGAR score, low birth weight, male sex, a recent viral infection and low family socioeconomic status. Prone sleeping seems to be a risk factor, one that should be responsive to office counseling [1].

> *Most of the risk factors described above are beyond the control of the parents, but at the very least, young parents should be encouraged not to place infants to sleep in a prone position. The mantra is: Back to sleep*

Reference

1. Adams SM, Good MW, Defranco GM. Sudden infant death syndrome. Am Fam Physician. 2009;79(10):870–874.

###

In One Large Study, Half of All Patients in Intensive Care Units Were Considered Infected and Receiving Antibiotics

The report described the analysis of 13,796 intensive care unit (ICU) patients on a single day. Of these, 7,087 (51%) were considered infected; 9,084 (71%) were receiving antibiotics. The respiratory tract was the most common site of infection reported [1].

> *I find two additional noteworthy items: One is that the number of patients receiving antibiotics (n = 9,084) well exceeded those considered infected (n = 7,087). Were 1,997 patients receiving prophylactic antibiotics? The second is the authors' observation that the risk of infection increases with duration of ICU stay [1].*

Reference

1. Vincent JL, Rello J, Marshall J, et al. International study of the prevalence and outcomes of infection in intensive care units. JAMA. 2009;302(21):2323–2329.

###

Clostridium difficile Is Now the Leading Cause of Nosocomial Infections in Community Hospitals

This conclusion comes from a report from Duke University, and is based on data from their network of 39 hospitals, involving more than three million patient-days [1].

> *The significance of this study is that C. difficile infection has surpassed methicillin-resistant Staphylococcus aureus infection as the chief cause of hospital-onset healthcare-facility-associated infections, with C. difficile infection occurring 25% more frequently than MRSA infections in the study reported [1].*

Reference

1. Miller BA. *Clostridium difficile* surpasses MRSA as the leading cause of nosocomial infections in community hospitals. Paper presented at the Fifth Decennial Conference on Healthcare-Associated Infections 2010: Abstract 386, presented March 20, 2010.

###

Methicillin-Resistant *Staphylococcus aureus*, No Longer Confined to the Hospital Setting, Has Become a Community Problem

Community-associated methicillin-resistant *Staphylococcus aureus*, first reported as recently as 1981, is the leading cause of skin and soft tissue infections seen in US emergency departments. The 2005 standardized mortality MRSA rate was 6.3 per 100,000 population. Recall from above for comparison that the current overall mortality rate in America is 776 per 100,000 US standard population. Among those at special risk are members of sports teams, prison inmates and child care attendees [1].

> *One physician from Dickson, Tennessee suggests a way to reduce the spread of MRSA. Trim the long fingernails. Subungual spaces make convenient hiding places for bacteria, from which they can be transferred to minor skin abrasions or the nasal mucosa [2].*

References

1. Klevens RM, Morrison MA, Nadle J, et al. Invasive methicillin-resistant *Staphylococcus aureus* infections in the United States. JAMA. 2007;298(15):1763–1771.
2. Jabr F. Practical pointers: short cut to preventing MRSA. Consultant, July 2009, page 437.

###

There Is Almost a 50:50 Chance that a Teenager in Your Office Is Sexually Active

According to the CDC, 47.8% of students in grades 9 through 12 have had sexual intercourse. Especially alarming in this report, considering the risks of sexually transmitted disease, is the fact 38.5% of the sexually active 9th to 12th graders failed to use condoms at the time of their last sexual encounter. What's more, 7.1% of children were reported to have had sexual intercourse before age 13 [1].

Physicians must be more willing than ever to raise the issues of sexual activity with teens. Failure to do so may result in unplanned pregnancy or unwanted communicable disease.

Reference

1. Eaton DK, Kann L, Kinchen S, et al and the CDC. Youth risk behavior surveillance – United States, 2007. MMWR Morb Mortal Wkly Rep. 2008;57(SS4):1–136.

###

Forced Sexual Intercourse Is More Common than We Have Thought

Approximately one in 15 US adults has been the victim of forced sexual intercourse, a figure which may actually be low owing to underreporting [1]. Furthermore, there seem to be what some may consider a surprisingly large number of adult survivors of childhood sexual abuse: 25% of women and 16% of men [2].

Asking about the possibility of a past history of forced sexual intercourse or some other type of sexual abuse may provide a clue to the cause of chronic pelvic pain, abdominal distress or some other persistent, elusive symptom. Another fact to keep in mind is that rape is the chief cause of post-traumatic stress syndrome (PSTD) in women, occurring in 25–50% of women who report a history of sexual assault [3].

References

1. Basile KC, Chen J, Black MC, Saltzman LE. Prevalence and characteristics of sexual violence victimization among US adults, 2001–2003. Violence Vict. 2007;22(4):437–448.
2. Dube SR, Anda RF, Whitfield CL, et al. Long-term consequences of childhood sexual abuse by gender of victim. Am J Prev Med. 2005;28(5):430–438.
3. Kessler RC. Posttraumatic stress disorder: the burden to the individual and to society. J Clin Psychiatry. 2000;61(suppl 5):4–12.

###

More than One Million Americans Are Infected with the Human Immunodeficiency Virus (HIV)

If the population of the United States is 300 million persons, more or less, then approximately 1 in every 300 Americans is HIV-infected. Furthermore, one in five of these HIV-infected individuals is unaware of being infected [1].

> *What's more, and this is a fact that I might have presented in Chap. 13 as an unforeseen finding, in certain areas of the United States, the prevalence of HIV infection is on a par with that found in some countries in Africa that we think of being hot-beds of disease. For instance, El-Sadr et al. report that 1 in 30 adults living in Washington, DC is HIV-infected, exceeding the prevalence rate in Ethiopia, Nigeria or Rwanda [1].*

Reference

1. El-Sadr WM, Mayer KH, Hodder SL. AIDS in America – forgotten but not gone. N Engl J Med. 2010;362(11):967–968.

###

The Centers for Disease Control and the U.S. Census Bureau Estimate that by the Year 2030, There Will Be Approximately 71 Million U.S. Adults Age 65 and Older, About Twice the Number in that Age Group as There Were in 2000

The report goes on to highlight the "unprecedented demands on public health senior services and the nation's health-care system" sure to result from this growing number of older adults [1].

> *The aging population also has implications for specialty choice by young physicians as we think ahead to a United States in which one in every five persons is age 65 or older.*

For example, two decades from now we are sure to need more physicians trained to provide comprehensive care for the elderly – family physicians and general internists – than today, and perhaps fewer pediatricians.

Reference

1. Centers for Disease Control and Prevention (CDC). Prevalence and most common causes of disability among adults – United States, 2005. MMWR Morb Mortal Wkly Rep. 2009;58(16):421–426.

###

Most US Pregnant Women Begin Prenatal Care During the 8th to 12th Week of Pregnancy

The significance of this figure, from a report by Mayer, is that many, perhaps most, of these women first see a physician *after* the period of organogenesis (4–10 weeks post-fertilization), thereby missing important opportunities for prenatal counseling regarding issues such as medication use, and consumption of coffee and alcohol [1]. Delay in initiating prenatal care may contribute to the 12% prematurity rate in the United States today [2].

There is much to discuss at the initial prenatal visit, and the earlier the better – to begin appropriate vitamin supplementation, perform vital screening tests, and review lifestyle choices. For example, restricting caffeine use to 200 mg or less daily may reduce the risk of miscarriage. In fact, there is so much the pregnant mother should know, and really should know before conception, that the ideal is a preconception visit for counseling to plan for the future pregnancy. Carl and Hill advocate making preconception counseling part of the annual exam for women of childbearing age [3].

References

1. Mayer JP. Unintended childbearing, maternal beliefs, and delay of prenatal care. Birth. 1997;24:247–252.
2. Proceedings of the Preconception Health and Health Care Clinical, Public Health and Consumer Workgroup Meetings, Atlanta, GA: Centers for Disease Control and Prevention, National Center on Birth Defects and Developmental Disabilities, 2006. Available at: http://www.cdc.gov/ncbddd/preconception/documents/Workgroup%20Proceedings%20June06.pdf. Accessed July 13, 2010.
3. Carl J, Hill A. Preconception counseling: make it part of the annual exam. J Fam Pract. 2009;58(6):307–313.

###

One in Four Pregnant Women Will Report Spotting in the First Few Weeks of Pregnancy, and Half of Those Who Bleed Will Miscarry

Thus, bleeding before 20 weeks of gestation is, by definition, threatened abortion [1].

I include these figures about early pregnancy bleeding just to remind us all to take such bleeding seriously. Deutchman et al. recommend reassurance and watchful waiting if – and this is an important "if" – fetal heart tones are detected, if the patient is medically stable, and if there is no adnexal mass or clinical sign of intraperitoneal bleeding [2].

References

1. Paspulati RM, Bhatt S, Nour SG. Sonographic evaluation of first-trimester bleeding. Radiol Clin N Am. 2004;42(2):297–314.
2. Deutchman M, Tubay AT, Turok DK. First trimester bleeding. Am Fam Physician. 2009;79(11):985–992, 993–994.

###

Almost One-Third of American Adults Are Obese

According to a 2009 review, 32.2% of adults and 17.1% of children and adolescents are obese [1]. As we look at what really causes people to die, Manson et al. estimate that 5–15% of US deaths each year can be attributed to obesity [2]. It is interesting to note that the obesity rate in the US is rising, while the rate of smoking is declining.

We don't need statistics to verify the reports of wide-spread obesity. Just sit on a bench in any shopping mall and do some people-watching. Our local newspaper tells that the average weight of a shopping mall Santa is 256 pounds [3]. I won't stand behind the data leading to this conclusion, but my intuition tends to support the estimate. All this is hugely important because obesity contributes to cardiovascular disease, diabetes, arthritis and more, and hence represents a huge health and economic burden for America.

References

1. Pi-Sunyer X. The medical risks of obesity. Postgrad Med. 2009;121(6):21–33.
2. Manson JE, Bussuk SS, Hu FB, Stampfer MJ, Colditz GA, Willett WC. Estimating the number of deaths due to obesity: can the divergent findings be reconciled? J Women's Health. 2007;16:168–176.
3. The Oregonian, Friday, December 11, 2009.

###

There Were More than Ten Million Aesthetic Procedures Performed in the U.S. in 2008

Of these 10.2 million treatments, 80% were minimally invasive procedures. These include injection of onabotulinumtoxin-A (Botox) and dermal filler, laser hair removal, laser skin resurfacing, intense pulsed light photorejuvenation and microdermabrasion. The American Society for Aesthetic Plastic Surgery reports a fivefold increase in the number of procedures done over the past decade [1].

Ten million aesthetic procedures is, in my opinion, a lot of procedures in a year, performed chiefly to deal with normal age-related facial changes. What's more, because of the high fees received for performing – or having one's assistant perform – appearance-enhancing treatments, some primary care physicians are being lured away from preventing and treating disease into the heady world of aesthetic practice. To quote one author writing for family physicians: "High patient and physician satisfaction have contributed to their (aesthetic treatments) growing popularity and availability in the primary care setting" [2]. As both a physician and patient aware of our limited health care resources, I must wonder if this is the best course for America.

References

1. The American Society for Aesthetic Plastic Surgery. Cosmetic Surgery National Data Bank 2008 Statistics. New York, NY: The American Society for Aesthetic Plastic Surgery; 2008. Available at: http://www.surgery.org/media/statistics/. Accessed December 13, 2009.
2. Small R. Aesthetic procedures in office practice. Am Fam Physician. 2009;80(11): 1231–1237.

###

Approximately One-Third of All Persons in the World Are Latently Infected With *Mycobacterium tuberculosis*

According to Inge and Wilson, this includes 11 million persons in the United States, most of these being born abroad in countries where tuberculosis is endemic [1]. There are approximately eight million new cases and two million disease-related deaths world-wide each year.

Tuberculosis, aka the white plague, is still with us. It causes the death of Mimi in Puccini's La Bohéme each time I see the opera. In the past the disease afflicted such notables as John Keats, Paul Gauguin, Washington Irving, Edgar Allen Poe, Ulysses S. Grant, Sarah Bernhardt, Nelson Mandela and Eleanor Roosevelt. First lady Eleanor Roosevelt, attended by the best and brightest physicians of her time, had her tuberculosis symptoms treated with corticosteroids [2]. Today we face the threat of multiple drug resistant tuberculosis, a specter which justifies thinking about TB in patients with symptoms of cough, fever and weight loss, especially if they have come to America from an endemic area.

References

1. Inge LD, Wilson JW. Update on the treatment of tuberculosis. Am Fam Physician. 2008;78(4):457–465.
2. Taylor RB. White coat tales: medicines' heroes, heritage, and misadventures. New York: Springer, 2008; page 218.

###

Inherited Cardiovascular Diseases Can Be Transmitted Through Voluntary Sperm Donation

Maron et al. report the saga of a 23-year old man with no knowledge of having underlying heart disease who, while under contract with a US sperm bank, donated sperm over a 2-year period in the early 1990s. The sperm bank seems to have made robust use of this donor's sperm. Of the 24 known offspring of this donor (including two conceived by his wife), nine have been found to have hypertrophic cardiomyopathy [1].

I found this a sad but true "Gee-Whiz" tale, one reminding us that the unexpected can always happen in medicine.

Reference

1. Maron BJ, Lesser JR, Schiller NB, Harris KM, Brown C, Rehm HL. Implications of hypertrophic cardiomyopathy transmitted by sperm donation. JAMA. 2009;302(15): 1681–1684.

###

The Most Common Things Occur Most Commonly

Because most of your day will be spend dealing with "horses," and not zebras, all physicians should be familiar with the *Most Common Things*. Here are some of these. Unless stated otherwise, all these most common things refer to incidence and prevalence in the United States:

- The most common type of skin cancer is basal cell cancer. In fact, it is the most common of all cancers.

- Leukemia is the most common cancer in children.
- The most common cancers in young men are testicular cancer and lymphoma.
- The most common cancers in young women are thyroid cancer and lymphoma.
- The most common cancer worldwide is lung cancer.
- The most common tumor of the anterior mediastinum is a thymoma.
- The most common neoplasm of the appendix is a carcinoid tumor.
- The most common sexually transmitted disease is chlamydia.
- The most common cause of visual loss in the elderly is age-related macular degeneration.
- The most common work-related disability is low back pain.
- The most common surgical emergency of the abdomen is acute appendicitis, which is also the most common surgical emergency during pregnancy.
- The most common cause of lower gastrointestinal bleeding is diverticular bleeding.
- The most common cause of anemia is iron deficiency, which may be due to poor intake, impaired absorption or blood loss.
- Alzheimer disease is the most common neurologic disorder.
- The most common cause of blindness in persons age 20–74 years is diabetic retinopathy.
- The most common cause of acute flaccid paralysis in healthy infants and children is Guillain–Barré syndrome.
- The most common cause of accidental death is motor vehicle crashes.

There are many more "most common causes." I suggest keeping an active list as you come across them.

#####

Chapter 4
Disease Prevention and Screening

> And lo! The starry folds reveal
> The blazoned truth we hold so dear.
> To guard is better than to heal –
> The shield is nobler than the spear.

Oliver Wendell Holmes, Sr. (1809–1894)
Songs in Many Keys,
For the 1860 Meeting of the National Sanitary
Association [1]

John L., a 72 year-old retired steelworker, came to our office last week for his first visit with our resident physician. He had several chronic diseases, but one acute problem had prompted him to call for an appointment. For 3 days, he had had a painful, bullous eruption on his right flank, just as he had experienced twice in the past, the latest occurrence about 6 years ago. Yes, the patient had herpes zoster. Somehow, he had ignored exhortations in the media and probably the advice of a previous physician. The resident treated the patient with antiviral medication, in an effort to reduce the duration of symptoms.

American physician and poet Oliver Wendell Holmes, Sr., quoted above, and reportedly the inspiration for the "Holmes" in the name Sherlock Holmes, was a champion of prevention. In a time when physicians had precious little to offer in the way of useful remedies, Holmes (Oliver Wendell, Sr., not Sherlock) once quipped that if the drugs of the day were tossed into the sea it would be better for mankind – but all the worse for the fishes. In 1843, Holmes published an article in the *New England Quarterly Journal of Medicine and Surgery*. His paper theorized that puerperal sepsis just might be transmitted by physician contact. If true, then puerperal sepsis might be prevented by the simple act of hand-washing, a notion that challenged the contemporary belief that physicians, being gentlemen, simply could not have contaminated hands [2]. Students of medical history will note that Holmes' report predated the 1847 findings of Ignaz Semmelweis (1818–1865) in Vienna by 4 years.

R.B. Taylor, *Essential Medical Facts Every Clinician Should Know: To Prevent Medical Errors, Pass Board Examinations and Provide Informed Patient Care,* DOI 10.1007/978-1-4419-7874-5_4, © Springer Science+Business Media, LLC 2011

In this chapter, I will present facts pertinent to disease prevention and screening, selected with an eye to avoiding errors of commission and omission, and to helping assure that our patients receive informed, up-to-date health care.

References

1. Strauss MB. *Familiar medical quotations*. Boston: Little, Brown; 1968; page 450.
2. Small MR. *Oliver Wendell Homes. Twayne's United States authors series*, 29. New York: Twayne Publishers; 1962.

###

There Are Approximately One Million New Cases of Herpes Zoster (HZ) Each Year

Let us begin with some prevention-oriented topics first. Given the example case cited above, zoster seems a good starting point. The high incidence of HZ – a million new cases annually – comes from a report by the Centers for Disease Control and Prevention, describing the disease as the "scourge of the elderly," and asking why every eligible older adult in America would not roll up his or her sleeve to receive the vaccine [1]. If most or all of America's seniors receive the vaccine, the incidence of HZ should drop precipitously.

> *Shingles seems to me to be the poster child disease for the comment by Louis Pasteur (1822–1895): "When meditating over a disease, I never think of a remedy, but, instead, a means of preventing it" [2]. Throughout most of my medical career, herpes zoster was a painful blistering affliction, typically striking for no apparent reason, often leaving a chronic postherpetic neuralgia to frustrate both patient and physician. Now, after decades of therapeutic impotence, we have an effective means of prevention.*
>
> *I like to think of numbers using visual imagery. Think of one million persons. That is the number of persons that crowd into Times Square on New Year's Eve. That is, more or less, 1 in every 300 Americans. Sharing these numbers with a patient may highlight the statistical risks of the unvaccinated and help persuade the reluctant ones to receive the HZ/ shingles vaccine.*

References

1. CDC seeks to protect older adults with shingles vaccine message. http://www.cdc.gov/vaccines/vpd-vac/shingles/dis-faqs.htm. Accessed January 2, 2010.
2. Pasteur L. Address to the Fraternal Association of Former Students of the *École Central des Artes et Manufactures*, Paris, May 15, 1884. Quoted in Strauss MB. *Familiar Medical Quotations*. Boston: Little, Brown; 1968; page 451.

###

If All U.S. Adults Became Nonsmokers of Normal Weight by 2020, We Forecast that the Life Expectancy of an 18-Year-Old Would Increase by 3.76 Life-Years or 5.16 Quality-Adjusted Years

I use a direct quote here to be sure I got the authors' words right [1]. The article by Stewart et al. especially highlights the increasing trends toward obesity, i.e., elevated body mass index (BMI), and relates this to the health gains we have enjoyed as less and less persons smoke. Here is another memorable quote from the paper: "If past obesity trends continue unchecked, the negative effects on the health of the U.S. population will increasingly outweigh the positive effects gained from declining smoking rates."

There is hope! A generation ago, schoolchildren learned of the dangers of smoking and pleaded, often successfully, with their parents to cease tobacco use. Today, my granddaughter will not set foot in a fast food restaurant. Her epiphany seemed to have occurred with a school experiment in which the class purchased a fast food burger, homogenized it, and viewed the amount of fat it contained. Score one for the public school system.

Reference

1. Stewart ST, Cutler DM, Rosen AB. Forecasting the effects of obesity and smoking on U.S. life expectancy. N Engl J Med. 2009;361;2252–2260.

###

Obesity Brings a Fourfold Higher Relative Risk of Fatal Cardiovascular Disease when Compared with Normal Weight Persons

The report upon which this conclusion is based also tells that obesity brings a two-fold greater risk of non-fatal heart attack [1]. In this study of 20,000 Dutch men and women, the authors found that in persons who were overweight or obese, half of all fatal cardiovascular events and a quarter of nonfatal cardiovascular disease could be attributed to overweight and obesity.

If the obesity trend continues, and smoking rates decline further, obesity may soon displace smoking as the leading actual cause of death.

Reference

1. Van Dis I, Kromhout D, Geleijnse JM, Boer JM, Verschuren WM. Body mass index and waist circumference predict both 10-year nonfatal and fatal cardiovascular disease risk: study conducted in 20,000 Dutch men and women aged 20–65 years. Eur J Cardiovasc Prev Rehabil. 2009;16(6):729–734.

###

Breastfeeding May Help to Prevent Obesity in Children

Obesity in childhood tends to predict adult obesity, and breastfeeding may lessen the risk of childhood obesity. This conclusion from the American Academy of Pediatrics is just one more reason why infants should be breastfed whenever possible [1].

> *How long the infant is breast fed matters, as well. A study of 918 children followed from birth until age 6 years revealed that early introduction of bottle feeding "brings forward the obesity rebound, predictive of obesity in later life" [2].*

References

1. Gartner LM, Morton J, Lawrence RA, et al. for the American Academy of Pediatrics Section on Breastfeeding. Breastfeeding and the use of human milk. Pediatrics. 2005;115:496–506.
2. Bergmann KE, Bergmann RL, Von Kries R, et al. Early determinants of childhood overweight and adiposity in a birth cohort study: role of breastfeeding. Int J Obes Relat Metab Disord. 2003;27(2):162–172.

Three Percent of American Women Take Potentially Teratogenic Medications

Here are just a few of the medications your preconceptual patient may be taking. All are rated pregnancy category X, indicating that studies in animals or pregnant women have shown positive evidence of fetal abnormalities or risk [1]:

Drug	Potential harm to fetus
Isotretinoin	Microcephaly, hydrocephalus, limb abnormalities
Methotrexate	Fetal malformations
Statins	Cleft lip, club foot, polydactyly
Warfarin	Intrauterine growth restriction, neurologic and skeletal defects

Furthermore, two thirds of women do not take folic acid supplementation [2]. The key here is that these numbers describe "women," even though they are not necessarily pregnant. The simple addition of folate to the diet of pregnant woman during the first trimester can reduce the incidence of neural tube defects such as spina bifida and anencephaly by as much as 70% [3].

> *These facts highlight the need for anticipatory guidance for all women of childbearing age. In short, consider that every sexually active woman of childbearing age may become pregnant next month. And sometimes it is even difficult to discern who will or will not be sexually active next month. Thus for all such women, ask about any potentially harmful medications that they might be taking. In addition to the category X drugs listed above,*

think about benzodiazepines, serotonin-selective reuptake inhibitor antidepressants, tetracyclines, antiepileptic drugs or lithium. Think about all the young women taking SSRI drugs for depression or valproate for migraine headache [4]. And do not forget to recommend folate supplementation, or at least a daily multivitamin that contains folate.

References

1. Physicians' Desk Reference. Montvale, NJ: Thomson Reuters; 2010.
2. Carl J, Hill A. Preconceptional counseling: make it part of the annual exam. J Fam Pract. 2009;58(6):307–309.
3. Lumley J, Watson L, Watson M, et al. Periconceptional supplementation with folate and/or multivitamins for prevention of neural tube defects. Cochrane Database Syst Rev. 2001;(3):CD1056.
4. Pedersan LH, Henriksen TB, Vestergaard M, Olsen J, Bech BH. Selective serotonin reuptake inhibitors in pregnancy and congenital malformations: population based cohort study. BMJ. 2009;339:b3569.

###

Many Otherwise Healthy Infants and Toddlers Have Low Vitamin D Levels

Here I continue on a vitamin theme, given that adequate levels of vitamins can guard against a number of preventable diseases. Gordon et al. studied 380 infants and toddlers seeking care in a primary care clinic in Boston. The researcher found that 12.1% of children tested had a vitamin D deficiency (20 ng/mL or less) while 40.0% had sub-optimal levels (30 ng/mL or less). Of the children with vitamin D deficiency, 7.5% had rachitic changes on imaging, and another 32.5% had signs of demineralization [1]. The authors found a strong association between low vitamin D levels and breastfeeding without vitamin supplementation.

I found the high prevalence of suboptimal vitamin D levels a little surprising, especially since the study was conducted in Boston, and not in a third world country. Granted that Boston, like my hometown of Portland, Oregon, does not have as many sunny days as Miami or San Diego. But that cannot be the entire answer. Dark skin pigmentation can be a factor, but this also is not the sole cause. I suspect that we, as a society, have become less than diligent about providing our children with the vitamins and the vitamin-D fortified milk they need. Just as an example, I cite a recent trip to Florida where I watched children consuming cola drinks for breakfast and washing down lunchtime burgers with presweetened ice tea.

Reference

1. Gordon CM, Feldman HA, Sinclair L, et al. Prevalence of vitamin D deficiency among healthy infants and toddlers. Arch Pediatr Adolesc Med. 2008;162(6):505–512.

###

Vitamin D Supplementation in Children May Help Prevent Seasonal Influenza A

A report from Japan describes a randomized, double-blind, placebo-controlled trial in which schoolchildren received either 1,200 IU Vitamin D3 supplementation or placebo daily. In the vitamin D cohort (n = 167), 18 children (10.8%) developed influenza A compared with 31 (18.6%) in the control group (n = 167) [1].

In the study cited, the reduction in influenza A was especially prominent in those children who had taken no prior vitamin D supplements [1].

Reference

1. Urashima M, Segawa T, Okazaki M, Kurihara M, Wada Y, Ida H. Randomized trial of vitamin D supplementation to prevent seasonal influenza A in schoolchildren. Am J Clin Nutr. 2010;91(5):1255–1260.

In Adults, Adequate Vitamin D Levels Can Help Prevent Fractures

Suboptimal vitamin D levels are common in adults as well as in children. Such deficiencies are clinically significant because adequate vitamin D levels achieved through supplementation have been shown to reduce hip fractures by 26% and all fractures by 23% [1]. In addition to preventing fractures, vitamin D can help relieve chronic back pain [2]. According to Stechschulte et al., other attributes of vitamin D are favorable effects on autoimmune diseases, heart disease cancer and cognitive function [1].

In the University Hospital Clinic where I work, there is more attention to patients' vitamin D levels than ever in the past. As for me, just the chance to enhance my cognitive function would be enough to determine my blood levels and take any needed supplementation. One must ask: Will the determination of a vitamin D level become a recommended part of the periodic health examination?

While we are on the topic of vitamin D and fractures, a recent study showed an increased incidence of falls and fractures in older community-dwelling women, but only in one specific circumstance: the annual administration of a single high dose (500,000 IU orally) of cholecalciferol. The authors speculate "that high serum levels of vitamin D or metabolites resulting from the annual dose, subsequent decrease in the levels, or both might be causal" [3].

References

1. Stechschulte SA, Kirsner RS, Dederman DG. Vitamin D: bone and beyond, rationale and recommendations for supplementation. Am J Med. 2009;122(9):793–802.

2. Schwalfenerg G. Improvement of chronic back pain or failed back surgery with vitamin D repletion: a case series. J Am Board Fam Med. 2009;22(1):69–74.
3. Sanders KM, Stuart AL, Williamson EJ, et al. Annual high-dose oral vitamin D and falls and fractures in older women. JAMA. 2010;303(18):1815–1822.

Vitamin D May Help Prevent Colorectal Adenomas and Cancer, as Well as Other Tumors

A meta-analysis of 17 epidemiological studies revealed that circulating 25-hydroxyvitamin D (25[OH]D) levels and vitamin D intake were inversely associated with colorectal adenoma incidence and recurrent adenomas [1]. In fact, high levels of circulating vitamin D are associated with lower rates of breast, ovarian, renal, pancreatic, and aggressive prostate cancers [1]. Garland et al. conclude, "There are no unreasonable risks from intake of 2,000 IU per day of vitamin D [2], or from a population serum 25(OH)D level of 40 to 60 ng/mL. The time has come for nationally coordinated action to substantially increase intake of Vitamin D and calcium."

> I consider the data above and the suggestion by Garland et al. to be a **practice changer**.
> Certainly given what we know, should we not consider supplementary vitamin D use to be the standard of care for anyone with a history of colorectal adenoma or a family history of colorectal cancer?
> In fact, in a review article published in the American Journal of Lifestyle Medicine, Lenz reports, "Several observational studies and a few prospective randomized controlled trials have demonstrated that adequate levels of vitamin D can decrease the risk and improve survival rates for several types of cancers including breast, rectum, ovary, prostate, stomach, bladder, esophagus, kidney, lung, pancreas, non-Hodgkin lymphoma, and multiple myeloma" [3].

References

1. Wei MY, Garland CF, Gorham ED, Mohr SB, Giovannucci E. Vitamin D and prevention of colorectal adenoma: a meta-analysis. Cancer Epidemiol Biomarkers Prev. 2008;17(11):2958–2569.
2. Garland CF, Gorham ED, Mohr SB, Garland FC. Vitamin D for cancer prevention. Ann Epidemiol. 2009;19(7):468–483.
3. Lenz TL. Vitamin D supplementation and cancer prevention. Am J Lifestyle Med. 2009;3(5):365–368.

Aspirin May Help Prevent Colorectal Cancer Deaths

Aspirin, like vitamin D, can help prevent colorectal cancer. It can also lower the risk of colorectal cancer specific and overall mortality in patients diagnosed with colorectal cancer, especially those with tumors that overexpress cyclooxygenase 2

(COX-2). This statement is based on a study of 1,279 men and women diagnosed with colorectal cancer. Noteworthy is the finding that aspirin's protective tendency did not include primary tumors with weak or absent expression of COX-2 [1].

Thus the immunohistochemical expression of COX-2 by the patient's cancer cells becomes significant when considering ongoing aspirin use, given that daily aspirin use carries its own risks, notably gastrointestinal bleeding, as described in the next topic.

Reference

1. Chan AT, Ogino S, Fuchs CS. Aspirin use and survival after diagnosis of colorectal cancer. JAMA. 2009;302(6):649–658.

###

Aspirin, While of Benefit for Many with Occlusive Vascular Disease, Is of Uncertain Benefit in the Primary Prevention of Occlusive Cardiovascular Disease in Persons Without Previous Disease when Weighed Against the Risk of Major Bleeds

In a metaanalysis of six trials involving 95,000 persons at low average risk for serious vascular events (myocardial infarction, stroke, or vascular death), Biagent et al. found that aspirin use was associated with a 12% reduction in serious vascular events, chiefly in non-fatal myocardial infarction, without significant change in stroke incidence or vascular mortality. However, and this is a noteworthy qualification, aspirin can cause major bleeds. Balancing the small benefit of aspirin use in the study was a significant increase in gastrointestinal and extracranial bleeds [1].

The key phrase used by Biagent and the Antithrombotic Trialists' (ATT) Collaboration to describe aspirin in the primary prevention of vascular disease was "uncertain net value." And so, when queried by our patients who have read about daily aspirin use in the Sunday Supplement, we, like our colleagues in the ATT, will continue to duck our heads, shuffle our feet, and offer noncommittal comments. Unless, of course, the patient is at risk of colorectal cancer or metastasis from a known colorectal tumor.

The Biagent/ATT trial conclusion is supported by the findings of a 2010 report by Fowkes et al. They describe the outcome of 3,350 participants in a randomized controlled trial with a mean follow-up of 8.2 years. These subjects all had a low ankle brachial index, suggesting atherosclerosis, and an increased risk of cardiovascular and cerebrovascular events. Patients received 100 mg of aspirin or placebo daily. There was no significant difference in the aspirin vs. the placebo groups in the incidence of vascular events or in all-cause mortality. There was one difference, however. Major hemorrhages requiring hospital admission occurred more often in the aspiring group (2.5 per 1,000 person/years) compared with the placebo group (1.5 per 1,000 person/years) [2].

References

1. Antithrombotic Trialists' Collaboration, Baigent C, Blackwell L, Collins R. Aspirin in the primary and secondary prevention of vascular disease: collaborative meta-analysis of individual participant data from randomized trials. Lancet. 2009;373(9678):1821–1822.
2. Fowkes FGR, Price JF, Stewart MCW, et al. Aspirin for prevention of cardiovascular events in a general population screened for a low ankle brachial index: a randomized controlled trial. JAMA. 2010;303(9):841–848.

###

Close Contacts of Immunocompromised Persons Can Be Immunized Safely, with Two Exceptions: Oral Polio Vaccine and Some Instances Involving Varicella Vaccine

It is generally safe to immunize close contacts, including household members, of immunocompromised persons, using recommended age-appropriate schedules [1]. The major exception is the use of live oral polio vaccine, which can be shed in feces for as long as 4 weeks following administration. Varicella vaccine has as asterisk on its use when an immunocompromised person is in the picture: The vaccine can be administered to close contacts, but if a person receiving the vaccine develops a rash, that person should not have contact with an immunocompromised patient until the rash subsides [2].

> *Of course, in an ideal world, vaccines are administered to the patient and close contacts prior to splenectomy, radiation therapy, chemotherapy, or use of immunosuppressive drugs.*

References

1. Garvin M, Kraus C. What is the best way to manage immunizations in patients on immunosuppressive therapy? Evid Based Pract. 2009;12(9):13.
2. Kroger AT, Atkinson WL, Marcuse EK, Pickering LK, Advisory Committee on Immunization Practices (ACIP), Centers for Disease Control and Prevention. General recommendations on immunization. MMWR Recomm Rep. 2006;55(RR-15):1–48.

###

Immunocompromised Patients Require Extra Attention when Receiving Immunizations

Of course, we would not give a live vaccine – such as live oral polio vaccine – to an immunocompromised patient. On the other hand, there are some vaccines that should be given that might not be indicated for the otherwise healthy person.

For example, the Centers for Disease Control and Prevention (CDC) recommends that when adult vaccination is indicated, the splenectomized patient should receive three vaccinations [1]:

- *Streptococcus pneumoniae*: Polyvalent pneumococcal vaccine
- *Haemophilus influenzae* type B: Haemophilus influenzae b vaccine
- *Neisseria meningitidis*: Meningococcal vaccine type varies with age group

I include this here because of a case I reviewed a few years ago. The patient was an Asian man who, after living in the United States for decades, decided to visit the land of his birth. Before his trip, he visited his physician to be sure he was medically ready to travel. In his past history was a record of splenectomy following an injury during his youth. But not to worry; the patient had received Pneumovax in the past. The physician administered the usual travel shots, gave the patient a prescription for malaria prophylaxis and wished him a pleasant journey. Several weeks into his trip, he contracted Haemophilus influenzae type B pneumonia and, after a stormy course in a local hospital, died of the disease.

Reference

1. Post-splenectomy vaccine prophylaxis. http://www.surgicalcriticalcare.net/Guidelines/splenectomy_vaccines.pdf. Accessed January 3, 2010.

The Surgical Mask Is Comparable – "Non-inferior" – to the Fit-Tested N95 Respirator in Preventing Influenza

Loeb et al. compared the effectiveness of surgical masks vs. fit-tested N95 respirators in preventing influenza in 446 nurses randomly assigned to use one or the other during the influenza season. Laboratory-confirmed influenza infection occurred in 23.6% of the surgical mask group and 22.9% of those in the N95 group – not much of a difference.

The authors conclude that, "the use of the surgical mask compared with an N95 respirator resulted in non-inferior rates of laboratory-confirmed influenza" [1].

This is a great study, looking at a question that affects what we do each day.

The outcome – not much difference in the two methods – which validates the use of surgical masks for protection in many settings, can save health care systems a lot of money, and may just increase compliance with reasonable precautions for the self-protection of health professionals.

Reference

1. Loeb M, Dafoe N, Mahoney J, et al. Surgical mask vs N95 respirator for preventing influenza among health care workers: a randomized trial. JAMA. 2009;302(17):1865–1871.

###

Warfarin Seems to Be No Better than Aspirin or Even Placebo in Preventing Recurrent Strokes

Let us look at two studies. The Warfarin–Aspirin Recurrent Stroke Study (WARSS) randomized 2,206 persons with cerebrovascular disease to therapy with warfarin or aspirin. After 2 years there was no difference between the two groups in the incidence of recurrent stroke [1].

Then what about warfarin vs. placebo? A Cochrane meta-analysis reviewed 11 randomized controlled trials involving 2,487 patients taking warfarin (or one of its analogues) or placebo after a transient ischemic attack (TIA) or presumed non-cardioembolic stroke. The authors report no statistical difference in regard to subsequent nonfatal stroke, recurrent ischemic stroke, myocardial infarction, or death. When it came to adverse events, however, warfarin anticoagulation resulted in a higher incidence of fatal intracranial hemorrhage and major extracranial hemorrhage [2].

As for me, when and if I have my first TIA, please don't give me warfarin. The drug was developed as a synthetic form of bishydroxycoumarin, an anticoagulant known to cause bleeding in cattle eating spoiled sweet clover silage [3].

References

1. Mohr JP, Thompson JL, Lazar RM, et al. A comparison of warfarin and aspirin for the prevention of recurrent ischemic stroke. N Engl J Med. 2001;345(20):1444–1451.
2. Sandercock PAG, Mielke O, Liu M, Counsell C. Anticoagulants for preventing recurrence following presumed non-cardioembolic ischaemic stroke or transient ischaemic attack. Cochrane Database Syst Rev. 2003;(1):CD000248.
3. Haubrich WS. Medical meanings: a glossary of word origins. Philadelphia: American College of Physicians; 1997; page 247.

###

Breast Cancer and Prostate Cancer Account for One Quarter of All Cancers in the United States

The incidence is remarkably close, with an estimated 194,000 breast cancer and 192,000 prostate cancer new cases diagnosed annually. (See Chap. 3 for the full list of cancers in America.) What's more, the 5 year survival rates are not too different: 98% for breast cancer and a remarkable 100% for prostate cancer [1]. I highlight the high incidence here to emphasize the need for diligent, and appropriate, detection efforts for these two common and treatable cancers.

At this point in the chapter, we move to screening, and the major screening controversies of the day have to do with early detection of breast and prostate cancer. We next look at these two issues, in an attempt to present some actual facts.

Reference

1. Esserman L, Shieh Y, Thompson I. Rethinking screening for breast cancer and prostate cancer. JAMA. 2009;302(15):1685–1692.

The US Preventive Services Task Force (USPSTF) Has Recommended that Mammography No Longer Be Considered a "Standard" Test for Women 40–49 Years of Age and that Mammography Be Performed Biennially Rather than Annually in Women from 50 to 74 Years of Age

The revised recommendations, released November, 2009, were based on careful statistical modeling [1]. They will not only save vital health care dollars; they will also reduce the number of false positive results that can lead to unwarranted tests and emotional stress. Not everyone, however, agrees with the changes, which have sparked heated controversy both in the medical community and in the federal government, as well as anger among breast cancer patients and women's advocacy groups [2]. Part of the uproar can be attributed to the somewhat unclearly phrased recommendation: "The USPSTF recommends against routine screening mammography in women aged 40 to 49 years. The decision to start… should be an individual one and take patient context into account, including the patient's values regarding specific benefits and harms" [1].

Controversy was inevitable, given that breast cancer is projected to strike one in every ten women during their lifetimes, and that the disease causes a half million deaths annually. In the face of a firestorm of criticism, the USPSTF did some hasty explaining of their recommendations, and reminded all that the clinical context must guide decisions for individual patients.

References

1. Preventive Services Task Force. Screening for breast cancer: U.S. Preventive Services Task Force recommendation statement. Ann Intern Med. 2009;151:716–726.
2. Partridge AH, Winer EP. On mammography – more agreement than disagreement. N Engl J Med. 2009;361(26):2499–2502.

###

There Is Controversy Over the Net Benefits of Adding Clinical Breast Examination (CBE) to Screening Mammography

Two well-designed studies have shown slightly higher breast cancer detection rates when clinical breast examination is used to supplement mammography, but at the cost of an increased number of false positive reports – with all the follow-up these entail [1, 2]. The study by Bancej et al. found, "On average, CBE increased the rate of detection of small invasive cancers by 2–6 percent over rates if mammography was the sole detection method. Without CBE, programmes would be missing 3 cancers for every 10,000 screens and 3–10 small invasive cancers for every 100,000 screens" [2].

A cost analysis of this issue would be informative, although I suspect that many screening decisions are often based on intuition, advocacy, or fear of litigation.

References

1. Chiarelli AM, Majpruz V, Brown P, Theriault M, Shumak R, Mai V. The contribution of clinical breast examination to the accuracy of breast screening. J Natl Cancer Inst. 2009;101(18):1223–1225.
2. Bancej C, Decker K, Chiarelli A, Harrison M, Turner D, Brisson J. Contribution of clinical breast examination to mammography screening in the early detection of breast cancer. J Med Screen. 2003;10(1):16–21.

###

There Is No Clear Consensus About Screening for Prostate Cancer Using Prostate Specific Antigen (PSA) Determinations in Men Under Age 75

A 2009 report of an 8-year study of 76,693 men, half who received annual screening including a PSA test compared with half who received usual care, tells that the death rate from prostate cancer was very low and did not differ significantly between the two groups [1].

A logical conclusion is that most older men with prostate cancer will die of something else – dying with their cancer, rather that because of it – making early detection unnecessary, not to mention the mischief cause by over-detection of tiny tumors and premature surgical intervention. It all seems very clear. That is, until we consider the results of the European Randomized Study of Screening for Prostate Cancer, which included 182,000 men ages 50–74 years. The authors of this study conclude, "PSA-based screening reduced the rate of death from prostate cancer by 20% but was associated with a high risk of over diagnosis" [2]. To me, a 20% reduction in rate of death seems noteworthy, until we remember that the 5-year survival rate for prostate cancer is quite high. Hence just a few deaths can lead to large changes in percent [3]. The authors of the European study estimate "that 1,410 men would need to be screened and 48 additional cases of prostate cancer would need to be treated to prevent one death from prostate cancer" [2].

In order to provide needed guidance, the USPSTF courageously [4]:

- Concludes that the current evidence is insufficient to assess the balance of benefits and harms of prostate cancer screening in men younger than age 75 years. And
- Recommends against screening for prostate cancer in men age 75 years or older. (Grade: D recommendation, meaning that there is moderate or high certainty that the service has no net benefit or that the harms outweigh the benefits.)

Just to put this in a clinical context in the setting of today's medicolegal environment, here is a true story, as reported in JAMA [5]. The doctor was a third year resident and the patient was a highly educated 53-year old man presenting for a routine physical examination. After a discussion of the benefits and risks of prostate cancer screening, a decision was made to forgo a PSA screening test. Then, somehow inevitably, the patient subsequently went to another physician who ordered PSA screening and diagnosed prostate cancer. The patient sued. Following a lengthy and contentious trial involving dueling prostate cancer experts, the jury reached a verdict. The resident physician was exonerated; the residency program was found liable for $1 million.

References

1. Andriole GL, Crawford ED, Grubb RL et al. Mortality results from a randomized prostate cancer screening trial. N Engl J Med. 2009;360(13):1310–1319.
2. Schroder FH, Hugosson J, Roobol MJ. Screening and prostate-cancer mortality in a randomized European study. N Engl J Med. 2009;360(13):1320–1328.
3. Esserman L, Shieh Y, Thompson I. Rethinking screening for breast cancer and prostate cancer. JAMA. 2009;302(15):1685–1692.
4. U.S. Preventive Services Task Force. Screening for prostate cancer: recommendation statement. http://www.ahrq.gov/clinic/uspstf08/prostate/prostaters.htm#clinical. Accessed January 5, 2010.
5. Merenstein D. Winners and losers. JAMA. 2004;291:15–16.

###

Electrocardiography May Have a Role in Screening College Athletes Before Sports Participation

Baggish et al. in Boston conducted a revealing study. They screened 510 college athletes with routine history, limited physical examination and electrocardiography. They also performed transthoracic echocardiography (TTE) to detect or exclude cardiac disease that might be relevant to participation in sports. TTE revealed cardiac abnormalities in 11 of the 510 athletes. History and physical exam screening picked up 5 of these 11 abnormalities. The addition of electrocardiography detected five more [1].

There was one down-side. The addition of electrocardiography increased the false-positive rate from 5.5% for history/physical exam only to 16.9% when electrocardiography was added [1].

Reference

1. Baggish AL, Hutter AM, Wang F, et al. Cardiovascular screening in college athletes with and without electrocardiography: a cross-sectional study. Ann Intern Med. 2010;152(5):269–275.

###

Obesity Is the Best Predictor of Undiagnosed Diabetes

Americans born in the twenty-first century have a one in three chance of developing diabetes mellitus during their lifetimes [1]. In Chap. 3, I reported that diabetes ranks number six as the cause of death in America and, by a coincidence of statistical reporting, is also the sixth leading cause of disability. (Also see Chap. 3) Given the high prevalence of the disease and the opportunity to help avoid some complications if diagnosed early, screening for diabetes seems logical.

Woolthuis et al. screened 3,724 high-risk patients and 465 low risk patients in a primary care setting. Screening detected undiagnosed diabetes in 2.2% of high risk patients and in 0.4% of low risk patients. Among various risk factors considered, obesity was the best predictor of undiagnosed diabetes [2].

Perhaps the USPSTF will consider the Primary Prevention Working Group study finding regarding obesity as a predictor when they next update their recommendations for diabetes screening. Currently the USPSTF recommends only screening for type 2 diabetes in asymptomatic adults with sustained blood pressure (either treated or untreated) greater than 135/80 mmHg. This advice is a Grade B recommendation, indicating that there is high certainty that the net benefit is moderate or there is moderate certainty that the net benefit is moderate to substantial [3].

References

1. Williamson DF, Vinicor F, Boman BA, Center for Disease Control and Prevention Primary Prevention Primary Prevention Working Group. Primary prevention of type 2 diabetes mellitus by lifestyle intervention: implications for health policy. Ann Intern Med. 2004;140(11):951–957.
2. Woolthuis EP, de Grauw WJ, van Gerwen WH, et al. Yield of opportunistic targeted screening for type 2 diabetes in primary care: the diabscreen study. Ann Fam Med. 2009;7(5):422–430.
3. U.S. Preventive Services Task Force. Screening for type 2 diabetes mellitus in adults. Available at: http://www.ahrq.gov/CLINIC/uspstf/uspsdiab.htm. Accessed January 5, 2010.

###

Men Age 65–75 Years Old Who Have Ever Smoked Should Be Screened for Abdominal Aortic Aneurysm (AAA)

This USPSTF recommendation for a one-time ultrasound screening is based on four studies showing benefit. A Cochrane Database metaanalysis of studies involving 127,891 men and 9,342 women showed a significant decrease in mortality from

AAA among screened men, but not among women [1]. In a fit of benevolence, the U.S. Congress voted to allow, as a Medicare benefit, a free one-time screening for men who have smoked and for men and women with a family history of AAA.

A century ago, give or take, Sir William Osler once quipped, "No disease is more conducive to clinical humility than aneurysm of the aorta" [2]. There is a prevalence of 5–10% in men aged 65–79 years. The aneurysm is silent, until rupture causes a surgical emergency – if the patient survives long enough to reach the operating room. Cosford reports a mortality rate of 80% among patients reaching a hospital, and 50% for those who receive emergency surgical repair [1].

As a note of historical interest, Albert Einstein died of a known aortic aneurysm, which eventually burst in 1955. Einstein refused emergency surgery, saying, "I do not believe in artificially prolonging life" [3].

References

1. Cosford PA, Leng GC. Screening for abdominal aortic aneurysm. Cochrane Database Syst Rev. 2007;(2):CD002945.
2. Osler W. Quoted in: Bean RB, Bean WB. *Aphorisms by Sir William Osler*. New York: Henry Schuman; 1950; page 134.
3. Einstein A. Quoted in: Meyers MA. *Happy accidents*. New York: Arcade; 2007; page 213.

###

There Is One Global Question that Is a Good Indicator of Unrecognized Hearing Loss in the Elderly: "Do You Have a Hearing Problem Now?"

Gates et al. studied 546 older persons receiving audiometry as part of a biennial examination. In addition to audiometric testing, they received two screening tests: The 10-item Hearing Handicap Inventory for the Elderly-Screening (HHIE-S) and the single global question: Do you have a hearing problem now? When compared to the results of audiometry for each person, the single, global question was found to be more effective than the 10-item HHIE-S in detecting unrecognized hearing loss [1].

From long ago, I recall a tale of how, in World War II, the medical corps was trying to predict which soldiers would crack under battle conditions owing to overwhelming anxiety. "Shell-shock" was a term used then. Many detailed surveys were tried. In the end, the best indicator was a single, global question: "Do you consider yourself to be a nervous person?" True or not, I think the story is instructive in its focus on simplicity.

Reference

1. Gates GA, Murphy M, Rees TS, Fraher A. Screening for handicapping hearing loss in the elderly. J. Fam Pract. 2003;52(1):56–62.

###

Sometimes the Patient's Ancestry Is the Key to Needed Preconceptual or Prenatal Screening

Here are some suggestions as to whom to consider for screening, especially when the family history is unknown or there is a possible history of genetic disease in the family [1].

Consider screening for genetic disorders in these settings:

Ancestry	Disorder to suspect
African-American	Sickle cell disease; thalassemia
Ashkenazi Jews	Tay–Sachs disease, Canavan disease
Caucasian	Cystic fibrosis
Mediterranean or Middle Eastern	Thalassemia
Southeast Asian	Thalassemia

With waves of immigrants arriving in America daily, many leaving their families of origin behind, we often lose the benefits of the multi-generational family history. In its place, however, we sometimes hear of ill-defined diseases in long-lost relatives. And in the instance of children adopted from abroad in infancy, there is likely to be no birth family history at all.

Reference

1. Carl J, Hill A. Preconceptional counseling: make it part of the annual exam. J Fam Pract. 2009;58(6):307–309.

Male Circumcision Reduces the Risk of Herpes Simplex Virus Type 2 (HSV-2) and Human Papillomavirus (HPV)

Male circumcision reduces the incidence of human immunodeficiency virus (HIV) infection. But what about other types of sexually transmitted infections? In a study of 5,534 HIV-negative and uncircumcised males ages 15–49, those also seronegative for HSV-2 were assigned to one of two groups. One received circumcision immediately; the control group received circumcision 2 years later. At 24 months the control group had higher rates of seroconversion for both HSV-2 and HPV. There was no significant difference between the two groups in the incidence of syphilis [1].

This is useful information, but I am not sure that knowing these facts alone will convince many of my adult male patients to elect circumcision.

Reference

1. Tobian AA, Serwadda D, Quinn TC, et al. Male circumcision for the prevention of HSV-2 and HPV infections and syphilis. N Engl J Med. 2009;360(13):1298–1309.

###

Just Because We Can Screen for a Disease Does Not Mean Everyone Needs to Be Screened

Sometimes we do a little too much, and we screen in instances that might best be ignored. Lobato et al. report the case of a 4-year-old girl at low risk for *Mycobacterium tuberculosis* infection who was found to have a positive skin test and hence treated with isoniazid. She developed fulminant isoniazid toxicity, eventually necessitating liver transplantation. The authors cite "the need to limit skin testing to persons who have a risk factor for infection" [1].

This seems to have been an instance in which clinical judgment should have trumped policy and protocol.

Reference

1. Lobato MN, Jereb JA, Starke JR. Unintended consequences: mandatory tuberculin skin testing and severe isoniazid hepatotoxicity. Pediatrics. 2008;121(6):e1732–e1733.

#####

Chapter 5
Risk Factors and Disease Correlates

*The only way to keep your health is to eat what you don't want,
drink what you don't like and, do what you'd druther not.*

Mark Twain (Samuel Clemens) [1835–1910]
Following the Equator, Chapter 13 [1]

Mark Twain seems to be saying that the best was to preserve health is to be aware of risks – and avoid them whenever possible.

Alonzo P, a 64 year old attorney and type 2 diabetic for more than a decade, had enjoyed good glycemic control with weight management and daily use of a sulfonylurea drug. He had noted some weight loss and vague abdominal and back pain for a few months. He decided to visit his physician after his wife reported that his eyes looked yellow – jaundiced. Blood tests and diagnostic imaging revealed carcinoma of the pancreas, already metastatic to the liver.

After coming to grips with the diagnosis and the grim prognosis, the patient set out to learn all he could about his disease. One of the things he discovered is that the very sulfonylurea drug he had been taking is correlated with an increased risk of solid cancers, including cancer of the pancreas. He also learned that another effective antidiabetic drug – metformin – is associated with a lower risk of pancreatic cancer, almost as if there were some protective effect.

At his next visit with his personal physician, Alonzo had wanted to know: "Why have I been taking a sulfonylurea and not metformin? And is it possible that, if I had taken metformin, I would not have this cancer today?"

Currie et al. studied the incidence of solid tumors in 62,809 patients taking various diabetes medications. They concluded that patients on insulin or insulin secretagogues were more likely to develop solid cancers than those taking metformin, and that metformin use alone was associated with a lower risk of cancer of the pancreas or colon [2]. This was consistent with the findings of Li et al., who conducted a case–control study of 973 patients with pancreatic cancer and 863 controls. They concluded: "Metformin use was associated with reduced risk, and insulin or insulin secretagogue use was associated with increased risk of pancreatic cancer in diabetic patients" [3].

Other studies support the thesis that chronic insulin therapy is associated with an increase risk of colorectal adenomas and cancer [4, 5]. On balance, after reviewing the available literature, Gerstein takes a contrary view, stating that randomized trials have not identified a consistent link between insulin use and cancers, and he

R.B. Taylor, *Essential Medical Facts Every Clinician Should Know: To Prevent Medical Errors, Pass Board Examinations and Provide Informed Patient Care,*
DOI 10.1007/978-1-4419-7874-5_5, © Springer Science+Business Media, LLC 2011

even suggests that "the evidence is also consistent with the hypothesis that insulin therapy targeting good glycemic control might actually reduce cancers" [6].

Despite Gerstein's thoughtful analysis, I wonder how long it will be until I see a television advertisement by an attorney soliciting diabetic patients who have developed pancreatic or colorectal cancer following treatment with insulin or an insulin secretagogue.

This chapter is about risks and clinical correlations – what sometimes accompanies or follows something. When looking at risks (such as the increased incidence of pancreatic cancer in diabetic patients using insulin or insulin secretagogues) and clinical correlations (such as the increased incidence of breast cancer in parkinsonism patients), I found that the two concepts often intersect. For that reason I have combined them – risk factors and disease correlates – in this chapter.

References

1. Strauss MB. Familiar medical quotations. Boston: Little, Brown, 1968, page 206.
2. Currie CJ, Poole CD, Gale EA. The influence of glucose-lowering therapies on cancer risk in type 2 diabetes. Diabetologia. 2009;52(9):1699–1708.
3. Li D, Yeung SJ, Hassan MM, Konopleva M, Abbruzzese JL. Antidiabetic therapies affect risk of pancreatic cancer. Gastroenterology. 2009;137(2):482–488.
4. Chung YW, Han DS, Park KH, Eun CS, Yoo KS, Park CK. Insulin therapy and colorectal adenoma risk among patients with type 2 diabetes mellitus: a case–control study in Korea. Dis Colon Rectum. 2008;51(5):593–597.
5. Yang YX, Hennessy S, Lewis JD. Insulin therapy and colorectal cancer risk among type 2 diabetes mellitus patients. Gastroenterology. 2004;127(4):1044–1050.
6. Gerstein HC. Does insulin therapy promote, reduce, or have a neutral effect on cancers? JAMA. 2010;303(5):446–447.

###

Beta-Blocker Use Increases the Risk of Severe Anaphylaxis

In 1987, Toogood described the increase in severity, and conceivably even the incidence, of acute anaphylaxis that can be seen in patients using beta-blockers. Why? Because beta blockade can limit the body's inability to mount a response to anaphylaxis. The author stated, "Allergy skin testing or immunotherapy is inadvisable in patients who take a beta-blocker orally or in the form of ophthalmic eyedrops" [1]. Then in 2009, Lang lent support to this concern, advising that while the literature during the years since 1987 does not support an increased incidence of anaphylaxis in patients taking beta-blockers, there is an increase risk of severe, prolonged anaphylaxis resistant to treatment [2].

Beta-blockers are prescribed for many reasons: hypertension, migraine prophylaxis, panic disorder, glaucoma (the eye drops citied by Toogood) and more. Then think about all the things that can trigger anaphylaxis in a susceptible person – skin testing, immunotherapy, insect sting, allergenic food or drugs, and injections of radiocontrast media. In an allergy-prone individual, I suggest that a prescription for a beta-blocker should be accompanied by a discussion of the possibility that anaphylaxis could occur in certain instances.

References

1. Toogood JH. Beta-blocker therapy and the risk of anaphylaxis. CMAJ. 1987;136(9):929–933.
2. Lang DM. Do beta-blockers really enhance the risk of anaphylaxis during immunotherapy? Curr Allergy Asthma Rep. 2008;8(1):37–44.

###

Perceived and Actual Overweight Increases the Risk of Suicide Attempts in Young Persons

Suicide ranks third as a cause of death among young Americans, and the rate seems to be rising, especially among young girls [1].

This report highlights the need to attend to mood changes in young persons who are – or even think they are – overweight. Should screening for suicide risk be part of weight control programs for adolescents and teens?

Reference

1. Swahn MH, Reynolds MR, Tice M, Miranda Pierangeli C, Jones CR, Jones IR. Perceived overweight, BMI, and risk for suicide attempts: findings from the 2007 Youth Risk Behavior Study. J Adolesc Health. 2009;45(3):292–295.

###

Risk Factors for Childhood Obesity Include Parental Obesity, Early Overweight, and Too Much Television Viewing

A longitudinal study of children in the United Kingdom identified key risk factors for obesity in childhood [1]. Of 25 putative risk factors, eight were found to be noteworthy:

- Parental obesity
- Very early (by 43 months) body mass index or adiposity rebound
- More than 8 h of television viewing per week at 3 years
- Catch-up growth
- Standard deviation score for weight at 8 and 18 months
- Amount of weight gain in the first year
- High birth weight
- Short sleep duration (less than 10.5 h) at 3 years

We cannot control parental obesity after the child is born; we can't influence birth weight; and I don't think we can do much about short sleep duration at 3 years. But we, as physicians, can certainly cite this study to parents, to discourage the all-too-common practice of baby-sitting by television.

Reference

1. Reilly JJ, Armstrong J, Dorosty AR, et al. Early risk factors for obesity in childhood: cohort study. BMJ. 2005;330(7504):1357.

Acetaminophen Use Increases the Risk of Asthma in Both Children and Adults

A meta-analysis of 19 studies by Etminan et al. found that the pooled odds ratio (OR) for asthma among subjects using acetaminophen was 1.63 [1]. There was also an increase in the risk of wheezing and asthma with prenatal use of the drug.

After reading this study, I will hesitate before recommending acetaminophen for symptom control in persons known to have episodic wheezing and asthma.

Reference

1. Etminan M, Sadatsavavi M, Jafari S, et al. Acetaminophen and the risk of asthma in children and adults: a systematic review and metaanalysis. Chest. 2009;136(5):1316–1323.

Aspirin Use After a Diagnosis of Breast Cancer May Reduce the Risk of Metastasis

A prospective observational study of 4,164 women with various stages of breast cancer revealed that, among those living at least 1 year after a breast cancer diagnosis, the use of aspirin afforded a decreased risk of distant metastasis and cancer death [1]. Those who fared best were the group who used aspirin 2–5 days a week.

Of course, with any regimen involving chronic aspirin use, as is sometimes prescribed in patients with coronary artery disease, the risk of acute gastrointestinal bleeding must be considered.

Reference

1. Holmes MD, Chen WY, Li L, Hertzmark E, Spiegelman D, Hankinson SE. Aspirin intake and survival after breast cancer. J Clin Oncol. 2010;28(9):1467–1472.

###

There Is an Especially High Risk of Venous Thromboembolism Following Hip or Knee Replacement

The prospective cohort *Million Women Study* highlighted the risks of venous thromboembolism following various surgical operations [1]. Subjects (all women; it was, after all the Million *Women* Study) were 70 times more likely to suffer venous thromboembolism in the 6-week post-operative period, and even 10 times more likely after a day-case procedure. Most at risk were patients undergoing knee or hip replacement, who experienced a 1 in 45 risk of post-operative venous thromboembolism. For cancer surgery patients, the risk was 1 in 85. The study cited involved only women, but men also suffer post-operative thromboembolism.

> *The following case was summarized in a medical journal: The patient, age 35, had knee surgery, and then 2 months late was hospitalized for diverticulitis. Ten days later he presented to the emergency room (ER) with symptoms of palpitations, chest pain, and dyspnea. Based in the clinical presentation and a normal electrocardiogram, the patient was diagnosed as having a panic attack, treated with a benzodiazepine and sent home.*
>
> *You can see where this is going. A few days later the patient experienced a pulmonary embolism, was life-flighted to another hospital, and died 8 h later. A subsequent lawsuit against the ER physician resulted in a $1.26 M verdict [2].*
>
> *The story highlights that venous thromboembolism, and specifically pulmonary embolism, should be in the differential diagnosis of any person with chest pain or dyspnea, and especially if that patient has had recent surgery, and even more especially if the surgery involved the hip or knee.*

References

1. Sweetland S, Green J, Liu B, et al: Million Women Study collaborators. Duration and magnitude of the postoperative risk of venous thromboembolism in middle aged women: prospective cohort study. BMJ. 2009;339:b4583.
2. What's the verdict? PE recognized too late. J Fam Pract. 2009;58(5):288.

###

Obese Adolescents Are at Increased Risk of Developing Multiple Sclerosis (MS)

This conclusion comes from the Women in the Nurses' Health Study and the Nurses' Health Study, involving a combined total of 238,371 women [1]. Although having a "large body size" at age 20 was associated with an increased risk of MS, there seemed to be no relationship between adult body size and MS risk.

The authors, who seem to make a distinction between age 20 and "adult," speculate that prevention of adolescent obesity may help reduce the risk of developing MS.

Reference

1. Munger KL, Chitnis T, Ascherio A. Body size and risk of MS in two cohorts of US women. Neurology. 2009;73(19):1543–1550.

###

High Consumption of Red Meat Increases the Risk of Early Age-Related Macular Degeneration (AMD)

In contrast, eating chicken is inversely associated with early AMD. These conclusions are based on an Australian study of 6,734 persons aged 58–69 years followed for more than a decade. The intake of meat was estimated from a food frequency questionnaire [1].

Other AMD risks include female sex, white race, obesity, and a family history of AMD. And so, if your patient has one or more of these risk factors, good advice might be: Eat more chicken. I hope that the next study will include fish.

Reference

1. Chong EW, Simpson JA, Robman JD, et al. Red meat and chicken consumption and its association with macular degeneration. Am J Epidemiol. 2009;169(7):867–876.

###

Vitamin D Deficiency Increases the Risk of Myocardial Infarction (MI)

Men with lower levels of plasma 25-hydroxyvitamin D (25[OH]D) are at increased risk of having a heart attack. This case–control study of 18,225 men ages 40–75 years revealed higher risk of heart attack in a graded manner with low levels of 25(OH)D, a finding that was independent of family history of myocardial infarction, ethnicity, lipid levels and other risk factors [1].

In a related study, researchers in New Zealand, analyzing data from 27,153 adults, concluded that "low serum 25[OH]D levels are associated with increased heart rate, systolic blood pressure, and rate-pressure product and suggest that low vitamin D status may increase cardiac work" [2].

With this finding, would it be useful to assay serum vitamin D levels in all patients with who have angina pectoris? Should we be prescribing vitamin D for all patients with risk factors for myocardial infarction?

References

1. Giovannucci E, Liu Y, Hollis BW, Rimm EB. 25-Hydroxyvitamin D and risk of myocardial infarction in men: a prospective study. Arch Intern Med. 2008;168(11):1174–1180.
2. Scragg RK, Camargo CA Jr, Simpson RU. Relation of serum 25-hydroxyvitamin D to heart rate and cardiac work (from the National Health and Nutrition Examination Surveys). Am J Cardiol. 2010;105(1):122–128.

###

Eating Chocolate May Reduce the Risk of Cardiovascular Disease

Our colleagues in Germany studied 19,357 initially healthy persons, of whom 166 developed myocardial infarctions and 136 experienced strokes over the following 8 years. The researchers found chocolate consumption associated with a lower cardiovascular disease risk, with the inverse association greater for stroke than for myocardial infarction [1]. Blood pressure reduction appeared to play an important role.

We have long known that chocolate is a "health food." Now here is evidence-based support for our intuitive belief.

Reference

1. Buijsse B, Weikert C, Drogan D, Bergmann M, Boeing H. Chocolate consumption in relation to blood pressure and risk of cardiovascular disease in German adults. Eur Heart J. 2010;31(13):1616–23.

###

Despite Earlier, Hopeful Studies, Selenium Does Not Seem to Reduce the Risk of Prostate Cancer

Several studies have suggested that selenium may help prevent the onset of prostate cancer and/or slow tumor progression, although none of these involved large numbers of subjects [1–3].

The conclusions of these earlier studies are challenged by the report of SELECT (a somewhat contrived acronym for the Selenium and Vitamin E Cancer Prevention Trial). This was a randomized, placebo-controlled trial involving 35,533 men age 50 and older in 427 sites with no initial evidence of prostate cancer. Doses used were selenium 200 μg and vitamin E 400 IU daily. There was a median follow-up of 5.46 years. The report concludes: "Selenium or vitamin E, alone or in combination at the doses and formulations used, did not prevent prostate cancer in this population of relatively healthy men" [4].

> The 2009 SELECT study, with an Olympic list of 33 co-authors (the prize-winner for this book) will be the definitive study on selenium prevention of prostate cancer for the foreseeable future. Almost incidentally, the study also showed no protection by vitamin E against prostate cancer.
>
> Also in 2009 we find a review of the studies examining the role of lycopene in prostate cancer progression. Although lycopene use may have been associated with some reduction in pain and urinary tract symptoms, data were considered "insufficient to draw a firm conclusion with respect to lycopene supplementation in prostate cancer patients" [5].

References

1. Clark LC, Dalkin B, Krongrad A, et al. Decreased incidence of prostate cancer with selenium supplementation: results of a double-blind cancer prevention trial. Br J Urol. 1998;81(5):730–734.
2. Duffield-Lillico AJ, Dalkin BL, Reid ME, et al. Selenium supplementation, baseline selenium status and incidence of prostate cancer: an analysis of the complete treatment period of the National Prevention of Cancer Trial. BJU Int. 2003;91(7):608–612.
3. Li H, Stampfer MJ, Giovannucci EL, et al. A prospective study of plasma selenium levels and prostate cancer risk. J Natl Cancer Inst. 2004;96(9):696–703.
4. Lippman SM, Klein EA, Goodman PJ, et al. Effect of selenium and vitamin E on risk of prostate cancer and other cancers: the Selenium and Vitamin E Cancer Prevention Trial (SELECT). JAMA. 2009;301(1):39–51.

5. Haseen F, Cantwell MM, O'Sullivan JM, Murray LJ. Is there a benefit from lycopene supplementation in men with prostate cancer? A systematic review. Prostate Cancer Prostatic Dis. 2009;12(4):316–324.

###

Multivitamin Use Just Might Increase the Risk of Advanced and Fatal Prostate Cancer

From the NIH AARP Diet and Heath Study comes the observation that men who reported using multivitamins more than seven times a week had an increased risk of advanced and fatal prostate cancer. Regular multivitamin use was not associated with the risk of early or localized prostate cancer [1].

> *The study merits attention because of the large number of subjects (10,241) and the relatively long period of follow-up (5 years). Nevertheless, intuition causes me to wonder about the conclusions. Multivitamin use influenced the incidence of advanced prostate cancer, but not early or localized cancers. But weren't advanced cancers once early or localized?*
>
> *And what about multivitamins? A multivitamin is not a single compound; it is a collection of various compounds. The Centrum brand of vitamins in my medicine cabinet contains, in addition to a potpourri of vitamins, calcium, phosphorus, iodine, magnesium, chromium, molybdenum, boron, nickel, silicon, lutein, lycopene, and more. All this is taken directly from the label. Why do I need to take boron? Silicon? Molybdenum? If there is indeed a connection with prostate cancer, could it be with a single ingredient and not with the entire multivitamin concoction? Or is there some evil synergistic action of two or more of the ingredients? Maybe nickel and lutein. I think we need to keep an eye on this.*

Reference

1. Lawson KA, Wright ME, Subar A, et al. Multivitamin use and the risk of prostate cancer in the National Institutes of Health – AARP Diet and Health Study. J Natl Cancer Inst. 2007;99(10):754–764.

###

Patients with Down Syndrome Are More Likely to Develop Hyperthyroidism than Those Without Down Syndrome

Note that we are subtly shifting from risk to clinical correlations. Yes, we have long recognized that Down syndrome patients have a high prevalence of hypothyroidism. But what about the presence of hyperthyroidism in these persons? Goday-Arno et al. reviewed 1,832 medical records of Down syndrome patients, finding 12 cases of hyperthyroidism. No gender preference was detected, and the hyperthyroidism was most likely to be caused by Graves's disease [1].

The lesson learned is that the Down syndrome patient's thyroid gland may be either hypo- or hyper-active.

Reference

1. Goday-Arno A, Cerda-Esteva M, Llores-Le-Rouix JA. Hyperthyroidism in a population with Down syndrome. Clin Endocrinol. 2009;71(1):110–114.

###

There Is an Increased Incidence of Cerebral Thromboembolism in Patients with Crohn Disease

Crohn disease patients are also at risk of developing arterial thromboembolism. Calderón et al. suggest a hypercoagulable state, with elevation of factors V, VII, fibrinogen and platelets, accompanied by decreased levels of antithrombin III [1]. Freilinger et al. describe a 39 year old patient who developed both ischemic stroke and peripheral thromboembolism [2].

In another report, a 37 year old woman visited a gastroenterologist for a postoperative consult. She reported blurred vision, dizziness, and tingling in the face and right arm. Her blood pressure was elevated. She had preexisting Crohn disease and she smoked. In spite of all the clues, the physician did not make the diagnosis. The next day the patient was diagnosed with a stroke, which resulted in right hemiplegia and aphasia [3].

Since many of our Crohn disease patients are young-to-middle aged, they may not seem to be in the stroke age group. In these individuals, we need to be extra vigilant for symptoms that may suggest an impending stroke.

References

1. Calderón R, Cruz-Correa MR, Torres EA. Cerebral thrombosis associated with active Crohn's disease. P R Health Soc J. 1998;17(3):293–295.
2. Freilinger T, Reidel E, Holtmannspötter K. Ischemic stroke and peripheral arterial thromboembolism in a patient with Crohn's disease: a case presentation. J Neurol Sci. 2008;266(1–2): 177–179.
3. What's the verdict? (No author listed) Failure to suspect stroke results in brain damage. J Fam Pract. 2009;58(11):620.

###

Migraine Patients Have a Higher Incidence of Patent Foramen Ovale (PFO) than Normal Persons

In fact, half of your migraine-headache-with-aura patients may have the heart defect. In a study of 121 patients, Domitrz et al. found PFO in 54% of patients with migraine-with-aura, in 25% of patients with migraine-without-aura, and in 25% of normal controls [1].

If half our patients with aura-associated migraine have PFO, what would happen if the septal defect were closed? Vigna studied 82 patients with moderate/severe migraine, PFO, a large right-to-left shunt and subclinical brain lesions on magnetic resonance imaging (MRI). Of these patients, 53 chose percutaneous closure of the defect, and 29 did not, and thus served as the control group whose migraine therapy was optimized. Postoperatively, migraine disappeared in 34% of the closure group, in contrast to 7% of the controls. There was a greater than 50% reduction in attacks reported by 87% of subjects in the closure group compared with only 21% of subjects in the control group [2].

> On the basis of these findings, should we be discussing elective closure of PFO in our migraine patients with this defect? As of today, the consensus seems to be "no" [3]. Stay tuned.
>
> Parenthetically, as one whose epispecialty has long been headaches, I am impressed with anything done that results in 34% rate of migraine disappearance; in my experience, migraine may improve but rarely disappears. Then there is the 87% of the study group reporting greater than 50% reduction in attacks; I tell my students – perhaps somewhat cynically – that whatever intervention is studied in migraine prophylaxis, the outcome will be more-or-less the same: Fifty percent of patients in the study group showed 50% improvement. By this reckoning, 87% of subjects showing a 50% improvement in symptoms is better than most approaches reported.

References

1. Domitrz I, Mieszkowski J, Kaminska A. Relationship between migraine and patent foramen ovale: a study of 121 patients with migraine. Headache. 2007;47(9):1311–1318.
2. Vigna C, Marchese N, Inchingolo V. Improvement of migraine after patent foramen ovale percutaneous closure in patients with subclinical brain lesions: a case–control study. JACC Cardiovasc Interv. 2009;2(2):107–113.
3. Carroll JD, Carroll EP. Is patent foramen ovale closure indicated for migraine? PFO closure is not indicated for migraine: "don't shoot first, ask questions later." Circ Cardiovasc Interv. 2009;2(5):475–481.

###

Migraine Headache with Aura Is Associated with a Twofold Increased Risk of Ischemic Stroke

This statement is based on a systemic review and meta-analysis of multiple studies relating migraine to ischemic stroke, myocardial infarction, and death due to cardiovascular disease. The report further suggested a higher risk for women than men, and for patients less than age 45, smokers and women who used oral contraceptives [1]. Other studies have extended the spectrum of associated cardiovascular problems to include angina, myocardial infarction, and ischemic cardiovascular death [2, 3].

> Bigal et al. remind us that migraineurs have a "higher prevalence of risk factors known to be associated with cardiovascular disease, including hypertension, diabetes, and hyperlipidemia" [4]. With all of this in mind, we should be especially diligent in identifying and attempting to modify cardiovascular risk factors in our migraine patients.

References

1. Schurks M, Rist PM, Bibal ME. Migraine and cardiovascular disease: systemic review and meta-analysis. BMJ. 2009;339:b3914.
2. Kurth T, Gazieno JM, Cook NR. Migraine and risk of cardiovascular disease in men. Arch Intern Med. 2007;167(8):795–801.
3. Kurth T, Schürks M, Logroscino G, Buring JE. Migraine and risk of cardiovascular disease in women. Neurology. 2009;73(8):581–588.
4. Bigal ME, Kurth T, Hu H, Santanello N, Lipton RB. Migraine and cardiovascular disease: possible mechanisms of interaction. Neurology. 2009;72(21):1864–1871.

###

A Third of Headache Patients Are Also Depressed

A case–control study of 200 patients by Marlow et al. showed that, upon screening with the PRIME-MD 9-item Patient Health Questionnaire, 32% of headache patients reported symptoms of depression. This compared with only 10% of patients without headache [1].

> We in primary care who care for both headache and depressed patients have long suspected this correlation. It is reassuring to see our hunch confirmed. This interesting correlation raises several questions. Are the patients depressed because of recurrent pain? Is headache a manifestation of primary depression in these individuals? Is there some common precursor? In any case, the co-existence of headache and depression can often influence the choice of medication for prophylaxis. Think of antidepressants as useful therapy for both.

Reference

1. Marlow RA, Kegowicz CL, Starkey KN. Prevalence of depression symptoms in outpatients with a complaint of headache. J Am Board Fam Med. 2009;22(6):633–637.

###

Prior Statin Use Is Correlated with Improved Outcomes in Patients with Community-Acquired Pneumonia (CAP)

Patients with community-acquired pneumonia who take statin drugs to lower cholesterol fare better when compared to those who do not take statins. Chalmers et al. examined records of patients admitted for CAP over a 2 year period, looking at 30-day mortality, the need for mechanical ventilation or inotropic support, and the development of complicated pneumonia. Compared with patients using other medications or no cardiovascular drugs, those using statins had reduced markers of systemic inflammation and improved outcomes [1].

This finding raises a question: If a patient diagnosed with community-acquired pneumonia is not taking statin drugs, should these be prescribed at that time?

Reference

1. Chalmers JD, Singanayagam A, Murray MP, Hill AT. Prior statin use is associated with improved outcomes in community-acquired pneumonia. Am J Med. 2008;121(11):1002–1007.

###

Parkinson Disease Is Associated with Less of Some Cancers, but Not All

An article in the journal *Neurology* reports that epidemiologic studies reveal that patients with Parkinson disease have, in general, lower cancer rates. As described in Chap. 12, parkinsonian patients have a relatively low incidence of smoking, but the authors conclude that the risk reduction cannot be ascribed to this non-smoking tendency. Also found was that, while Parkinson disease patients enjoyed a reduced risk for most cancers, they were at increased risk of developing breast cancer and melanoma. All of this is postulated to be related to involvement and mutations of common genes in both diseases [1].

Perhaps some extra diligence is warranted in screening for breast cancer and melanoma in Parkinson disease patients.

Reference

1. Inzelberg R, Jankovic J. Are Parkinson disease patients protected from some but not all cancers? Neurology. 2007;69(15):1542–1550.

###

In Patients with Colorectal Cancer, Physical Activity Is Correlated with a Lower Risk of Death

The Health Professional Follow-up Study included 668 men with a history of stage I to III colorectal cancer. In these patients, those who engaged in physical exercise had a lower risk of colorectal cancer-specific and overall mortality [1].

The study cited showed the benefit of exercise was not related to age, body mass index, tumor location, stage of disease, or even prediagnosis physical activity. For all who can do so, regular exercise is a good idea – for many reasons – and this is just one more.

Reference

1. Meyerhardt JA, Giovannucci IL, Ogino S, et al. Physical activity and male colorectal cancer. Arch Intern Med. 2009;169(22):2102–2108.

###

There Is a High Prevalence of Osteopenia and Osteoporosis in Patients with Chronic Obstructive Pulmonary Disease (COPD)

A study of 658 patients in 88 US medical centers revealed that, based on bone mineral density (BMD) testing, 41% of women and 42% of men had osteopenia, and 30% of women and 18% of men had osteoporosis [1].

The figures cited come from a study of the long-term effects on bone of inhaled corticosteroid (ICS) therapy in COPD patients. Following this 3-year trial, investigators report that "no significant effect on BMD was detected for ICS therapy compared with placebo" [1].

Reference

1. Ferguson GT, Calverley PM, Anderson JA, et al. Prevalence and progression of osteoporosis in patients with COPD: results from the TOwards a Revolution in COPD Health study. Chest. 2009;136(6):1456–1465.

###

Married Patients with Cancer Live Longer

In a review of an impressive 3.79 million records accessed through the Surveillance, Epidemiology and End Results (SEER) registry, Sprehn et al. found that among subjects who were not married, those separated at the time cancer was diagnosed had the shortest survival of all, followed by widowed, divorced, and never-married patients [1]. For those subjects separated at the time of cancer diagnosis the 5-year relative survival was 72% of that of married patients at 5 years, and 64% at 10 years.

I found noteworthy that the finding that the survival advantage of married vs separated persons "persists when data are analyzed by gender" [1].

Reference

1. Sprehn GC, Chambers JE, Saykin AJ, Konski A, Johnstone PA. Decreased cancer survival in individuals separated at time of diagnosis: critical period for cancer pathophysiology? Cancer. 2009;115(21):5108–5116.

###

Patients with Endometriosis Have a Higher Prevalence of Infection, Melanoma and Ovarian Cancer than the General Population

A survey by Gemmill et al. of 4,441 women with surgically diagnosed endometriosis revealed more instances of upper respiratory infection and vaginal infection then in those without the disease. There also was a higher rate of melanoma and ovarian cancer, although breast cancer was found to occur less commonly than in the general population [1].

This suggests that the immune system is somehow involved in endometriosis. It also means that we must pay attention to the patient's heightened risk of cancer in these patients.

Reference

1. Gemmill JA, Stratton P, Cleary SD, Ballweg ML, Sinaii N. Cancers, infections, and endocrine diseases in women with endometriosis. Fertil Steril. 2010;94:1627–1631.

###

There Seems to Be a Negative Correlation Between Alzheimer Disease (AD) and Cancer

By that I mean that, at least in a study of white older persons, there was a reduced risk of cancer in patients with AD and a reduced risk of AD in patients with a history of cancer [1]. The study involved 3,020 persons age 65 or more followed for dementia for a mean of 5.4 years and for cancer for a mean of 8.3 years, with adjustments for demographics, hypertension, diabetes and so forth. The relatively small number of minorities in the study group precluded the provision of "stable estimates," and thus the conclusion mentions only white patients.

> Behrens et al. suggest that the inverse relationship of cancer and Alzheimer disease is based in the mechanisms involved in cell survival/death regulation. Simply stated, in cancer there is augmentation of cell survival and proliferation, while in Alzheimer disease there is increased neuronal cell death [2]. That there is something specific to these two conditions seems reinforced by the finding of no relationship between cancer and vascular dementia [1].

References

1. Roe CM, Fitzpatrick AL, Xiong C, et al. Cancer linked to Alzheimer disease but not vascular dementia. Neurology. 2010;74:106–112.
2. Behrens MI, Lendon C, Roe CM. A common biological mechanism in cancer and Alzheimer's disease. Curr Alzheimer Res. 2009;6(3):196–204.

###

Higher Circulating Leptin Levels Are Associated with Reduced Incidence of Alzheimer Disease

As part of the ongoing Framingham Study, 785 persons had plasma leptin levels assayed and a subsample of 198 dementia-free survivors underwent volumetric brain MRI approximately 7.7 years later. The authors report finding a lower incidence of dementia and AD in individuals with higher leptin levels [1].

According to Carro, leptin is a peptide involved in lipid homeostasis. It has been shown to reduce amyloid beta levels and tau-related pathological pathways, the major pathological hallmarks of AD. Finding a way to increase circulating leptin levels may prove helpful in preventing or treating AD [2].

References

1. Lieb W, Beiser AS, Vasan RS. Association of plasma leptin levels with incident Alzheimer disease and MRI measures of brain aging. JAMA. 2009;302(23):2565–2572.
2. Carro EM. Therapeutic approaches of leptin in Alzheimer disease. Recent Pat CNS Drug Discov. 2009;4(3):200–208.

\#\#\#

Sleep Restriction May Correlate with Alzheimer Disease

A study in mice revealed that brain levels of amyloid increased during wakefulness and decreased during sleep. Taking things one step further, Kang et al. injected the brains of mice with orexin, a sleep inhibiting compound, and found that amyloid levels rose. When orexin was blocked, allowing sleep, amyloid levels fell [1].

Yes, this was a study in mice and, yes, the study measured levels of amyloid and not the actual development of Alzheimer disease. Nevertheless, this sort of basic research, like the study involving leptin described above, may prove to be the vanguard of future interventions for AD.

Reference

1. Kang JE, Lim MM, Bateman RJ, et al. Amyloid-beta dynamics are regulated by orexin and the sleep-wake cycle. Science. 2009;326(5955):1005–1007.

\#\#\#

There Is a Link Between Cardiovascular Disease (CVD) and Hip Fracture

Persons with a diagnosis of heart failure, stroke or coronary artery disease are at increased risk of hip fracture. Heart failure carries the greatest risk with a crude absolute rate of hip fracture ten times greater than persons without a CVD diagnosis [1].

One might logically jump to the conclusion that persons with CVD simply fall more often, explaining the increased incidence of hip fracture. Sennerby et al. suggest that this is not the case and, instead, that cardiovascular disease and osteoporotic fractures share a common cause. Their study examined identical twins. They found that when Twin A had a cardiovascular disease, there was a greater incidence of hip fracture in Twin B, even when Twin B did not have CVD. They conclude: "Increased risks (of hip fracture) in co-twins without an index diagnosis (CVD) suggest genetic factors in the association between CVD and osteoporotic fractures" [1].

Reference

1. Sennerby U, Melhus H, Gedeborg R, et al. Cardiovascular diseases and risk of hip fracture. JAMA. 2009;302(15):1666–1673.

There Is an Association Between Coronary Artery Disease and Major Depression

What is interesting is that the sustained effect of coronary artery disease on major depression is much stronger than the effect of major depression on coronary artery disease, according to a study of 30,374 twins. The risk of major depression co-occurring with coronary artery disease was increased if the diagnosis was myocardial infarction [1].

In this study involving twins, genetic factors in co-morbidity seemed to play greater roles in women than in men, and in younger rather than older individuals.

Reference

1. Kendler KS, Gardner CO, Fiske A, Ganz M. Major depression and coronary artery disease in the Swedish twin registry: phenotypic, genetic, and environmental sources of comorbidity. Arch Gen Psychiatry. 2009;66(8):857–863.

Depression Rivals Smoking as a Risk Factor for Death

Linking a large population survey of 61,349 persons and a comprehensive mortality database, Norwegian investigators found a profound link between depression and mortality. The authors concluded, "Depression as a risk factor for mortality was comparable in strength to smoking." Curiously, the presence of co-morbid anxiety lessened the incidence of death [1].

> Considering that smoking is the leading "actual cause of death," (See Chap. 3.) the mortality risk of having depression is high, indeed. And, parenthetically, I think that the reduced incidence of death with comorbid depression/anxiety reminds us that depression is not a single, monolithic disease. Now I wonder if treating depression actually lessens the risk of death.

Reference

1. Mykletun A, Bjerkeset O, Overland S, Prince M, Dewey M, Stewart R. Levels of anxiety and depression as predictors of mortality: the HUNT study. Br J Psychiatry. 2009;195(2):118–125.

###

There Are Some Diverse Clinical Findings Associated with an Increased Risk of Death

Here are a few of the disease manifestations that should worry the informed clinician:

- Major depressive disorder (MDD) within a few weeks of hospitalization for an acute coronary syndrome (ACS) or failure of MDD to improve during the 6 months following ACS predicted more than a doubling of mortality over the following 6.7 years [1].
- Ambulatory heart failure (HF) patients with low serum sodium and low standard deviation of all normal-to-normal RR intervals (SDNN) and high serum creatinine are at increased risk of fatal progressive HF [2].
- Anemia in elderly persons with atrial fibrillation increases the risk of death [3].
- A low thigh circumference, perhaps related to decreased muscle mass, is associated with an increased risk of heart disease and premature death [4].
- Sleep-disordered breathing is associated with all-cause mortality, notably due to coronary artery disease, and especially in men ages 40–70 years [5].
- Rheumatoid arthritis is associated with a 60% increase in cardiovascular mortality compared to those without the disease [6].
- Slow walking speed in older persons is associated with an increased risk of cardiovascular death [7].

> All of the above are correlates "associated with" premature death. None are absolute. Yet having one or two of the above, if accompanied by hypertension, diabetes, hyperlipidemia or other cardiovascular risk factors, could present a very worrisome picture indeed.

References

1. Glassman AH, Bigger JT, Gaffney M, et al. Psychiatric characteristics associated with long-term mortality among 361 patients having an acute coronary syndrome and major depression: seven year follow-up of SADHART participants. Arch Gen Psychiatry. 2009;66(9): 1022–1029.
2. Kearney MT, Fox KA, Lee AJ, et al. Predicting death due to progressive heart failure in patients with mild-to-moderate chronic heart failure. J Am Coll Cardiol. 2002;40(10): 1801–1818.
3. Sharma S, Gage BF, Deych E, Rich MW. Anemia: an independent predictor of death and hospitalizations among elderly patients with atrial fibrillation. Am Heart J. 2009;157(6): 1057–1063.
4. Heitmann BL, Frederiksen P. Thigh circumference and risk of heart disease and premature death: prospective cohort study. BMJ. 2009;339:b3292.
5. Punjabi NM, Caffo BS, Goodwin JL, et al. Sleep-disordered breathing and mortality: a prospective cohort study. PLoS Med. 2009;6(8):e1000132.
6. Meune C, Touze ER, Trinquart L, et al. Trends in cardiovascular mortality in patients with rheumatoid arthritis over 50 years: a systematic review and meta-analysis of cohort studies. Rheumatology. 2009;48(10):1309–1313.
7. Dumurgier J, Elbaz A, Ducimetière P, Tavernier B, Alpérovitch A, Tourio C. Slow walking speed and cardiovascular death in well functioning older adults: prospective cohort study. BMJ. 2009;339:4460–4463.

#####

Chapter 6
Practical Clinical Pearls

Diagnosis is founded upon observation of trifles

Hen JY, Rule number 53.
Quoted in Meador CK [1]

This chapter about how observing some trifles and recognizing what is seen is intended to help us become better diagnosticians.

> Caroline P., a 7-year old white girl, was brought to her physician because of repeated bouts of rhinosinusitis and bronchitis. Finally the physician sought consultation with an otolaryngologist, who diagnosed nasal polyps and recommended surgery. Before agreeing to surgery, the mother asked if there could be anything else causing the problem. This query prompted the physician to ask some more questions. Yes, Caroline had always seemed to have "fatty" stools. Also, her mother had long noted that when she kissed her child, she somehow tasted "salty." She had just never mentioned the "salty kisses" to the doctor. These findings prompted a sweat chloride test, which revealed a very high sodium chloride concentration, consistent with the diagnosis of cystic fibrosis (CF).

Nasal polyps in a child age 12 or under may be the tip-off to a diagnosis of cystic fibrosis, the most common fatal autosomal recessive disease affecting white children and adults. Mainz et al. estimate the incidence of chronic rhinosinusitis and/or nasal polyps in CF patients at up to 50% [2]. Robertson et al. state that paranasal and sinus disease is present in almost every patient with cystic fibrosis [3]. In a study of 23 children 5–18 years of age, Yung et al. found that 13 had endoscopic evidence of nasal polyposis [4]. All these figures compare with very uncommon incidence of nasal polyps in normal children [5].

Then there is the "salty kisses" clue to the diagnosis of cystic fibrosis. For 400 years there has been the belief that, "A child that tastes salty will die soon" [6]. Today sweat testing for sodium chloride levels is the cornerstone of cystic fibrosis diagnosis.

That nasal polyps (or for that matter "sweaty kisses") can be the tipoff to cystic fibrosis is a useful and time-honored clinical pearl. Lorin et al. have provided us with a handy definition of these treasured nuggets of wisdom: "Clinical pearls are best defined as small bits of free standing, clinically relevant information based on experience or observation." They fit in the "vast domain of experience-based

R.B. Taylor, *Essential Medical Facts Every Clinician Should Know: To Prevent Medical Errors, Pass Board Examinations and Provide Informed Patient Care*,
DOI 10.1007/978-1-4419-7874-5_6, © Springer Science+Business Media, LLC 2011

medicine, and can be helpful in dealing with clinical problems for which controlled data do not exist" [7]. The Lorin et al. description, however, fails to take into account today's easy access to medical evidence – randomized controlled trials, meta-analyses, and all the rest. Thus, when we encounter a pearl such as the nasal polyp–CF connection, we can readily seek data to verify or discredit the pearl. For most of the pearls presented in this chapter, I have been able to find some supporting data, in an effort to move from medical folklore to evidence-based fact. In some cases, I could find no pertinent studies, and these pearls for which we continue to rely on "experience and observation" are presented with this disclaimer.

How will you know when you come across a valuable pearl? First of all, it is not a well-known fact; there are "glass beads," perfectly good clinical facts, but they are not pearls. Secondly, they express some sort of truth; seemingly profound statements that lack clinical validity are "plastic pearls," the misconceptions and myths covered in Chap. 2. Something about a pearl is memorable, perhaps because the source is a venerated teacher, maybe because you acquired the knowledge through painful personal experience. Then there is generalizability – knowledge that can be useful in future clinical settings. And finally, the pearl is phrased in a succinct manner.

Sometimes the word "pithy" is used, but I like to reserve this word to describe aphorisms. For example, here are two of my favorite aphorisms: "Adhesions are the last refuge of the diagnostically destitute," by Sir William Osler (1849–1919), and "All that wheezes is not asthma," by Chevalier Jackson (1865–1958) [8]. Are these almost-poetic aphorisms also clinical pearls? Maybe. But most clinical pearls are simply statements, and we remember them because they help us in our daily practice. This chapter presents my string of clinical pearls – a few are lyrical, most are not – with literature citations whenever I could find them.

References

1. Meador CK. A little book of doctors' rules II. Philadelphia: Hanley & Belfus; 1999.
2. Mainz JG, Koitschev A. Management of chronic rhinosinusitis in CF. J Cyst Fibros. 2009;8(suppl 1):S10–S14.
3. Robertson JM, Friedman EM, Rubin BK. Nasal and sinus disease in cystic fibrosis. Ped Respir Rev. 2008;9(3):213–219.
4. Yung MW, Gould J, Upton GJ. Nasal polyposis in children with cystic fibrosis: a long-term follow-up study. Ann Otol Rhinol Laryngol. 2002;111(12 Pt 1):1081–1086.
5. Lund VJ. Diagnosis and treatment of nasal polyps. BMJ. 1995;311:1411–1414.
6. Quinton PM. Cystic fibrosis: lessons from the sweat gland. Physiology (Bethesda). 2007;22:212–225.
7. Lorin MI, Palazzi DL, Turner DL, Ward MA. What is a clinical pearl and what is its role in medical education? Med Teach. 2008;30(9–10):870–874.
8. Quoted in Taylor RB. White coat tales: medicine's heroes, heritage and misadventures. New York: Springer; 2008; pages 127–129.

###

It Is Not a Stroke Until the Patient Has Had 50 of D50

My evidence for this pearl is an essay on clinical pearls by Mangrulkar et al. [1]. I doubt that anyone has ever done a randomized, controlled trial of giving every other suspected stroke patient a quick trial of empiric 50 mL intravenously of 50% dextrose (D50) solution. Such a quick and harmless trial will, of course, revive the person in insulin-induced hypoglycemia but have no effect on stroke.

I present this pearl early in the chapter because, although I cannot find evidence-based support in the form of a randomized clinical study, it has the other key features of a useful clinical pearl: It is catchy, clinically relevant and time-tested. It has both face validity and the attribute, as described by Osler, of being like a burr that sticks in your memory [2].

References

1. Mangrulkar MD, Saint S, Chu S, Tierney LM. What is the role of the clinical "pearl?" Am J Med. 2002;113(7):1–7.
2. Reveno WS. Medical Maxims. Springfield IL: Charles C. Thomas; 1951.

###

A Handshake Can Be the First Step in Diagnosis

Shaking hands with a patient is not only a welcoming social gesture. It can also provide clues to a number of diagnoses:

- Anxiety may cause a sweaty palm.
- A very warm hand may indicate fever or even hyperthyroidism.
- A weak grip may indicate depression, fatigue, or neurologic deficit.
- A very cold hand may be a sign of Raynaud's phenomenon.
- A gnarled hand may indicate rheumatoid arthritis.
- A shaky hand, with an intention tremor, may indicate Parkinsonism.
- A "weaving" handshake may be seen in chorea.
- A contracture of the flexor tendons occurs with Dupuytren contracture, seen especially in persons of Celtic or Viking descent [1].
- A wrist drop occurs with "Saturday night palsy" or even lead poisoning [2].

This question, about what diseases can be suggested by a handshake, is one of my favorites when teaching medical students.

References

1. Brenner P, Krause-Bergmann A. Van VH. Dupuytren contracture in North Germany: epidemiological study of 500 cases. Unfallchirug. 2001;104(4):303–311.
2. Spinner RJ, Poliakoff MB, Tiel RL. The origin of "Saturday night palsy." Neurosurgery. 2002;51(3):737–74.

###

Drooping Eyelids and the "Peek" Sign May Signal the Presence of Myasthenia Gravis

These manifestations of extraocular muscle weakness occur in 90% of patients with myasthenia gravis, and represent the initial complaint in about half [1]. The "peek" sign occurs as the patient appears to peek at the examiner when, "after momentary opposition on gentle sustained lid closure, the lid margins separated, resulting in widening of the palpebral fissure and scleral exposure" [2].

> *Keep in mind that in about one patient in five with myasthenia gravis, the only manifestation of the disease will be the eye signs [1].*

References

1. Sommer N, Melms A, Weller M, Dichgans J. Ocular myasthenia gravis: a critical review of clinical and pathophysiological aspects. Doc Ophthalmol. 1993;84(4):309–333.
2. Osher RH, Griggs RC. Orbicularis fatigue: the "peek" sign of myasthenia gravis. Arch Ophthalmol. 1979;97:677–699.

###

Beware of Future Migraine when a Child Has Severe Motion Sickness

Childhood carsickness can be the first sign of what will become adult migraine. The phenomenon may even occur with virtual motion found in panoramic movies. Motion sickness occurs in approximately 50% of all migraine sufferers, and the childhood tendency may linger, even when the headaches begin in adult life [1].

> *When a parent mentions that a child has motion sickness, I inquire about a family history of migraine. Also, ask your current adult migraine patients if they recall carsickness in childhood; many of them will respond that they clearly recall nausea, especially when riding in the back seat of the car.*

Reference

1. Marcus DA, Furman JM, Balaban CD. Motion sickness in migraine sufferers. Expert Opin Pharmacother. 2005;6(15):2691–2697.

Three of Every Ten Patients with Subarachnoid Hemorrhage (SAH) Are Initially Misdiagnosed

How can this occur, when every third year medical student learns the significance of a sudden, severe, and worst-ever headache? The answer is that the telltale sudden, severe headache is absent in one fourth of all patients with SAH, and even if present, its presence may not be clearly communicated to the physician [1, 2].

Edlow attributes the 30% misdiagnosis rate to two general causes: failure to understand the full spectrum of manifestations of SAH and failure to know the limits of the key diagnostic tests – computed tomography and lumbar puncture [3]. For example, the sensitivity of computed tomography scanning of the brain declines after the first day of symptoms [2].

References

1. ACROSS Group. Epidemiology of aneurismal subarachnoid hemorrhage in Australia and New Zealand. Incidence and case fatality from the Australasian Cooperative Research on Subarachnoid Hemorrhage Study (ACROSS). Stroke. 2000;31(9):1843–1850.
2. Hankey GJ, Nelson MR. Easily missed? Subarachnoid hemorrhage. BMJ. 2009;339:b2874.
3. Edlow JA. Diagnosis of subarachnoid hemorrhage. Neurocrit Care. 2005;2(2):99–109.

When a Long Distance Runner Is Found to Be Anemic, Think of *Runner's Anemia*

When a long-distance runner presents with a mild anemia he or she may have "runner's anemia." In this setting, there is a relative macrocytosis resulting from the hemolysis of older, mature red blood cells. The hemolysis is the result of pounding of feet on pavement, and can be related to the number of miles run. Other factors may include plasma volume expansion and gastrointestinal blood loss [1]. Eichner suggests that runner's macrocytosis resulting from footstrike hemolysis may, by ridding the system of aging erythrocytes, actually benefit the athlete in some instances [2].

Awareness of the phenomenon of footstrike hemolysis and runner's anemia may save the patient the expense of a search for a deficiency state or myelodysplastic syndrome.

References

1. Dang CV. Runner's anemia. JAMA. 2001;286(6):714–716.
2. Eichner ER. Runner's macrocytosis: a clue to footstrike hemolysis. Runner's anemia as a benefit versus runner's hemolysis as a detriment. Am J Med. 1985;78(2):321–325.

###

A Patient with Early and Rampant Dental Caries May Have Sjögren Syndrome

Sjögren syndrome is an autoimmune disease manifested chiefly as dry eyes (keratoconjunctivitis sicca), dry mouth (xerostomia) and fatigue. The dry mouth, with decreased saliva produced, leads to the formation of dental caries [1].

This is just one more reason to examine each patient's mouth and teeth. To quote Lindsay, "For one mistake made for not knowing, ten mistakes are made for not looking" [2].

Ask these patients how they deal with the problem of dry mouth. The carious process is often hastened as patients use hard candy to relieve xerostomic symptoms.

References

1. Mathews SA, Kurien BT, Scofield RH. Oral manifestations of Sjögren syndrome. J Dent Res. 2008;87(4):308–318.
2. Lindsay JA. Medical axioms, aphorisms and clinical memoranda. London: H.K. Lewis Co.; 1923; page 7.

###

Behçet Syndrome May Present as Severe, Recurrent Aphthous Stomatitis

Also known as the oculo-oral-genital syndrome or malignant aphthosis, Behçet syndrome characteristically causes painful ulcers of the mouth, eyes and genital areas. Although posterior uveitis can be a prominent feature of the disease, oral ulcers occur in most patients and can be the only or earliest manifestation of the disease [1].

The highest prevalence of the Behçet syndrome is in Turkey, and the disease seems to be most common and most severe along the path of the old Silk Road traversed by Marco Polo in the thirteenth century and by others that subsequently followed in his footsteps [2, 3]. The geographic distribution of the disease suggests that genetics play a role, and that the source long ago may have been one or more peripatetic and highly fecund merchants traveling the trading routes connecting the Eastern Mediterranean and China. The eponymous name of the syndrome is of Turkish, not French, origin and is pronounced "bay-chet."

References

1. Oh SH, Han EC, Lee JH, Bang D. Comparison of the clinical features of recurrent aphthous stomatitis and Behçet's disease. Clin Exp Dermatol. 2009;34(6):e208–e212.
2. Alli N, Gur G, Yalcin B, Hayran M. Patient characteristics in Behçet disease: a retrospective analysis of 213 Turkish patients during 2001–2004. Am J Clin Dermatol. 2009;10(6):411–418.
3. Yurdakul S, Hamuryudan V, Yazici H. Behçet syndrome. Curr Opin Rheumatol. 2004;16(1):38–42.

###

The First Indication of Hyperthyroidism May Be the Onset of Atrial Fibrillation (AF)

The incidence of atrial fibrillation in the general population is 4% (a figure I find surprisingly high). Among persons with hyperthyroidism, there is a 15% incidence of AF. Subclinical hyperthyroidism causes a threefold increase in the incidence of AF [1].

Be especially suspicious of this possible connection in older patients. Also, here is a tip, one of those for which I have been unable to find evidence-based support. Reveno states, "The patient notices rapid heart action more promptly than irregularity" [2]. Of course, both cardiac manifestations – tachycardia and irregularity – can occur in hyperthyroidism.

References

1. Bielecka-Dabrowa A, Mikhailidis DP, Rysz J, Banach M. The mechanisms of atrial fibrillation in hyperthyroidism. Thyroid Res. 2009;2(1):4–8.
2. Reveno WS. 711 Medical maxims. Springfield IL: Charles C. Thomas; 1951; page 32.

###

A Patient with Chest Pain Relieved by Leaning Forward May Have Pericarditis

Specifically, patients with uncomplicated pericarditis have a "pleuritic" type of chest pain, sometimes radiating to the one or both shoulders that decreases in intensity when the patient sits up and leans forward. Occasionally, however, the patient will describe a dull, oppressive discomfort much like that of angina or myocardial infarction [1].

In this setting, listen carefully for a pericardial friction rub, specific for acute pericarditis. On the electrocardiogram, look for widespread ST elevation or PR depression.

Reference

1. Goyle KK, Walling AD. Diagnosing pericarditis. Am Fam Physician. 2002;66(9):1695–1702.

###

The Patient with Cough and Dyspnea Who Uses a Hot Tub Might Just Have *Hot Tub Lung*

Hot tub lung is a recently recognized lung disorder caused *Mycobacterium avium* complex. A study of 21 patients referred to a tertiary level center revealed a variety of (off-target) referral diagnoses, including asthma, bronchitis and sarcoidosis. In all instances, *M. avium* was isolated from the hot tub water, respiratory secretions and/or lung tissue [1].

> We have known about hot tub dermatitis due to Pseudomonas, and now we have hot tub lung to think about when enjoying a soak.

Reference

1. Hanak V, Kalra S, Aksamit TR, Hartman TE, Taxelaar HD, Ryu JH. Hot tub lung: presenting features and clinical course of 21 patients. Respir Med. 2006;100(4):610–615.

###

A Patient with Acute Appendicitis Usually Has a Loss of Appetite

If the patient is hungry, a diagnosis of acute appendicitis should be questioned. That patients with appendicitis have usually lost their appetites is a confirmed clinical pearl. In a study of 267 patients operated upon for acute appendicitis, Gonclaves et al. found that 86% had anorexia [1].

> Perhaps the "stick in the memory" pearl is: Beware of opening the belly of the hungry patient.

Reference

1. Gonclaves M, Martins AP, Leal MJ. Acute appendicitis in children. Acta Med Port (Portugal). 1993;6:377–382.

###

The Jump Test Can Help Clarify a Suspected Diagnosis of Appendicitis

Sometimes the abdominal examination in a child can be a challenge, especially if there is pain. The stakes are especially high when the child might have acute appendicitis or some other cause of a surgical abdomen. One way to test for peritoneal irritability is to ask the child to jump up and down. The child with simple stomach cramps or other non-surgical problem will generally comply readily. In contrast, the child with a peritoneal irritability suggesting a surgical abdomen, however, is likely to resist the "jump test" because of pain [1].

> Why not? As a diagnostic maneuver, the jump test is safe and cheap. Even with modern imaging technology, the diagnosis of appendicitis is often not clear-cut.
>
> On a historical note regarding appendicitis, in 1909 the Journal of the American Medical Association (JAMA) published an essay speculating that some of the deaths that have shaped history and that have been attributed to poisoning – such as that of Britannicus, son of Roman emperor Claudius – might well have been caused by appendicitis. Consider, as described a century ago: "After all, the story of appendicitis, if one has not the key to it reads very much like that of poison. The symptoms develop suddenly, not long after a meal; there is apt to be intense pain; general peritonitis develops, and the abdominal tenderness indicates some intense irritant within, which, of course, would be thought to be the poison at work" [2].

References

1. Holtry L. Practical Pointers. Consultant, July 2009; p. 437.
2. Pathology and History, April 17, 1909. Reiling J, series editor. JAMA. 2009;301(16):1721.

###

Painless Jaundice in a Patient with a Palpable Gall Bladder Is Probably Not Caused by Gallstones

Sometimes in our fascination with technologic diagnosis, we forget about the time-honored methods of physical diagnosis. Presented here is Courvoisier's Law, extrapolated from the work of Swiss surgeon Ludwig Courvoisier (1843–1918), who pioneered removal of gallstones from the common bile duct. Upon studying 187 cases of common bile duct obstruction, the surgeon observed that an obstructing stone in the bile duct seldom causes gall bladder distention. There is a simple reason for this: Gallstones develop gradually, typically causing a fibrotic gall bladder that cannot distend with back-pressure. According to Fitzgerald et al., chronicity is the key [1, 2].

> Thus when a patient has both jaundice and a palpable gall bladder, think of something else – such as cancer of the pancreas.

And, oh yes, this finding has nothing to do with Courvoisier brand of cognac, favorite libation of Emperor Napoleon Bonaparte. The name of the beverage dates to an early wine and spirit maker named Emmanuel Courvoisier, who lived about a century before the surgeon with the same surname.

References

1. Parmar MS. "Courvoisier's law". CMAJ. 2003;168(7):876–877.
2. Fitzgerald JE, White MJ, Lobo DN. Courvoisier's gall bladder: law or sign? World J Surg. 2009;33(4):886–891.

###

A Patient with Flushing that Does Not Respond to Usual Therapy May Have Carcinoid Syndrome

This may be the menopausal woman whose severe hot flushes are resistant even to estrogen therapy. Diarrhea, bronchospasm and valvular heart lesions are other manifestations of carcinoid syndrome.

If carcinoid syndrome is suspected, consider obtaining a urinary level of 5-hydroxy indole acetic acid (5-HIAA).

References

1. Van der Lely AJ, de Herder WW. Carcinoid syndrome: diagnosis and medical management. Arq Bras Endocrinol Metabol. 2005;49(5):850–860.
2. Jabboour SA, Dividovici BB, Wolf R. Rare syndromes. Clin Dermatol. 2006;24(4):299–316.

###

Sarcoidosis Is an Unlikely, but Possible, Cause of Joint Symptoms in Children

Ukae et al. report sarcoidosis in preschool children mimicking juvenile rheumatoid arthritis [1].

The authors describe findings in three areas: joints, eyes and skin.

The authors note that this presentation of sarcoidosis differs from that in older children, and recommend skin biopsy to clarify the picture when there is diagnostic uncertainty.

Reference

1. Ukae S, Tsutsumi H, Adachi N, Takahashi H, Kato F, Chiba S. Preschool sarcoidosis manifesting as juvenile rheumatoid arthritis: a case report and a review of the literature of Japanese cases. Acta Paediatr Jpn. 1994;36(5):515–518.

###

The Spleen Must Triple in Size Before Becoming Palpable

This pearl is from Reveno's book of medical maxims [1]. Unfortunately Reveno does not provide documentation for this assertion, and I have been unable to find confirming evidence. Nevertheless, we all recall the difficulty of detecting enlargement of an organ tucked up under the left costal margin, and if the threefold size increase pearl is true, than it would seem that any disease accompanied by splenomegaly is not in its early stages.

Kraus et al. studied 122 patients undergoing diagnostic splenectomy and identified a specific disease in 116 of these specimens. The most common cause of unexplained splenomegaly was malignancy; in 25% of cases the cause was a reactive disorder or benign neoplasm [2].

The list of possible causes of splenomegaly is long [3]. Here are some entities that have been reported:

Category	Example
Congestive splenomegaly	Portal vein thrombosis
Acute infectious disease	Infectious mononucleosis
Chronic infectious disease	Malaria
Blood cell destruction	Hereditary spherocytosis
Myeloproliferative disease	Polycythemia vera
Neoplastic disease	Acute or chronic lymphocytic leukemia
Infiltrative splenomegaly	Amyloidosis
Other causes	Cyst, sarcoidosis, occult splenic rupture

References

1. Reveno WS. 711 Medical maxims. Springfield IL: Charles C. Thomas; 1951; page 112.
2. Kraus MD, Fleming MD, Vonderheide RH. The spleen as a diagnostic specimen: a review of 10 years' experience at two tertiary care institutions. Cancer. 2001;91(11):2001–2009.
3. Taylor RB. Difficult diagnosis. Philadelphia, PA: Saunders; 1985; page 493.

###

Varicocele Generally Occurs on the Left, and a Unilateral Right-Sided Varicocele Is a Worrisome Finding

Most varicoceles are on the left, owing to the anatomy of the left spermatic vein [1]. In up to a third of patients the abnormality will be bilateral. A unilateral right varicocele should raise the suspicion of a mass lesion obstructing the right inferior vena cava [1, 2].

> *Biyani et al. report that varicocele affects 10–15% of men and adolescent boys; I have not found the incidence to be nearly that high. They conclude that, although found in 25% of men with abnormal semen analysis, "there is little evidence that varicocele affects male fertility." Given the 25% prevalence in men with abnormal semen [2], I must wonder about the conclusion.*

References

1. Evaluation of nonacute pathology in adult men. Available at: http://www.uptodateonline.com/online/content/topic.do?topicKey=primneth/7784&linkTitle=VARICOCELE&source=preview&selectedTitle=3~11&anchor=4#4. Accessed March 31, 2009.
2. Biyani CS, Cartledge J, Janetschek G. Varicocele. Clin Evid (Online). 2009 Jan 6; 2009;pii:1806.

###

When a Male with Scrotal Pain Has an Intact Cremasteric Reflex, the Diagnosis May Be Something Other than Testicular Torsion

A study of 245 boys with acute scrotal swelling found a 100% correlation between the presence of the ipsilateral cremasteric reflex and the absence of testicular torsion. The cremasteric reflex was absent in all 56 boys in the study found to have testicular torsion [1].

> *A review of available evidence by Schmitz and Safraned, however, turned up some case reports of testicular torsion in the presence of an intact cremasteric reflex. They state, "Neither the presence or absence of any particular physical sign conclusively rules out testicular torsion" [2]. Here I believe that the key word is "conclusively." Based on these two reports, I would rank the stated clinical pearl as useful, but imperfect.*

References

1. Rabinowitz R. The importance of the cremasteric reflex in acute scrotal swelling in children. J Urol. 1984;132(1):89–90.
2. Schmitz D, Safraned S. How useful is a physical exam in diagnosing testicular torsion? J Fam Pract. 2009;58(8):433–434.

###

The Best Test to Detect Diabetic Peripheral Neuropathy Is the 128-Hz Tuning Fork

The supporting study included 24 patients with diabetic foot ulcers, 24 diabetics without known neuropathy and a non-diabetic control group. Upon comparison of various testing methods, the 128-Hz tuning fork was found to be best, and specifically was superior to monofilament testing [1].

From my neuroanatomy study days, I seem to recall that vibratory sense, as measured by the tuning fork, reflects the function of the posterior columns in the spinal cord, these being the longest nerves in the body and thus the most vulnerable to injury, e.g. diabetic neuropathy.

Reference

1. Meijer JWG, Smit AJ, Lefrandt JD, et al. Back to basics in diagnosing diabetic polyneuropathy with the tuning fork! Diabetes Care. 2005;28(9):2201–2205.

When a Patient with Back Pain Experiences Decreased Pain with Forward Flexion of the Spine, Think of Lumbar Spinal Stenosis

In evaluating the possibility of this disease, largely affecting older individuals, it is also important to ask about radicular pain or sciatica, present in 95% of persons with disk herniation [1].

Here is another tip: Patients with lumbar spinal stenosis may describe decreased discomfort when climbing stairs, and activity in which we all flex the trunk. In contrast, patients with vascular claudication may report increased pain with stair-climbing [1].

Reference

1. Chad DA. Lumbar spinal stenosis. Neurol Clin. 2007;25:407–418.

###

A Schoolchild with Backache: Think Backpack

Today schoolchildren carry around remarkably heavy backpacks, often amounting to 10–20% of their body weight. A group at the University of California – San Diego assessed the impact of backpack weight-bearing using upright magnetic resonance imaging. Five girls and three boys were scanned while hoisting backpacks of various weights. Increasing backpack loads caused significant compression of lumbar disc heights, significantly increased lumbar asymmetry, and back pain that increased with increased weight loads [1].

According to the authors, 37% of US children ages 11–14 report back pain, and over 92% of US children carry backpacks that equal 10–20% of their body weight. Could there actually be a connection? Yes, there can, as demonstrated in this nicely designed study, despite the small number of subjects.

As a personal observation, in this age of computers, flash memory drives and smart phones, why is a stack of heavy textbooks needed? Or are there other items in the heavy backpacks?

Reference

1. Neuschwander TB, Cutorne J, Macias BR, et al. The effect of backpacks on the lumbar spine in children: a standing magnetic resonance imaging study. Spine. 2010;35(1):83–88.

Patients Who Cannot Fully Extend the Elbow Following an Injury Have a 50:50 Chance of Fracture

This pearl comes from a study of 1,740 patients with elbow trauma. Of 602 able to fully extend the elbow, 17 had a fracture. Of 1,138 patients lacking full elbow extension, there were fractures in 521 individuals [1].

Here is another instance in which a knowledgeable physical examination, grounded on an evidence-based fact, can predict what will be found on imaging. Such skills prove especially useful in settings, such as disaster relief work, when ready imaging is unavailable.

Reference

1. Appelboam A, Reuben AD, Benger JR, et al. Elbow extension test to rule out elbow fracture: multicentre, prospective validation and observational study of diagnostic accuracy in adults and children. BMJ. 2008;337:a2428

###

The Patient with Bone Pain at Night Relieved by Aspirin May Have Osteoid Osteoma

Osteoid osteoma is an uncommonly-occurring benign bone tumor that typically occurs in children and young adults. The femur and spine are common tumor sites. Plain roentgenograms may show a lucency surrounded by cortical thickening. Sometimes plane films are unrevealing, and computed tomography, a bone scan, or magnetic resonance imaging may be needed to confirm the diagnosis.

The pain may be relieved by aspirin or another nonsteroid anti-inflammatory drug (NSAIDs). In my lifetime series of two patients, both reported dramatic – almost magical – relief with these medications.

References

1. Cohen MD, Harrington TM, Ginsburg WW. Osteoid osteoma: 95 cases and a review of the literature. Semin Arthritis Rheum. 1983;12(3):265–281.
2. Azouz EM, Kozlowski D, Marton D, Sprague P, Zerhouni A, Asselah F. Osteoid osteoma and osteoblastoma of the spine in children: report of 22 cases with brief literature review. Pediatr Radiol. 1986;16(1):25–31.

###

Plantar Fasciitis Is Like Pregnancy; It Goes Away in About 9 Months

The pearl is restated from Meador's *A Little Book of Doctors' Rules II* [1]. In this instance I was able to find evidence to support the lore. Davis et al. followed 105 heel pain patients for an average of 29 months. They received the usual: NSAIDs, relative rest, heel cushions, stretching exercises and occasionally injections. Of the 105 patients, 89.5% experienced resolution of the heel pain within 10.9 months [2].

It is true that 10.9 months is a little longer than the typical pregnancy, but not that much. I think what we have here is a useful pearl.

References

1. Meador CK. A little book of doctors' rules II. Philadelphia: Hanley & Belfus; 1999, Rule number 51.
2. Davis PF, Severud E, Baxter DE. Painful heel syndrome: results of non-operative treatment. Foot Ankle Int. 1994;15(10):531–535.

###

Not Every Person Has a Dorsalis Pedis Pulse

The dorsalis pedis pulse, important in the diagnosis of peripheral vascular disease, can be difficult to locate and, in fact, is bilaterally absent in 1.8% of individuals. Robertson et al. sought the dorsalis pedis pulse in 547 healthy young persons using both digital palpation and a Doppler probe (the latter a method most of us don't use on routine examination). They found congenitally absent dorsalis pedis pulses bilaterally in nine subjects and unilaterally absent in another six subjects. Of course, if you cannot find the dorsalis pedis artery, you can go to the posterior tibial artery, found just where its name suggests and absent in only one of the 547 subjects examined [1].

Assuming it is present, the artery can be found on the dorsum of the foot by considering that, more or less, it forms an equilateral triangle with the medial and lateral malleoli.

Reference

1. Robertson GS, Ristic CD, Bullen BR. The incidence of congenitally absent foot pulses. Ann R Coll Surg. 1990;72(2):99–100.

###

The First Sign of Parkinson Disease (PD) May Be Micrographia

This pearl is from the on-line book by Rice, *Wisdom of the Ageds: Clinical Pearls*, in which he presents a string of experience-based, intuitive pearls collected from professional colleagues [1].

In a review article based on a search for studies describing the clinical characteristics of PD, Jankovic described the cardinal signs of the disease as rest tremor, bradykinesia, rigidity, and loss of postural reflexes [2]. Of the many secondary motor symptoms – which include dysarthria, sialorrhea, and festination (walking with quick, small steps as if hurrying to avoid losing balance) – micrographia (literally, small writing) may be the earliest manifestation of PD. In looking at this phenomenon, Gangadhar et al. describe PD handwriting as showing both smaller size and larger velocity fluctuation compared to normal handwriting [3].

Once in the days before electronic medical records, I noted the onset of micrographia in the handwritten hospital chart notes of an aging colleague. Within a few years, he had gradually developed the full picture of Parkinson disease.

References

1. Rice RE. Wisdom of the ageds: clinical pearls. Page 35. Available at: http://www.familymedicine. us.edu/ricer/ClinicalPearls.pdf. Accessed January 16, 2010.
2. Jankovic J. Parkinson's disease: clinical features and diagnosis. J Neurol Neurosurg Psychiatry. 2008;79(4):368–376.
3. Gangadhar G, Joseph D, Srinivasan AV, et al. A computational model of Parkinsonian handwriting that highlights the role of the indirect pathway in the basal ganglia. Hum Mov Sci. 2009;28(5):602–618.

Parkinsonism that Begins with a Tremor Runs a Slower Course than Disease that Starts with Rigidity or Hypokinesia

This finding comes from an evidence-based meta-analysis in which the authors conclude: "Patients whose initial symptom is tremor may experience slower disease progression and may have a longer duration of response to levodopa therapy" [1].

Hackney and Earhart advocate for short duration, intensive tango dancing for Parkinson patients, holding that this activity, completed within a short time period appears to be appropriate and effective for the individuals with mild-moderately severe Parkinson disease [2]. Could tremor, apparently the more benign of the initial symptoms, be more amenable to tango dancing than rigidity or hypokinesia?

References

1. Suchowersky O, Reich S, Perlmutter J, Zesiewicz T, Gronseth G, Weiner WJ. Practice parameter: diagnosis and prognosis of new onset Parkinson disease: an evidence-based review. Neurology. 2006;66(7):968–975.
2. Hackney ME, Earhart GM. Short duration, intensive tango dancing for Parkinson disease: an uncontrolled pilot study. Complement Ther Med. 2009;17(4):203–207.

Patients with Drug-Induced Parkinsonism Tend Not to Exhibit Tremor

This differs from patients with idiopathic Parkinson disease in which unilateral rest tremor is an early manifestation in 75% of patients [1].

Idiopathic parkinsonism is a not-uncommon disease. It occurs in more than one in a hundred persons age 65 and older, making it the second most common neurodegenerative disease in America. Alzheimer disease holds the number 1 spot [1].

Reference

1. Blount BW, Robbins L. Parkinson disease. CME Bull. 2010;9(2):1–6.

###

Auditory Hallucinations Are Usually Psychotic in Origin, While Visual Hallucinations Are More Likely to Be Caused by Chemicals, Including Drugs of Various Types

This is another one of Meador's "doctors' rules" [1]. Hugdahl describes auditory hallucinations – "hearing voices" in the absence of external acoustic input – as a key characteristic of schizophrenia [2]. In the case of visual hallucinations think of known hallucinogenic drugs such as lysergic acid diethylamide (LSD), phencyclidine (PCP, angel dust), and mescaline. Even stopping a drug, as in the case of alcohol withdrawal on those who are physically dependent, can lead to visual hallucination and delirium tremens [3].

> I have witnessed the onset of delirium tremens on what began as an uneventful post operative day 3, when a young woman – whom we would soon learn was a closet alcoholic – began seeing "strange little men" perched on the foot of her bed, not long before she descended into full-blown delirium tremens.

> Meador also states that olfactory hallucinations are unusual, but when present are usually organic [1]. Possibilities include temporal lobe seizures, brain injury, Alzheimer disease and as the prelude to a migraine headache.

References

1. Meador CK. A little book of doctors' rules II. Philadelphia: Hanley & Belfus; 1999, Rule number 157.
2. Hugdahl K. "Hearing voices": auditory hallucinations as failure of top-down control of bottom-up processes. Scand J Psychol. 2009;50(6):553–560.
3. Alcohol withdrawal syndrome: how to predict, prevent, diagnose and treat it. (No authors listed). Prescribe Int. 2007;16(87):24–31.

###

When a Patient with Dementia Suddenly Develops Coexistent Delirium, Suspect a Urinary Tract Infection

This is likely to be an Alzheimer disease patient who may have an indwelling catheter or be the recipient of repeated "straight" catheterization [1].

> Urinary tract infections are very common in nursing homes, in both demented and non-demented patients, and sometimes can become life-threatening. A clinical mentor working

in a nursing home setting once stated graphically, "When you approach a patient while holding a catheter, it is like having a loaded gun in your hand." He was alluding to the risk of infection, and although the metaphor was perhaps a little hyperbolic, the image has persisted in my mind.

Reference

1. Rice RE. Wisdom of the ageds: clinical pearls. Page 41. Available at: http://www.familymedicine. us.edu/ricer/ClinicalPearls.pdf. Accessed January 16, 2010.

###

The Characteristics of Bruising Can Help Differentiate Between Accidental and Abusive Trauma in Children

In a case control study of children admitted for trauma – both physical abuse and accidental trauma – the total numbers and body regions of bruises were found to differ in the two groups.

Characteristics predictive of physical abuse trauma were bruises on the ear, neck or torso in a child age 4 or less and bruising on any area in an infant less than 4 months of age. Also, abused children tended to have more bruises than those who suffered accidental trauma [1].

Of course, being sensitive to the possibility of child abuse is part of any encounter involving childhood trauma. With that said, is there any active grade-school child – especially boys – who has no bruises on his shins?

Here is another intuitive tip from Meador: The child with a strange injury who is very quiet and well behaved may be an abused child [2].

References

1. Pierce MC, Kaczor K, Aldridge S, O'Flynn J, Lorenz DJ. Bruising characteristics discriminating physical child abuse from accidental trauma. Pediatrics. 2010;125(1):67–74.
2. Meador CK. A little book of doctors' rules II. Philadelphia: Hanley & Belfus; 1999, Rule number 175.

###

A Patient with Slate Blue, Silvery Discoloration of the Skin May Have Argyria

Argyria is a gray-blue discoloration of the skin, most noticeable in sun exposed areas, which can also involve the conjunctiva, gums, and nail beds. The disease was seen in the early nineteenth century, when treatment with silver preparations was common for various maladies [1]. The incidence waned in the twentieth century, as more effective and disease-specific medicine became available. Argyria, however, has not disappeared and a number of sporadic cases have been reported, largely attributed to ingestion of silver-containing alternative health products [2, 3].

From my childhood, I recall my mother painting my sore throat with Argyrol, a silver protein solution sold as an anti-infective. My recollection is from the days when penicillin was a newly-discovered wonder drug. But what about today? On a long airport layover recently, I came across a magazine, Mental_Floss. In it was the story of a 58 year old man who used colloidal silver to treat a dermatitis, turned blue, and appeared on the Today show. The article also described a Montana politician who took colloidal silver beginning in 1999 in anticipation of a Y2K lack of antibiotic availability. His blue skin did not deter him from running, twice, for the U.S. senate [4].

This morning, in early 2011, I found the web site for Argyrol, reportedly still indicated: "to cleanse mucous membrane tissues, especially of the eyes, nose, upper sinuses, throat (access to inner ear); also genito-urinary tracts; hygiene protocol to remove germs, mucous and debris that can cause infection" [5].

References

1. Lambert EC. Modern medical mistakes. Bloomington, IN: Indiana University Press; 1978; page 70.
2. Chang AL, Khosravi V, Egbert B. A case of argyria after colloidal silver ingestion. J Cutan Pathol. 2006;33(12):808–811.
3. Kim Y, Suh HS, Cha HJ, Kim SH, Jeong KS, Kim DH. A case of generalized argyria after ingestion of colloidal silver solution. Am J Ind Med. 2009;52(3):246–250.
4. Blue in the face. (No author listed). Mental_Floss. 2010;9(1):16.
5. Argyrol SS. Mild Silver Protein Home. Available at: http://argyrol.com/agprotein.phtml. Accessed July 14, 2010.

Premature Whitening of the Hair Can Be Due to Vitamin B$_{12}$ Deficiency

Cobalamin deficiency can provide two visible clues: depigmentation of the hair and hyperpigmentation of the skin [1]. In our quest for the classic macrocytosis, anemia and vitamin B12 deficiency of pernicious anemia (PA) we sometimes fail to attend to other clues such as skin and hair changes, mental changes, and peripheral neuropathy [2]. In a study of 70 consecutive patients diagnosed with pernicious anemia, 19% did not have anemia, and 33% lacked macrocytosis [3].

Mori et al. propose that the dominant mechanism in hyperpigmentation in an increase in melanin synthesis [1]. It seems curious that the disease can cause an increase in skin pigment and a decrease in hair color.

References

1. Mori K, Ando I, Kukita A. Generalized hyperpigmentation of the skin due to vitamin B12 deficiency. J Dermatol. 2001;28(5):282–285.
2. Puri V, Chaudhry N, Goel S, et al. Vitamin B12 deficiency: a clinical and electrophysiological profile. Electromyogr Clin Neurophysiol. 2005;45(5):273–284.
3. Carmel R. Pernicious anemia. The expected findings of very low serum cobalamin levels, anemia, and macrocytosis are often lacking. Arch Intern Med. 1988;148(8):1712–1714.

###

A Skin Lesion Showing the "Dark Dot Sign" Is Most Likely to Be a Basal Cell Carcinoma

First of all, of course, basal cell is the most common of the skin cancers, and so the odds are on your side. (See Chap. 3.) Notwithstanding, the presence of one or more "dark dots" or pigmented speckling gives a strong hint that a suspicious lesion is a basal cell cancer [1, 2].

> *On the other hand, Fox cautions that hyperpigmented dots or blotches can occur in squamous cell carcinoma or melanoma [1]. For this reason, the "dark dot sign" pearl must be, as all maxims should be, considered in the clinical context.*

References

1. Fox GN. An aid for spotting basal cell carcinoma. J Fam Pract. 2009;58(2);73–75.
2. Goldberg LH, Friedman RH, Silapunt S. Pigmented speckling as a sign of basal cell carcinoma. Dermatol Surg. 2004;30:1553–1555.

###

The "Ugly Duckling" Sign May Signal the Presence of a Melanoma

Simply stated, the "ugly duckling" is a skin lesion that looks different from all the patient's other moles. In a study of the "ugly duckling" theory, back skin images of 12 patients were shown to a variety of health workers: 13 dermatologists, 5 dermatology nurses, and 8 non-clinical medical staff. All 5 melanomas in the images and only 3 of 140 benign moles were identified as "ugly," that is, different from the others on the patient's skin [1].

> *I consider this a brilliant study, confirming the validity of the "ugly duckling" pearl. I am especially impressed with the diagnostic acumen of the non-medical clinical staff. With this high level of performance, do we need dermatologists to screen for "ugly ducklings?"*

Reference

1. Scope A, Dusza SW, Halpern AC. The "ugly duckling" sign: agreement between observers. Arch Dermatol. 2008;144(1):58–64.

###

Sudden, Effortless Smoking Cessation May Indicate Lung Cancer

When a patient with long-term nicotine addiction, such as the three-pack a day smoker, spontaneously decides to stop smoking in the absence of a vigorous tobacco cessation effort by the physician, suspect lung cancer. Campling, reporting at the 13th World Conference on Lung Cancer, San Francisco, July 31–August 4, 2009, suggested that spontaneous smoking cessation may be a presenting feature of lung cancer. She speculates that the cause is tumor secretion of a factor interfering with nicotine addiction [1].

> These were not coughing, wheezing, dyspneic patients. Of the 55 patients reported to quit before being diagnosed with lung cancer, 49 (89%) were asymptomatic at the time [1].
>
> In another study regarding smoking cessation and lung cancer, Parsons et al. performed an extensive systematic review of the literature with meta-analysis, finding "preliminary evidence that smoking cessation after diagnosis of early stage lung cancer improves prognostic outcomes." This seems to affirm the truism that it is never too late to stop smoking [2].

References

1. Campling B. Easy smoking cessation may signal lung cancer. Pulmonary Med. September 1, 2009;9:47.
2. Parsons A, Daley A, Begh R, Aveyard P. Influence of smoking cessation after diagnosis of early stage lung cancer on prognosis: systematic review of observational studies with meta-analysis. BMJ. 2010;340:b5569.

###

Sometimes Clinicians Can Be Part of the Infection Problem

Three Pittsburgh physicians conducted a nice study of what lurks on our stethoscope heads. They imprinted stethoscope heads onto culture agar plates before and after cleaning the stethoscope heads with an alcohol based hand foam. There were 184 cultures, from 92 stethoscopes. Colony counts of bacteria were significantly lower after the washes, and three methicillin-resistant *Staphylococcus aureus* (MRSA) colonies were found in the pre-wash cultures, but not in the post-wash cultures [1].

> *Have we, all these years, simply assumed that handwashing was enough, and that our stethoscope heads somehow resisted bacterial contamination? To what extent are our diagnostic instruments, and our clothing, part of the MRSA problem?*

Reference

1. Schroeder A, Schroeder MA, D'Amico FD. What's growing on your stethoscope? And what you can do about it. J Fam Pract. 2009;58(8):404–405.

#####

Chapter 7
Laboratory Testing, Electrocardiography and Imaging

> *I have been surprised to note the readiness with which high-grade young physicians, graduates from medical institutions which are models for our time, yield to the temptation of machine-made diagnoses.*
>
> American Physician William J. Mayo (1861–1939) [1]

Testing – blood determinations, urine analysis, electrocardiography, various types of body imaging and all the rest – represent a two-edged sword for physicians. On one hand a test result can provide the key piece of data that clinches a diagnosis; an example is the detection of a malarial crescent on a blood smear. On the other hand, easy access to laboratory testing can foster dependence, and even a little intellectual laziness, in the clinician. After all, it is easier to order a test than listen to a patient, although, given such a forced choice, eliciting a thorough medical history is generally the best option.

Nevertheless, laboratory testing and imaging are part of twenty-first century practice, and often can play a pivotal role in the clinical scenario. Consider the following case, a true story – except that key facts have been changed to protect the innocent. For the record, I was not among the cast of physicians described below.

Shirley J, age 69 and a type 2 diabetic returned from a visit to her sister in Connecticut with vague symptoms, including fatigue, fever, joint achiness and stiffness, headache, and weight loss. She visited an emergency physician, received a complete blood count and chemistry screen, and was discharged with a diagnosis of persistent viral infection symptoms.

Ten days later, she had some annoying visual symptoms. She was examined by an ophthalmologist, who found evidence of fairly early cataracts, normal ocular tension levels, and an unremarkable retinal examination. He wondered if she might be experiencing episodes of hyperglycemia.

A few weeks later, with her symptoms unchanged, Shirley visited her diabetologist, who reviewed her medications and confirmed that her glycosylated hemoglobin was within the normal range.

Finally she decided to see her generalist physician, whom she had last seen for a routine physical examination a few years earlier. He elicited a history, performed an examination

R.B. Taylor, *Essential Medical Facts Every Clinician Should Know: To Prevent Medical Errors, Pass Board Examinations and Provide Informed Patient Care*, DOI 10.1007/978-1-4419-7874-5_7, © Springer Science+Business Media, LLC 2011

and embarked on a diagnostic quest, determined to find the source of the problem. Testing included a repeat of the blood count and screening chemistry tests including liver function tests, a test for Lyme disease, various tests for rheumatologic diseases, including an erythrocyte sedimentation rate (ESR). He also obtained a chest X-ray and magnetic resonance imaging (MRI) of the head.

One by one, the test reports arrived. (This was in the days before most of us had electronic medical records.) Everything was unremarkable, with one exception – an ESR of 105 mm/h. This was – or should have been – the tipoff to the elusive diagnosis of giant cell (temporal) arteritis.

For completeness, I must tell the rest of the story. The physician reviewed all the laboratory reports, all, that is, except the ESR report, which somehow was overlooked or lost. Or perhaps he suffered a moment of inattention as it crossed his desk. Whatever happened, the disease continue to be undiagnosed for a few more weeks, until one evening the patient presented to the emergency room with sudden loss of vision in her left eye, a defect from which she would not recover.

The lessons to be learned from this story are several. One is that a battery of negative tests does not mean that the patient is disease-free. The second, in the case of the diabetologist, is that just because "your" disease is well controlled does not mean that the patient does not need further testing or referral. Finally, when you finally do happen to order the key test, be sure that you see the result and act promptly.

Reference

1. Mayo WJ. Aphorisms. In: Aphorisms of Dr. Charles Horace Mayo and Dr. William James Mayo, Willius FA, editor. Rochester, MN: Mayo Foundation for Medical Education and Research, 1988, page 55.

Policy Edicts Can Influence Diagnostic Testing Decisions

In its zeal to assure quality even in the most basic patient care activities, the Joint Commission issued stringent regulations governing waived laboratory testing. These regulations include point-of-care testing for fecal occult blood, with a new requirement requiring physicians to manually document testing control data. Adams et al. performed a before-and-after of 788 patient charts, looking at the number of digital rectal exams and fecal occult blood tests performed. They found that following the implementation of the new policy, physicians performed 16.7% fewer rectal examinations and that fecal occult blood testing declined by 18.7% [1].

In the current clinical climate in which a rectal examination with fecal occult blood testing is already an uncommon event, do we need one more deterrent to this useful and inexpensive test? In our quest for quality assurance, are we missing the diagnosis of some colorectal carcinomas?

Reference

1. Adams BD, McHugh KJ, Bryson SA, Dabulewicz J. The law of unintended consequences: The Joint Commission regulations and the digital rectal examination. Ann Emerg Med. 2008;51(2):197–201.

Elevated Red Blood Cell Distribution (RWD) Is Associated with an Increased Risk of Death

A part of a complete blood count (CBC), the RWD is a measure of variability in the size of circulating red blood cells. A high RWD level is characteristic of iron deficiency anemia. In addition, high RWD levels in persons with symptomatic cardiovascular disease (CVD) have been found to be associated with an increased risk of death. Now a recent study has shown the association between elevated RWD and death to extend to persons free of CVD. Patel et al. studied the RWD levels of 8,175 adults age 45 and older who were enrolled in the 1988–1994 National Health and Nutritional Examination Survey, and compared these values to mortality data through the end of year 2000. They found that higher RDW values strongly associated with an increased risk of death from all causes, making the finding a "strong predictor of mortality in the general population of adults 45 years or older." The all-cause mortality risk increased by 22% for every 1% increment in RWD.

The clinical utility of this finding is yet to be fully determined. However, because the RWD is widely available as a byproduct of CBC testing, and because of the power of the study described, knowing about the high RWD-risk of death association may occasionally be informative.

Reference

1. Patel KV, Ferrucci L, Ershler WB. Red blood cell distribution width and the risk of death in middle aged and older adults. Arch Intern Med. 2009;169(5):515–523.

Glycosylated Hemoglobin (HbA1c) Is a Useful Screening Test for Diabetes Mellitus

For years, the gold standard for diabetes screening and diagnosis has been fasting plasma glucose (FPG) and the glucose tolerance test. Despite cost issues, there is an increasing tendency to screen for diabetes using HbA1c levels. In a study of 6,890 adults from the 1999–2006 National Health and Nutrition Examination

Survey, Carson et al. found that HbA1c levels of 6.5% or greater demonstrate reasonable agreement with fasting glucose for diagnosing diabetes [1].

An Australian study of clinical and general populations led to the conclusion that HbA1c levels of 5.5% or less predicted absence of and levels of 7.0% or greater predicted the presence of type 2 diabetes. Finding an HbA1c level between 6.5 and 6.9% made diabetes "highly probable in clinical and population settings" [2].

> *Is the use of HbA1c as a screening test a good idea? Because of the cost differential between FPG and HbA1c, for many of us the decision will be made by who pays the bill, whether government or an insurance company. But what if we approached the issue logically? Following a systematic review of primary cross-sectional studies, Bennett et al. concluded that, because HbA1c has less intra-individual variation and better predicts both micro- and macrovascular complications, "the additional benefits in predicting costly preventable clinical complications may make this a cost-effective choice" [3]. Also, HbA1c determination does not require that the patient be fasting, a practical consideration in everyday practice.*

References

1. Carson AP, Reynolds K, Fonseca VA et al. Comparison of A1C and fasting glucose criteria to diagnose diabetes among U.S. adults. Diabetes Care. 2010;33(1):95–97.
2. Lu ZX, Walker KZ, O'Dea K, Sikaris KA, Shaw JE. HbA1c for screening and diagnosis of Type 2 diabetes in routine clinical practice. Diabetes Care. 2010;33(4):817–819.
3. Bennett CM, Guo M, Dharmage SC. HbA1c as a screening tool for detection of Type 2 diabetes: a systematic review. Diabet Med. 2007;24(4):333–343.

###

Decreasing Low Density Lipoprotein Cholesterol (LDL-C) Is the Key to Lowering the Risk of Cardiovascular Disease, and Simply Increasing High Density Lipoprotein Cholesterol (HDL-C) Levels Does Not Seem to Help

From McMaster University in Canada comes a report of an ambitious meta-regression analysis of 108 randomized clinical trials involving 299,310 subjects. The result: "All analyses that adjusted for changes in low density lipoprotein cholesterol showed no association between treatment-induced change in high density lipoprotein cholesterol and risk ratios for coronary heart disease deaths, coronary artery disease events, or total deaths" [1].

The Canadian study is more-or-less consistent with a 2007 systematic review of a mere 31 randomized trials that also found only modest evidence to support aggressively increasing high density cholesterol levels by methods other than what can be achieved by sensible lifestyle changes [2].

> *For those who strive to elevate HDL-C levels beyond what can be achieved by lifestyle modifications, the agent used are niacin and fibrates, although the primary emphasis continues to be on LDL-C reduction.*

References

1. Briel M, Ferreira-Gonzalez I, You JJ, et al. Association between change in high density lipoprotein cholesterol and cardiovascular disease and mortality: systematic review and meta-
regression analysis. BMJ. 2009;338:b92.
2. Singh IM, Shishehbor MH, Ansell BJ. High-density lipoprotein as a therapeutic target: a systematic review. JAMA. 2007;298(7):786–798.

###

HbA1c Levels of 5.5% or Greater Are Associated with an Increased Risk of Diabetic Retinopathy

A study of 1,066 adults from the 2005–2006 National Health and Nutrition Examination Survey revealed a steep increase in retinopathy prevalence among individuals with HbA1C levels of 5.5% or more. A similar increased risk was noted with FPG levels of 126 mg/dL or greater, but the HbA1c "discriminated prevalence of retinopathy better than FPG" [1].

This is another study documenting the merits of HbA1c testing, especially pertinent, given that retinopathy has a prevalence of 36% in people with diagnosed diabetes [1].

Reference

1. Cheng YJ, Gregg EW, Geiss LS, et al. Association of A1c and fasting plasma glucose levels
with diabetic retinopathy prevalence in the U.S. population: Implications for diabetes diagnostic thresholds. Diabetes Care. 2009;32(11):2027–2032.

###

Lipid Studies Can Be Done Without the Need for Fasting

Di Angelantonio et al. studied lipid assessment in vascular disease, studying major lipids and apolipoproteins and their predictive value in cardiovascular disease. This was a truly epic review of 68 long-term prospective studies involving 302,430 persons and 2.79 million person-years of follow-up. The authors conclude: "Lipid assessment in vascular disease can be simplified by measurement of either total and HDL cholesterol levels or apolipoproteins without the need to fast or without regard to triglyceride" [1].

I present this study to highlight the fact that we can now obtain lipid studies when the patient is not fasting. As a bonus, tucked away in this data-laden study is the following finding: Persons with the lowest HDL levels had nearly a three times greater risk of cardiovascular events when compared with those with the highest levels [1].

Reference

1. Emerging Risk Factors Collaboration: Di Angelantonio E, Sarwar N, Kaptoge S, et al. Major lipids, apolipoproteins, and the risk of vascular disease. JAMA. 2009;302(18):1993–2000.

###

Elevated C-Reactive Protein (CRP) Levels Are Associated with an Increased Risk of Diabetes Mellitus

A number of studies have shown a relationship between low-grade systemic inflammation and diabetes. Data from the Multi-Ethnic Study of Atherosclerosis, involving 5,571 subjects, showed a higher incidence of type 2 diabetes in persons with elevated levels of C-reactive protein, fibrinogen and interleukin 6 in white, black and Hispanic populations [1]. In a study of 1,754 persons from the University of Medical Sciences in Iran, Nabipour et al. found that, "beyond traditional cardio-vascular risk factors, elevated CRP is significantly correlated with diabetes in the general population of the northern Persian Gulf" [2].

The findings of these two studies was collaborated by Chen et al., who measured their subjects' CRP values over an average of 16 years apart. They concluded that the long- and intermediate-term variability of CRP values was not great, and was specifically less than the variability of plasma cholesterol levels in these same subjects. They also reported that while "CRP over the intermediate term did not predict new-onset metabolic syndrome at the final examination, CRP did predict an increase in glucose and new-onset diabetes" [3].

Increased levels of inflammatory markers, and specifically CRP, are also linked to increased risks of cardiovascular disease and depression [4]. Will we soon see a recommendation for CRP determinations as part of routine health maintenance examinations?

Parenthetically, kudos to the authors of ref. [2], who succinctly state the outcome of their findings in the title of the article: Elevated high sensitivity C-reactive protein is associated with type 2 diabetes. *Such clarity is a great courtesy to those of us searching for important bits of new information.*

References

1. Bentoni AG, Burke GL, Owusu JA, et al. Inflammation and the incidence of type 2 diabetes: the Multi-Ethnic Study of Atherosclerosis (MESA). Diabetes Care. 2010;33(4):804–810.
2. Nabipour I, Vahdat K, Jafari SM, et al. Elevated high sensitivity C-reactive protein is associated with type 2 diabetes: the Persian Gulf Healthy Heart Study. Endocr J. 2008;55(4):717–722.
3. Chen TH, Gona P, Sutherland PA, et al. Long-term C-reactive protein variability and prediction of metabolic risk. Am J Med. 2009;122(1):53–61.
4. Dinan TG. Inflammatory markers in depression. Curr Opin Psychiatry. 2009;22(1):32–36.

###

Elevated Serum Uric Acid (SUA) Levels Are Associated with an Increased Risk of Death

High levels of serum uric acid are associated with poor prognosis in a variety of conditions, including hypertension, heart failure, cardiovascular disease, and renal failure. Recently Wasserman et al. examined the prognostic significance of an elevated SUA in 650 adult patients consecutively admitted to an internal medicine hospital service. In addition to the diseases listed above, they also found higher SUA levels in patients with diabetes and, of course, gout, as well as those using diuretics. They did not find SUA significantly correlated with current diagnoses of malignancy or infection, or with elevated CRP levels. They conclude, "Initial SUA is an independent predictor of mortality in admitted medical patients." Furthermore, the authors graciously define what they mean by "high" and "normal" levels of SUA. Persons with a SUA less than 6 mg/dL had a 5% mortality, while those with a SUA above 12 mg/dL had a 27% mortality [1].

Perhaps this study is not about serum uric acid levels at all, but rather about the mortality risk of clusters of diseases which just happen to be associated with different uric acid profiles. Also, given that malignancies with a high rate of proliferation or high sensitivity to treatment can have lysis of tumor cells and a subsequent hyperuricemia (owing to catabolism of purine nucleic acids), I was surprised to note that in this study malignancies were generally not associated with elevated SUA levels.

We must ask if the elevated SUA levels are simply a marker of increased risk of mortality, of cell damage of some sort, or if the hyperuricemia plays some sort of pathologic role in the various disease processes. If the latter is true, should the elevated serum uric acid levels be treated?

Reference

1. Wassermann A, Shnell M, Boursi B, Guzner-Gur H. Prognostic significance of serum uric acid in patients admitted to the Department of Medicine. Am J Med Sci. 2010;339(1):15–21.

###

Elevated Serum Tumor Necrosis Factor Alpha (TNF-Alpha) Is Associated with Increased Cognitive Decline in Alzheimer Disease

In a brilliant study of 300 community-dwelling Alzheimer patients, care givers were asked to record the incidence of acute inflammatory events, which were then correlated with measurement of TNF-alpha levels. I find the results, quoted here, to be remarkable: "Acute systemic inflammatory events, found in around half of all subjects, were associated with an increase in the serum levels of proinflammatory cytokine TNF-alpha and a twofold increase in the rate of cognitive decline over a

6-month period. High baseline levels of TNF-alpha were associated with a fourfold increase in the rate of cognitive decline. Subjects who had low levels of serum TNF-alpha throughout the study showed no cognitive decline over the 6-month period" [1].

> *Again, of course, I wonder if we are making too much of a marker, and that what is really happening is that the cognitive decline is related to the impact of intercurrent flu, pneumonia, gastroenteritis, vasculitis and so forth? Or are we on to something that might have implications for disease surveillance regarding, as in the discussion of CRP above, low-grade systemic inflammation?*
>
> *Then there is the classic consideration that applies to many clinical situations. When contemplating ordering a test, ask yourself what you will do if the result is (a) positive, or (b) negative. If the two answers are the same, is the test really needed?*

Reference

1. Holmes C, Cunningham C, Zotova E, et al. Systemic inflammation and disease progression in Alzheimer disease. Neurology. 2009;73(10):768–774.

###

Fluoroquinolone Use Can Cause a False Positive Opiate Urine Drug Screen

There are actually several drugs that can cause false positive results on urine drug screening [1]. These include:

Gatifloxacin and other fluoroquinolones – opiates
Nonsteroidal anti-inflammatory drugs (NSAIDs) – cannabinoids and barbiturates
Vicks VapoInhaler (which contains L-methamphetamine) – amphetamines

Knowing these confounders is important, because a false positive screen can cause a person to lose a job or be dismissed from a treatment program.

> *There are also ways to game the urine drug screening process to yield a false negative result. A drug abuser might dilute the specimen by drinking massive volumes of water or taking diuretics, add household bleach to the submitted urine specimen, or even submit a bogus specimen provided by a non-drug-using accomplice.*

Reference

1. Vincent EC, Zebelman A, Goodwin C, Stephens MM. What common substances can cause false positives on urine screens? J Fam Pract. 2006;55(10):893–897.

###

Tricyclic Antidepressants Can Cause a False Positive Test for Pheochromocytoma

Testing for the possible presence of pheochromocytoma yields a surprisingly high number of abnormal results. In a study by Yu and Wei of 1,896 patients tested for pheochromocytoma, there was at least one elevated test result in 417 individuals (22%) [1]. In this study the highest false positive rate was found in tests for urine metanephrines (50%), and the lowest false positive rate occurred in vanillylmandelic acid determinations.

In fact, tricyclic antidepressants are only one class of drugs that can cause falsely high levels of catecholamines and metanephrines [2]. Others include:

Acetaminophen
Amphetamines
Buspirone
Ethanol
Levodopa
Prochlorperazine
Pseudoephedrine and other adrenergic agonists
Reserpine

> *Pheochromocytoma may be a zebra diagnosis, but pheochromocytoma testing is not uncommon. Yu and Wei hold that such testing is becoming more frequent in clinical practice, underscoring the need to know the drugs which might confound reported results.*

References

1. Yu R, Wei M. False positive test results for pheochromocytoma from 2000 to 2008. Exp Clin Endocrinol Diabetes. 2010;118:577–585
2. Bravo EL, Gifford RW Jr. Pheochromocytoma. Endocrinol Metab Clin North Am. 1993;22(2):329–341.

###

Vitamin C Can Cause False Negative Dipstick Tests for Urinary Hemoglobin and Glucose

A study of 4,379 routine urine specimens tested using dipsticks revealed a high rate of falsely negative determinations for hemoglobin in specimens containing ascorbic acid. In this study, 22.8 of specimens examined were positive for vitamin C. The authors went on to study the effect of various doses of vitamin C from 100 to 1,000 mg, and also vitamin C containing fruit juices. The found that "even the lowest doses of oral vitamin C or juice resulted in sufficient urinary vitamin C to produce false-negative dipstick results in hemoglobin or glucose testing" [1].

Given that many persons take vitamin C for prevention or treatment of colds, this effect on dipstick testing could have clinical significance, especially in regard to diseases such as diabetes or bladder cancer. We must keep in mind that the dipsticks used in daily practice do not tell us whether or not there is ascorbic acid in the specimen.

Reference

1. Brigden ML, Edgell D, McPherson M, Leadbeater A, Hoag G. High incidence of significant urinary ascorbic acid concentrations in a west coast population – implications for routine urinalysis. Clin Chem. 1992;38(3):426–431.

###

Digital Rectal Examination (DRE) of the Prostate Can Increase the Level of Prostatic Specific Antigen (PSA), but Not Very Much

Does DRE have an effect on PSA testing? That is, if I am worried about a man's prostate, perform a robust digital examination, and then send him down the hall to have a PSA determination drawn, can I trust the result? To address this question, three urologists at the Mayo Clinic recruited 143 patients for a prospective, randomized controlled trial. Half the men had two PSA determinations with an intervening DRE; the other half also had two PSA determinations without DRE. Overall the study group (with DRE) had showed a second PSA value that was 0.4 ng/mL higher than the first, while the control group had a -0.1 change. Furthermore, the second PSA reading was higher in 76% of the study group but only in 32% of the control group. The authors opine that a 0.4 ng/mL median increase appears inconsequential. They conclude: "Based on these findings, physicians should be confident that the serum PSA concentration in the immediate post-digital rectal examination is accurate and does not compromise clinical use of the tumor marker" [1].

All this is well and good as far as median increases are concerned. In the study reported, "only" four patients with an initial PSA value in the reference range (0.0–4.0 ng/mL) had a post-digital rectal examination value greater than 4.0. This just might be a good time to recall that the individual patient in your office is not the average from which statistics are derived.

The questions swirling around DRE and PSA have led to the question: Is there any role at all for DRD in the detection of prostate cancer? A recent study found that the positive predictive value of DRD was not impressive: 48.6% in the first round of screening, 29.9% in the second round and 21.2% in the third. However, the value of the DRE is in the useful prognostic information provided by the fact that an abnormal DRE is associated with a greater increased risk of very high-grade disease [2].

References

1. Chybowski FM, Bergstralh EJ, Oesterling JE. The effect of digital rectal examination on the serum prostate specimen antigen concentration: results of a randomized study. J Urol. 1992;148(1):83–86.
2. Loeb S, Catalona WJ. What is the role of digital rectal examination in men undergoing serial screening of serum PSA levels? Nat Clin Pract Urol. 2009;6(2):68–69.

There May Be a Role for Glucose Oxidase Strip Testing for Cerebrospinal Fluid (CSF) Rhinorrhea, After All

Glucose oxidase strip testing for CSF rhinorrhea, an alleged plastic pearl that found its way into generations of medical reference books, fell into disuse following several studies showing that it lacked specificity. In one study, glucose was found in 15 of 17 samples of nasal discharge in normal children [1]. In another article, the authors report finding positive results for glucose in the nasal secretions of 44% of 50 normal individuals studied [2].

Now from London comes an algorithm which just might breathe new life into the glucose oxidase strip CSF rhinorrhea test. Baker et al. propose the following: "In patients at risk of CSF leak, nasal discharge is likely to contain CSF if glucose is present in the absence of visible blood, if blood glucose is less than 6 mmol × L(-1), and if there are no symptoms of upper respiratory infection" [3].

The settings in which skull fracture management decisions are made often do not allow for leisurely laboratory investigations, and such tests may not even be available. Hence, to support our clinical judgement, we have relied on the best tests available. In some situations, this test just might be the proposed algorithm-guided glucose oxidase strip test for CSF rhinorrhea.

References

1. Huff HF, Morrow G. Glucorrhea revisited. Prolonged promulgation of another plastic pearl. JAMA. 1975;234(10):1052–1053.
2. Steedman DJ, Gordon M. CSF rhinorrhea: significance of the glucose oxidase strip test. Injury. 1987;18(5):327–328.
3. Baker EH, Wood DM, Brennan AL, Baines DL, Philips BJ. New insights into the glucose oxidase stick test for cerebrospinal fluid rhinorrhea. Emerg Med J. 2005;22(8):556–557.

###

A Normal d-Dimer Test Does Not Always Rule Out Pulmonary Embolism (PE)

Evaluate the patient before considering the results of a d-dimer test. This is the advice of Gibson et al., following a study of 1,722 consecutive patients suspected of having PE. Before paying attention to the d-dimer result, the clinician should determine the likely or unlikely clinical probability for PE, based on the Wells clinical decision rule. In their study, the authors found venous thromboembolism (VTE) in 1.1% of persons with an unlikely clinical probability and a normal d-dimer concentration, and in 9.3% or patients with a likely clinical probability and a normal d-dimer test. They advise that patients with a likely clinical probability for PE undergo further testing, regardless of the d-dimer test outcome [1].

> Given that pulmonary embolism is, in my opinion, one of the "must never miss" diagnoses, the reported study highlights the importance of guideline-based clinical assessment tempered by experience and intuition, and then, only then, by consideration of the results of blood testing.

Reference

1. Gibson NS, Sohne M, Gerdes VE, Nijkeuter M, Buller HR. The importance of clinical probability assessment in interpreting a normal d-dimer in patients with suspected pulmonary embolism. Chest. 2008;134(4):789–793.

###

If You See an Inverted P Wave on an Electrocardiogram (ECG), Think First of Electrode Misplacement

Reversed arm leads are the most likely cause of what would be a confusing electrocardiographic finding. Other possibilities are dextrocardia and the very uncommon retrograde atrial depolarization [1, 2].

> Reversed arm leads are highly unlikely to occur in an ECG laboratory, but are a very real possibility in a teaching hospital, where inexperienced learners are sent to do an emergency bedside ECG tracing in the middle of the night.

References

1. Bean JR. Evaluating an abnormal ECG: reversed leads or cardiac trouble? JAAPA. 2000;13(9):55–56, 59.
2. Glancy DL, Jones M. ECG of the month. Reversal of the arm leads or situs inversus with mirror-image dextrocardia? Reversal of the limb leads and of the precordial leads. J La State Med Soc. 2007;159(2):63–65.

###

First Degree Heart Block (FDHB) Is Not a Benign Incidentaloma

We have long seemed to treat first degree atrioventricular block with a ho-hum attitude. Defined as a PR interval exceeding 200 ms, FDHB is frequently encountered on electrocardiograms. Although often found in healthy persons without cardiovascular risk factors, there is actually a long list of possible causes. These include: acute myocarditis, Lyme disease, ankylosing spondylitis, hemochromatosis, diphtheria, hyper- and hypokalemia, hypomagnesemia, athletic heart and old age.

Not surprisingly, then, Cheng et al. have published a study that challenges our traditional dismissive approach to FDHB. Their subjects were 7,575 persons from the Framingham Heart Study, followed for 12 years. They examined the associations of PR interval with the incidence of arrhythmic events and death. They found that persons with FDHB had a 2-fold adjusted risk of atrial fibrillation, a 3-fold adjusted risk of having a pacemaker implanted, and a 1.4-fold adjusted risk of all-cause mortality [1].

> Let me take a moment to review some of the medications that can cause FDHB:
> Beta blockers
> Digitalis
> Flecainide (Tambocor)
> Lithium
> Disopyramide (Norpace)
> Procainamide (Pronestyl)
> Quinidine (Quinaglute, Cardioquin)
> Verapamil (Calan, Isoptin)

Reference

1. Cheng S, Keyes MJ, Larson MG, et al. Long-term outcomes in individuals with prolonged PR interval or first-degree atrioventricular block. JAMA. 2009;301(24):2571–2577.

###

Low-Dose Computed Tomography (CT) Screening for Lung Cancer Has a High Rate of False-Positive Results

In a randomized controlled trial involving 3,190 current or former adult smokers who received low-dose computed tomography or chest radiography to screen for lung cancer, the probability of a false positive result with one low-dose CT screening examination was 21%, rising to 33% in patients who had two screenings. By comparison, the rates of false positives with chest radiography were 9% with one examination and 15% with two [1].

> Low dose CT lung cancer screening is actively promoted directly to consumers, and yet it is not altogether harmless. The high rate of false positive is significant because in the study described here 7% of patients with a false positive CT examination and 4% of those with a false positive chest X-ray subsequently underwent an invasive diagnostic procedure [1].

Reference

1. Croswell JM, Baker SG, Marcus PM, et al. Cumulative incidence of false positive test results in lung cancer screening: a randomized trial. Ann Intern Med. 2010;152(8):505–512.

Don't Count on a Normal Chest Radiograph to Rule Out Pneumonia in a Bedridden Patient

In a study of chest radiography to assess 58 bedridden patients for pneumonia, the sensitivity was found to be 65%, the specificity 93% and the positive and negative predictive values were 83 and 65%, respectively. The overall accuracy of pneumonia diagnosis was 69% [1].

> The figures above are clearly not as high as one would wish. In the setting of suspected pneumonia in a bedfast patient, the gold standard continues to be non-contrast-enhanced high-resolution computed tomography of the chest [1].

Reference

1. Esayag Y, Nikitin I, Bar-Ziv J, et al. Diagnostic value of chest radiographs in bedridden patients suspected of having pneumonia. Am J Med. 2010;123(1):88.e1–e5.

###

There Is Some Cancer Risk Associated with Every Computed Tomography Scan

Two 2009 reports looked at the data. Smith-Bindman et al., following a retrospective cross-sectional study of 1,119 consecutive adults receiving various types of CT scanning at four different institutions, found a 13-fold variation in radiation received. In projecting the risk of future cancer, the authors estimate that 1 in 270 women who underwent CT coronary angiography at age 40 will develop cancer as a result of that scan [1].

In a separate report from the National Cancer Institute in Bethesda, Maryland, there is the estimate that CT scans performed in the year 2007 will result in 29,000 future cancers. The greatest risk follows scans of the abdomen and pelvis, followed by those of the chest and head [2].

Just to put things in perspective, there are approximately 70 million CT scans performed in the United States annually [2]. If we agree that the US population is just a little over 300 million persons, then theoretically 23% of all Americans are scanned each year.

References

1. Smith-Bindman R, Lipson J, Marcus R, et al. Radiation dose associated with common computed tomography examinations and the associated lifetime attributable risk of cancer Arch Intern Med. 2009;169(22):2078–2086.
2. Berrington de González A, Mahesh M, Kim KP, et al. Projected cancer risks from computed tomographic scans performed in the United States in 2007. Arch Intern Med. 2009;169(22):2071–2077.

###

Thoracoabdominal Calcifications Noted on Roentgenograms Are Significant Predictors of Cardiovascular Disease and Total Mortality

In a study done in Finland, 833 adults with type 2 diabetes and 1,292 without diabetes and without prior evidence of cardiovascular disease were followed for 18 years. In these individuals and after adjustment for known risk factors, the presence of roentgenographically visible thoracicoabdominal calcifications were associated with an increased incidence of cardiovascular disease and total mortality, most notable in type 2 diabetic and non-diabetic women with elevated CRP levels [1].

This seems to be one more incidental finding, previously considered unimportant, that has acquired some new clinical significance.

Reference

1. Juutilainen A, Lehto S, Suhonen M, Ronnemaa T, Laakso M. Thoracoabdominal calcifications predict cardiovascular disease mortality in type 2 diabetic and nondiabetic subjects: 18-year follow-up study. Diabetes Care. 2010;33(3):583–585.

###

Routine Lumbar Imaging for Low Back Pain Is Unhelpful Unless There Is an Indication of a Serious Underlying Condition

Chou et al. looked at outcomes in six studies of low back pain involving patients who had immediate imaging (plain films, computed tomography or magnetic resonance imaging) versus those patient with similar symptoms who did not. The bottom line, according to the authors: "Lumbar imaging for low-back pain without indications of serious underlying conditions does not improve clinical outcomes" [1].

Such a recommendation has immense implications, considering that 5.6% of US adults have low back pain each day [2]. Of course, if we do less imaging for low back pain, we just might find fewer insignificant spinal abnormalities, and perform less unnecessary surgery to fix them.

References

1. Chou R, Fu R, Carrino JA, Deyo RA. Imaging strategies for low-back pain: systematic review and metaanalysis. Lancet. 2009;373(9662):463–472.
2. Loney PL, Stratford PW. The prevalence of low back pain in adults: a methodological review of the literature. Phys Ther. 1999;79:384–396.

###

Newly Proposed Prediction Rules Allow Avoidance of Computed Tomography Head Imaging in Children at Very Low Risk of Clinically-Important Brain Injury After Head Trauma

Following a study of 42,412 children presenting to 25 North American emergency departments within 24 h of head trauma with Glasgow Coma Scale scores of 14–15, Kuppermann et al. have validated prediction rules to identify children at very low risk for clinically important traumatic brain injury for whom CT can be avoided. The following is their proposal to identify children younger than age 2 and age 2 years and older in whom a head CT is unnecessary:

- *Prediction rule for children under age 2*: normal mental status, no scalp hematoma except frontal, no loss of consciousness or loss of consciousness for less than 5 s, non-severe injury mechanism, no palpable skull fracture, and acting normally according to the parents.
- *Prediction rule for children age 2 years and older*: normal mental status, no loss of consciousness, no vomiting, non-severe injury mechanism, no signs of basilar skull fracture, and no severe headache.

The authors report that neither rule missed a neurosurgical problem in validation populations [1].

> *Computed tomography is not only costly; there is also significant radiation exposure, with some risk of radiation-induced malignancy. As I ponder these prediction rules, I find myself thinking about football injuries, not uncommon in the teenage population, and how "loss of consciousness" will be defined in practice [2]. Is being "dazed" or "dinged" a loss of consciousness? If so, will this indicate a need for imaging under the prediction rules?*

References

1. Kuppermann N, Holmes JF, Dayan PS, et al. Identification of children at very low risk of clinically-important brain injuries after head trauma: a prospective cohort study. Lancet. 2009;374(9696):1160–1170.
2. Reddy CC, Collins MW. Sports concussion: management and predictors of outcome. Curr Sports Med Rep. 2009;8(1):10–15.

###

Imaging May Be Helpful in Selected Instances of Newly Diagnosed Epilepsy in Children

Following a review of published studies, the International League Against Epilepsy (ILAE) Subcommittee for Pediatric Neuroimaging found that nearly half of imaging studies in children with localization-related new-onset epilepsy were reported as abnormal. Conversely, in the absence of a history of a localization-related seizure, abnormal neurologic examination or focal electroencephalography (EEG), the detection of a significant imaging abnormality is rare. They conclude: "Imaging is recommended when localization-related epilepsy is known or suspected, when the epilepsy classification is in doubt, or when an epilepsy syndrome with remote symptomatic cause is suspected" [1].

> *In the study described, 2–4% of imaging studies provided potentially management-changing information. Also, although the authors use the word "imaging," they specify that, because of its versatility, better resolution, and lack of radiation, magnetic resonance imaging (MRI) is preferred to CT [1].*

Reference

1. Gaillard WD, Chiron C, Cross JH, et al. Committee for Neuroimaging, Subcommittee for Pediatric. Guidelines for imaging infants and children with recent-onset epilepsy. Epilepsia. 2009;50(9):2147–2153.

###

In Suspected Acute Appendicitis, Computed Tomography Use Can Lower the Rate of Negative Appendectomies: Especially in Young Women

There are some curious gender differences when it comes to appendicitis. In a study of 308 consecutively enrolled "possible appendicitis" patients, abdominal CT studies were used when the diagnosis was uncertain. In patients selected for surgery on the basis of high clinical suspicion alone – no CT study performed – the negative appendectomy rate for men was 7% and 24% for women. With the selective use of CT, the overall (both men and women) negative appendectomy rate was 16%. These authors advise that "CT be performed routinely in women with suspected appendicitis and selectively in men" [1].

A more recent study evaluated suspected appendicitis adult patients at Duke University Medical Center over a 10 year period. Of these, 925 underwent urgent appendectomy. Significantly, during the 10 years – 1998–2007 – the use of preoperative CT rose from 18.5 to 93.2%. During this time, the negative appendectomy rate for women age 45 and younger decreased from 42.9 to 7.1%. A similar trend toward a lower negative appendectomy rate with increasing use of preoperative CT was not noted for men or for women older than age 45 years [2].

In a related study, Santos et al. asked: How often does computed tomography change the management of acute appendicitis? They studied 100 "possible appendicitis" patients, of whom 70 went on to appendectomy, concluding that CT rarely changes management in patients highly suspicious for appendicitis, but frequently changes management when the clinical diagnosis of appendicitis is in doubt [3].

References

1. Hershko DD, Sroka G, Bahouth H, Ghersin E, Mahajna A, Krausz MM. The role of selective computed tomography in the diagnosis and management of suspected acute appendicitis. Am Surg. 2002;68(11):1003–1007.
2. Coursey CA, Nelson RC, Patel MB, et al. Making the diagnosis of acute appendicitis: do more preoperative CT scans mean fewer negative appendectomies? A 10-year study. Radiology. 2010;254(2):460–468.
3. Santos DA, Manunga J Jr, Hohman D, Avik E, Taylor EW. How often does computed tomography change the management of acute appendicitis? Am Surg. 2009;75(10):918–921.

###

In the Setting of Possible Appendicitis During Pregnancy, an Ultrasound (US) Determination Read as Positive May Require No Further Confirmatory Test Other than Surgery

The statement above is the conclusion of a study of 47 patients with suspected appendicitis during pregnancy. Of these, 43 had US, of which 86% were nondiagnostic studies; six patients with positive US studies all had appendicitis at surgery. Also, during this study 13 patients had CT, with no false-positive or false-negative results [1].

I have some random thoughts about this study. It would seem that 47 patients is not a huge sample, until one considers that the authors needed patients with the confluence of two conditions – pregnancy and suspected appendicitis. Secondly, this was a record review, and not a randomized, controlled trial. Because this was a chart review, clinical assessment of appendicitis risk was a factor in the decision-making regarding each patient, representing a confounding variable in the study. And finally, this is another setting in which radiation exposure is a consideration.

Reference

1. Freeland M, King E, Safcsak K, Durham R. Diagnosis of appendicitis in pregnancy. Am J Surg. 2009;198(6):753–758.

###

Migraine Patients Are at Increased Risk for Subclinical Brain Infarcts, Detectable on Magnetic Resonance Imaging

A cross-section, prevalence study of migraineurs with aura (n = 161), migraineurs without aura (n = 134), and controls (n = 140) revealed a greater incidence of infarcts in the migraine patients than in controls. The chief region in which a difference was noted was the cerebellar region of the posterior circulation territory, where the prevalence of infarcts in migraineurs, both those with and without aura, was 5.4% compared to 0.7% in controls [1].

A more recent study by Scher et al. of 4,689 persons in Iceland found that migraine with aura was associated with late-life prevalence of cerebellar infarct-like lesions on MRI, but that the association was statistically significant only for women [2].

From studies such as these we are learning that migraine is more than just a headache. In fact, however, migraine is not the only headache that can cause abnormalities visible on MRI. De Benedittis et al. studied 63 headache patients – 28 migraineurs and 35 with tension type headache – and 54 headache-free controls, looking for focal white matter abnormalities on MRI [3]. Here is what they found:

Patient group	Incidence of white matter abnormalities (%)
Migraine patients	32.1
Tension type HA patients	34.3
Headache-free patients	7.4

References

1. Kruit MD, van Buchem MA, Hofman PA, et al. Migraine as a risk factor for subclinical brain lesions. JAMA. 2004;291(4):427–434.
2. Scher AI, Gudmundsson LS, Sigurdsson S, et al. Migraine headache in middle age and late-life brain infarcts. JAMA. 2009;301(24):2563–2570.
3. De Benedittis G, Lorenzetti A, Sina C, Bernasconi V. Magnetic resonance imaging in migraine and tension-type headache. Headache. 1995;35(5):264–268.

###

Transdermal Patches Containing Metal in the Backing Can Cause Burns During an MRI Scan

The Food and Drug Administration has issued a Public Health Advisory, alerting physicians and patients that transdermal patches containing aluminum or other metals in the backing can overheat if worn during an MRI scan. The result can be a burn at the site of the patch [1].

According to the FDA, patches to be considered as part of this alert include the following [2]:

Proprietary name	Generic/established name
Androderm	Testosterone transdermal system
Catapres TTS	Clonidine
Fentanyl	Fentanyl
Habitrol	Nicotine transdermal system
Nicotrol TD	Nicotine transdermal system
ProStep	Nicotine transdermal system
Neupro	Rotigotine
Lidoprel	Lidocaine HCl and epinephrine
Synera	Lidocaine and tetracycline
Transderm-Scop	Scopolamine

References

1. Guidelines for Screening Patients for MR Procedures and Individuals for the MR Environment, Institute for Magnetic Resonance Safety, Education, and Research. http://www.imrser.org. 2009.

2. Public Health Advisory: Risk of burns during MRI scans from transdermal drug patches with metallic backings. Available at: http://www.fda.gov/drugs/drugsafety/publichealthadvisories/ucm111313.htm. Accessed February 10, 2010.

###

After Starting a Potent Bisphosphonate in a Postmenopausal Woman with Osteoporosis, Wait 3 Years Before Monitoring Response Using a Bone Mineral Density Determination

The recommendation to wait 3 years before monitoring the effect of bisphosphonate therapy in postmenopausal osteoporosis may be considered a **practice-changer**, based on a study by Sharma [1]. The advice is based on a study from Australia, based on secondary analysis of data involving 6,459 postmenopausal women with low bone density involved in the Fracture Intervention Trial. The authors compared the effects of alendronate and placebo, using bone mineral densities obtained at baseline and at 1, 2, and 3 years after treatment with alendronate. They concluded that monitoring therapy before 3 years may be misleading and should be avoided [2].

> *I find any recommendation advocating for less imaging to be heartwarming. Is there significance to the fact that it comes from the School of Public Health at the University of Sydney in Australia?*

References

1. Sharma U. Bisphosphonate therapy: when not to monitor BMD. J Fam Pract. 2009;58(11):594–596.
2. Gell KJ, Hayen A, Macaskill P, et al. Value of routine monitoring of bone mineral density after bisphosphonate treatment: secondary analysis of trial data. BMJ. 2009;338:b2266.

###

Be Alert to the Seductive Power of Testing, Tracings, and Images

I began this chapter with a quote from Dr. William J. Mayo, cautioning against the temptation of the "machine-made diagnosis." Do not become enchanted with the wonder, charm and apparent certainty of our "testing" devices. Always use your logic, experience, and intuition to interpret the findings of any report.

#####

Chapter 8
Alarming Symptoms and Red Flag Findings

> *Disease often tells its secrets in a casual parenthesis.*
>
> British surgeon and social scientist Wilfred Trotter
> (1872–1939) [1]

Trotter, whose interests extended from neurosurgery to development of the herd instinct theory, the latter based on observing flocks of sheep, packs of wolves, and hives of bees, suggests that we should pay close attention to clinical symptoms and signs – the often-subtle clues to diagnosis. Some of these clues – such as back pain after heavy lifting or the painful blisters of a zoster infection – will be mundane. Others, however, may be both understated – the "casual parenthesis" – and alarming. These are the red flags of medicine, calling for prompt attention. This chapter examines some of these.

Oscar L., a 54-year-old anthropology professor who, from time to time, visited archeological sites in exotic places, had mild hypertension and was a strong advocate of herbal remedies. Oscar used allopathic medicine with great reluctance and only as a last resort.

One day Oscar visited his family physician, whom he saw from time to time for checkups, and with whom he had periodic skirmishes about taking medicine for his high blood pressure. At this visit, however, Oscar had specific symptoms – fever as high as 102° and muscle aches. "Doctor, I think I have the flu. I'm sure I got it on that plane ride; you know how they don't properly filter the air in the passenger cabin. And I don't want to take any antibiotics."

An alarm bell sounded in the doctor's subconscious. Fever and travel, notably travel to exotic destinations, is a red flag combination. He asked, "Oscar, have you been on one of your overseas trips recently?"

"Yes, as a matter or fact, I have. I returned from a trip to Cambodia a few weeks ago."

"And did you take any pills to prevent malaria?"

"Doctor, you know I don't like those things."

The physical exam revealed an enlarged spleen, and blood tests showed thrombocytopenia and hyperbilirubinemia. The clincher was a blood smear for malaria, which revealed the presence of intracellular malaria parasites.

Faced with this diagnosis, and the risks associated with non-treatment, Oscar consented to therapy and made a full recovery.

Approximately 1 of every 12 visitors to developing world countries will require medical care during or following travel. Fever without localizing signs is a frequent

R.B. Taylor, *Essential Medical Facts Every Clinician Should Know: To Prevent Medical Errors, Pass Board Examinations and Provide Informed Patient Care,* DOI 10.1007/978-1-4419-7874-5_8, © Springer Science+Business Media, LLC 2011

complaint, especially in visitors to southeast Asia or sub-Saharan Africa. Of these persons presenting with fever, malaria is a leading cause, although visitors to Central America and areas other than sub-Saharan Africa often were found to have dengue [2]. Each year, approximately 1,300 U.S. travelers return with malaria, and 10 of them die of the disease [3]. The cause of most of these deaths is *Plasmodium falciparum* [4]. Most of these illnesses and deaths are preventable; a study by Dorsey et al. of patients with imported malaria led to the conclusion that "a standard chemoprophylaxis regimen is highly effective in preventing falciparum malaria, but that many American travelers do not receive it" [5].

References

1. Trotter W. Art and science in medicine, Section 6. In: The collected papers of Wilfred Trotter, F.R.S. London: Oxford University Press. 1941.
2. Freedman DO, Weld LH, Kozarsky PE, et al. Spectrum of disease and relation to place of exposure among ill returned travelers. N Engl J Med. 2006;354(2):119–130.
3. Isturiz RE, Torres J, Besso J. Global distribution of infectious diseases requiring intensive care. Crit Care Clin. 2006;22(3):469–488.
4. Magill AJ. Malaria: diagnosis and treatment of falciparum malaria in travelers during and after travel. Curr Infect Dis Rep. 2006;8(1):35–42.
5. Dorsey G, Gandhi M, Oyugi JH, Rosenthal PJ. Difficulties in the prevention, diagnosis, and treatment of imported malaria. Arch Intern Med. 2000;160(16):2505–2510.

###

Four General Alarm Symptoms Are: Rectal Bleeding, Hematuria, Dysphagia, and Hemoptysis

In study of 763,325 patients age 15 and older, the four clinical presentations mentioned were especially likely to indicate either cancer or non-cancer diagnoses. After studying first episodes of these symptoms, investigators calculated, "For every four to seven patients evaluated for hematuria, hemoptysis, dysphagia or rectal bleeding, relevant diagnoses will be identified in one patient within 90 days" [1].

Another study sought to identify red flag signs that might confirm or exclude the presence of serious infection in children. Following a systematic review of 30 studies and calculation of likelihood ratios, Van den Bruel et al. identified three noteworthy red flag signs suggesting the presence of serious infection in children: cyanosis, poor peripheral perfusion and a petechial rash [2].

Van den Bruel et al. also cite one primary care study in which strong red flags were parental concern and clinician instinct, two factors that other studies seemed to ignore [2].

The rest of this chapter discusses more specific alarm symptoms and red flag signs. I continue first with the infectious diseases. Then I will describe diseases of children, diseases we generally associate with adults, and some potentially perilous situations in health care delivery.

References

1. Jones R, Charlton J, Latinovic R, Gulliford MC. Alarm symptoms and identification of non-cancer diagnoses in primary care: cohort study. BMJ. 2009;339:b3094.
2. Van den Bruel A, Haj-Hassan T, Thompson M, Buntinx F, Mant D; for the European Network on Recognizing Serious Infection Investigators. Diagnostic value of clinical features at presentation to identify serious infection in children in developed countries: a systematic review. Lancet. 2010;1375(9717):834–845.

###

Fever, Headache and a Centripetal Rash Suggest Rocky Mountain Spotted Fever (RMSF)

Recognition of manifestations suggesting RMSF, one of the Rickettsial infections transmitted by arthropod vectors, is important because early empiric treatment can prevent serious complications or even death [1, 2]. Think of this possibility in settings where RSMF is endemic, such as North Carolina or Oklahoma, and in situations in which the patient may have experienced a tick bite [3].

When we consider RMSF, we think of fever and rash. Don't forget about headache, which Glaser et al. state is "often the earliest and most common reported symptom in rickettsial infections, present in more than 80% of cases" [4].

References

1. Lacz NL, Schwatz RA, Kapila R. Rocky Mountain spotted fever. J Eur Acad Dermatol Venereol. 2006;20(4):411–417.
2. Dantas-Torres F. Rocky Mountain spotted fever. Lancet Infect Dis. 2007;7(11):724–732.
3. Chen LF, Sexton DJ. What's new in Rocky Mountain spotted fever? Infect Dis Clin North Am. 2008;22(3):415–432.
4. Glaser C, Christie L, Bloch KC. Rickettsial and ehrlichial infections. Handb Clin Neurol. 2010;96C:143–158.

###

In a Patient with Fever or Other Evidence of Infection, There Are Three Manifestations that May Be Early Signs of Sepsis: Leg Pain, Cold Hands and Feet, and Skin Color Abnormalities Such as Mottling or Pallor

The conclusion described here is from a study of 448 children age 16 and younger admitted to hospital with a diagnosis of meningococcal disease. Of these children, 72% had the clues to sepsis – leg pain, cold extremities, and skin color changes – present hours before the onset the classic manifestations of meningitis: fever, neck stiffness, and altered mental state [1].

Based on the red-flag triad suggesting sepsis, I will look specifically for these manifestations when examining children with signs of systemic infection and/or possible meningococcemia.

Reference

1. Thompson MJ, Ninis N, Perera R. Clinical recognition of meningococcal disease in children and adolescents. Lancet. 2006;367(9508):397–403.

###

A Rash with Central Clearing Could Be Erythema Migrans (EM), the Tip-Off to Lyme Disease

The rash, generally found within a month following the infecting tick bite, occurs in up to 80% of patients with Lyme disease. Erythema migrans and some non-specific manifestations suggesting a viral syndrome may be the earliest signs of the disease. There can occasionally be multiple EM lesions, indicating the presence of spirochetemia. Early recognition and treatment of the infection is ideal because late manifestations can include neurologic or cardiac involvement [1, 2].

Note that the earliest manifestations of Lyme disease may occur several weeks following the tick bite, which may well have been forgotten, even if ever noticed in the first place.

References

1. Wormser GP, Dattwyler RJ, Shapiro ED. The clinical assessment, treatment, and prevention of Lyme disease, human granulocytic anaplasmosis, and babesiosis: clinical practice guidelines by the Infectious Diseases Society of America. Clin Infect Dis. 2006;43(9):1089–1134.
2. Halperin JJ. Nervous system Lyme disease. Infect Dis Clin North Am. 2008;22(2):261–274.

###

A Skin Lesion with an Area of Anesthesia in a Person with a Suspicious Exposure History Could Be a Sign of Hanson Disease/Leprosy

Other cutaneous manifestations of leprosy include loss of eyebrows and lashes, as well as plantar ulcers [1]. Areas of the world where leprosy is endemic include Brazil, India, Madagascar, Mozambique, Myanmar, and Nepal [2].

Just in case we become complacent that leprosy cannot occur in America, there is a report of leprosy in three individuals, none of whom had ever been outside the country, knew one another, or had contact with a known leprosy patient. The common thread in their stories is a history of armadillo exposure [3].

References

1. Elinav H, Palladas L, Applbaum YH, et al. Plantar ulcers and eyebrow-hair paucity. Clin Infect Dis. 2006;42(5):684–685.
2. World Health Organization Technical Advisory Group. Report on the first WHO Technical Advisory Group on the Elimination of Leprosy. WHO/CDS/CPE/CEE/2000.4, Geneva: World Health Organization. 2000.
3. Abide JM, Webb RM, Jones HL, Young L. Three indigenous cases of leprosy in the Mississippi delta. South Med J. 2008;101(6):635–638.

###

A Child with an Unexplained Fever for 5 Days or More Just Might Have Kawasaki Disease (KD)

Kawasaki disease, aka mucocutaneous lymph node fever, is a systemic inflammatory disease of childhood [1]. The most common manifestation is fever. Other findings may be erythema of the oral mucosa and lips, a pleomorphic rash, and bilateral nonexudative conjunctivitis and uveitis [2].

KD, like RMSF and Lyme disease, is best detected early, when therapy (in this case, intravenous gamma globulin) has the best chance of preventing complications, such as coronary artery aneurysms, ischemic heart disease, or sudden death [3].

References

1. Burns JC, Glode MP. Kawasaki syndrome. Lancet. 2004;364(9433):533–544.
2. Smith LB, Newburger JW, Burns JC. Kawasaki syndrome and the eye. Pediatr Infect Dis J. 1989;8(2):116–118.

3. Newburger JW, Takahashi M, Gerber MA, et al. Diagnosis, treatment and long-term management of Kawasaki disease. A statement for health professionals from the Committee on Rheumatic Fever, Endocarditis, and Kawasaki Disease, Council on Cardiovascular Disease in the Young, American Heart Association. Circulation. 2004;110(17):2747–2771.

###

A History of a Penetrating Injury, Increasing Wound Pain and Soft Tissue Crepitus Strongly Suggest the Diagnosis of Gas Gangrene

Deep penetrating injury – gunshot, knife or crushing injury – is involved in approximately three quarters of cases of gas gangrene, and the most common organism is *Clostridium perfringens* [1]. In addition to local findings, signs of systemic toxicity and shock may be seen.

> *As a sign of the times, there have been reports of gas gangrene following tar heroin injections [2].*

References

1. Awad MM, Bryant AE, Stevens DL, Rood JI. Virulence studies on chromosomal alpha-toxin and theta-toxin mutants constructed by allelic exchange provide genetic evidence for the essential role of alpha-toxin in Clostridium perfringens-mediated gas gangrene. Mol Microbiol. 1995;15(2):191–202.
2. Christie B. Gangrene bug killed 35 heroin users. West J Med. 2000;173(2):82–83.

###

Bloody Diarrhea, Vomiting and Abdominal Pain May Be the Precursors to the Hemolytic Uremic Syndrome (HUS)

HUS, often related to consumption of undercooked beef, occurs chiefly in children. Most cases are caused by Shiga-toxin producing *Escherichia coli*. The classic triad of HUS – hemolytic anemia, thrombocytopenia and acute renal damage – typically follows the onset of diarrhea by 5–10 days [1, 2].

> *The disease is most common in summer and is especially likely to occur in rural settings. In addition to undercooked beef, HUS can be transmitted by water, fruits, vegetables or unpasteurized milk. This all speaks to the importance of careful food and beverage hygiene, especially during summer picnics. In order to make a timely diagnosis and plan therapy, Slutsker et al. recommend that all patients with acute bloody diarrhea have stools cultured for E. coli 0157:H7 [2].*

References

1. Gerber A, Karch H, Allerberger F, Verweyen HM, Zimmerhackl LB. Clinical course and the role of shiga toxin-producing Escherichia coli infection in the hemolytic-uremic syndrome in pediatric patients, 1997–2000, in Germany and Austria: a prospective study. J Infect Dis. 2002;186(4):493–500.
2. Slutsker L, Ries AA, Greene KD, Wells JG, Hutwagner L, Griffin PM. Escherichia coli 0157:H7 diarrhea in the United States: clinical and epidemiologic features. Ann Intern Med. 1997;126(7):505–513.

###

The Patient Who Travels and Who Reports Linear or Clustered Bites Might Have Bedbugs

The common bed bug, *Cimex lectularius*, once ubiquitous in earlier times ("Don't let the bedbugs bite.") has made a comeback. The patient may have had a short stay in a hotel, and return with bedbugs in his luggage. Staying at a luxury hotel or on an elegant cruise ship is no guarantee that there will be no bedbugs; is has to do with who occupied your bed the night before you [1, 2].

Ask patients about small, flat, oval, wingless insects that may lurk in bedding, easy chairs or any soft furniture.

References

1. Davis RF, Johnston GA, Sladden MJ. Recognition and management of common ectoparasitic diseases. Am J Clin Dermatol. 2009;10(1):1–8.
2. Sutton DL, Thomas DJ. Don't let the bedbugs bite. Nursing. 2008;38(1):24–26.

###

Think of Wilms Tumor in a Child with a Painless Abdominal Mass or Swelling

A painless abdominal mass and/or swelling are often the only findings a child with Wilms tumor will have, although some will manifest abdominal discomfort, hypertension or hematuria [1]. Early detection leading to prompt therapy has allowed us to consider Wilms tumor, in the words of Spreafico and Bellani, "one of the successes of pediatric oncology, with an overall cure rate of over 85%, using relatively simple therapies" [2].

For those who value precision in medical terminology, the correct wording is Wilms tumor, not Wilm's tumor; the disease is named for German surgeon Max Wilms (1867–1918).

Finding an abdominal mass suspicious of Wilms tumor is not a time to invite an army of medical students to examine the belly. Energetic palpation can lead to tumor cell spillage, potentially changing disease staging, therapy and prognosis.

References

1. D'Angio GJ. The National Wilms Tumor Study: a 40 year prospective. Lifetime Data Anal. 2007;13(4):463–470.
2. Spreafico F, Bellani FF. Wilms tumor: past, present and (possibly) future. Expert Rev Anticancer Ther. 2006;6(2):249–258.

###

A Child with Purpura, Joint Symptoms and Abdominal Pain May Have Henoch–Schönlein Purpura

The clincher will be finding evidence of renal impairment. Most cases of this immune-mediated vasculitis occur in children, and they usually follow upper respiratory infections, often ones caused by streptococci. Although the presenting manifestations generally subside, there can be long-lasting renal involvement [1, 2].

Because early treatment with steroids and sometimes also immunosuppressants can reduce the risk of ongoing renal disease, early identification of Henoch–Schönlein purpura is imperative [3].

References

1. McCarthy HJ, Tizard EJ. Clinical practice: diagnosis and management of Henoch-Schönlein purpura. Eur J Pediatr. 2009;169(6):643–50.
2. Rivera F, Anaya S. Henoch-Schönlein nephritis and persistent hypocomplementemia: a case report. J Med Case Reports. 2010;4(1):50–52.
3. Reamy BV, Williams PM, Lindsay TJ. Henoch-Schönlein purpura. Am Fam Physician. 2009;80(7):697–704.

###

The "Red Flag" Findings for Osteogenesis Imperfecta Are Excessive Numbers of Fractures, Perhaps Associated with Hearing Loss, Blue Sclera, and Teeth that Seem to Wear Down Readily

A positive family history is very helpful in identifying this genetic disorder, which can have a variety of other manifestations, including short stature, spinal scoliosis, and increased laxity of ligaments [1, 2].

One important reason to be aware of this disease is that, with multiple and sometimes atypical fractures, it could be mistaken for child abuse.

References

1. Rauch F, Glorieux FH. Osteogenesis imperfecta. Lancet. 2004;363(9418):1377–1385.
2. Byers PH. Disorders of collagen biosynthesis and structure. In: The metabolic and molecular bases of inherited disease, 8th ed. Scriver C, Beaudet AL, Valle D, Sly W (Eds), New York: McGraw-Hill. 2001;Page 5241.

Fever, Irritability and Bone Hyperplasia in an Infant Suggest the Presence of Caffey Disease, aka Infantile Cortical Hyperostosis

This disease, transmitted as an autosomal dominant trait, can cause a fever as high as 104°F. In addition to the findings noted above, there may be an elevated alkaline phosphatase, a high erythrocyte sedimentation rate, and a leukocytosis [1, 2].

Here is another disease that could be misdiagnosed as child abuse. In Caffey disease, the mandible is typically involved, which can help differentiate this disease from inflicted trauma.

References

1. Kamouon-Goldrat A, le Merrer M. Infantile cortical hyperostosis (Caffey disease). J Oral Maxillofac Surg. 2008;66(10):2145–2150.
2. Bernstein RM, Zaleske DJ. Familial aspects of Caffey's disease. Am J Orthop. 1995;24(10):777–781.

###

A Young Child with a Fracture Attributed to Falling Out of Out of Bed Is a Red Flag for Child Abuse

More than half of physically abused children have fractures [1]. Yet, there is one scenario that should sound alarm bells: a fracture attributed to a fall from bed. Three studies looked at this situation, and all reached the same conclusion, that falling out of bed seldom results in fractures [2, 3, 4].

I measured and my bed, with one of those new thick mattresses, is still only 30 in. high. Of course, the height is a little greater if the child climbs over a crib rail. The three studies cited chiefly involved small children, age 6 years and younger. At that age, in a fall from a relatively low height, children will tend to get bruised and scraped, but not suffer broken bones. That statement is not necessarily true for older children with more rigid bones, especially those who fall from upper levels of double-decker bunk beds and land on their outstretched hands.

References

1. Sinal SH, Stewart CD. Physical abuse of children: a review for orthopedic surgeons. J South Orthop Assoc. 1998;7(4):264–276.
2. Helfer RE, Slovis TL, Black M. Injuries resulting when small children fall out of bed. Pediatrics. 1977;60(4):533–535.
3. Nimityongskul P, Anderson LD. The likelihood of injuries when children fall out of bed. J Pediatr Orthop. 1987;7(2):184–186.
4. Lyons TJ, Oates RK. Falling out of bed: a relatively benign occurrence. Pediatrics. 1993;92(1):125–127.

###

Herpes Zoster Involving the Tip of the Nose Can Presage a Sight-Threatening Herpes Zoster Ophthalmicus Inflammation of the Eye

The rash involves the external branch of the fifth cranial nerve, and its association with herpes zoster of the eye was first described in 1864 by Sir James Hutchinson [1, 2]. A study by Zaal et al. of 83 non-immunocompromised adults with acute herpes ophthalmicus over a 2-year period, with a skin rash with a duration of less than 1 week led to the conclusion that the presence of herpes zoster skin lesions affecting the dermatomes of both nasociliary branches – the external nasal and the infratrochlear – was "invariably associated with the development of ocular inflammation" [3].

This nineteenth century observation is the basis for the current eponymous designation Hutchinson's sign. As for the 2003 study by Zaal et al., we seldom see use of the word "invariably" in a research report. Every physician should know about this "red flag" sign, which should prompt a prompt ophthalmologic referral.

References

1. Hutchinson J. Clinical report on herpes zoster frontalis ophthalmicus (shingles affecting the forehead and nose). Ophthalmic Hospital reports and Journal of the Royal London Ophthalmic Hospital, London, 1864;3(72);865–866, 1865;5:191.
2. Tomkinson A, Roblin DG, Brown MJ. Hutchinson's sign and its importance in rhinology. Rhinology 1995;33(3):180–182.
3. Zaal MJ, Völker-Dieben HJ, D'Amaro J. Prognostic value of Hutchinson's sign in acute herpes zoster ophthalmicus. Graefes Arch Clin Exp Ophthalmol. 2003;241(3):187–191.

###

A Painful Red Eye Associated with Headache, Nausea and Vomiting Is Often Seen with Acute Angle Closure Glaucoma

Other possible manifestations are decreased vision, corneal edema and a somewhat dilated pupil that reacts poorly to light [1, 2, 3]. There is also chronic angle closure glaucoma, with a gradual rise in intraocular pressure, which may have few symptoms.

Acute angle closure glaucoma is an ocular emergency, necessitating urgent referral to an ophthalmologist experienced in managing this problem.

References

1. Liebowitz HM. The red eye. N Engl J Med. 2000;343(5):345–351.
2. Sutherland JE, Mauer RC. Selected disorders of the eye. In: Family medicine: principles and practice, ed. 6. Taylor RB (Ed). New York: Springer, 2003;Page 598.
3. Pokhrel PK, Loftus SA. Ocular emergencies. Am Fam Phys. 2007;76(6):829–836.

###

The Sudden Appearance or Increase in Retinal Floaters in One Eye May Herald the Onset of Retinal Detachment

Byer studied 350 consecutive patients with posterior vitreous detachment of the eye, the most common precursor of retinal detachment. Of patients who complained initially of having one or two floaters, with or without light flashes, 7.3% went on to develop a retinal tear. In patients with phakic eyes with secondary retinal tears on initial examination, 29% reported that their only symptoms were one to two floaters and light flashes [1].

A colorful description of an especially large floater may be a resemblance to a "large housefly." In a separate study, Go et al. found some familial risk of retinal detachment that could not be explained by the presence or absence of myopia in the families [2].

Retinal detachment is especially prevalent in boxers and others who suffer head trauma [3]. Following his welterweight title fight versus Thomas Hearns in 1981, boxer Sugar Ray Leonard was found to have a retinal detachment, causing him to retire – temporarily – from boxing. Retinal detachment can also follow cataract surgery.

References

1. Byer NE. Natural history of posterior vitreous detachment with early management as the pre-mier line of defense against retinal detachment. Ophthalmology. 1994;101(9):1503–1513.
2. Go SL, Hoyng CB, Klaver CC. Genetic risk of rhegmatogenous retinal detachment: a familial aggregation study. Arch Ophthalmol. 2005;123(9):1237–1241.
3. Macguire JI, Benson WE. Retinal injury and detachment in boxers. JAMA. 1986;255(18): 2451–2453.

###

A Patient Taking Alpha-Adrenergic Receptor Blockers and Headed for Cataract Surgery Is at Risk for Floppy Iris Syndrome (FIS)

Two problems are common in older men: benign prostatic hypertrophy and cata-racts. When hesitancy and nocturia become a problem, the patient often receives a prescription for tamsulosin (Flomax) or another alpha-adrenergic receptor blocker. This combination can lead to an intraoperative complication: floppy iris syndrome. Neff et al. reviewed cataract extraction surgery in 899 eyes of 660 patients, finding intraoperative FIS in 4.1% of patients; tamsulosin and other alpha(1)-antagonist use (other than tamsulosin) were strongly correlated with intraoperative FIS in their study [1].

A study reported by Bell et al. looking at tamsulosin and serious ophthalmic adverse events in older men following cataract surgery had similar results. They calculated an estimated number needed to harm (NNH) of 255. This group, looking at a variety of adverse events, found "no significant associations with exposure to other alpha-blocker medications used to treat BPH" [2].

A report from the Altos Eye Physicians in California, following a study of 167 consecutive eyes in 135 patients, offers the opinion: "When experienced surgeons could anticipate intraoperative FIS and employ compensatory surgical techniques, the complication rate from cataract surgery was low and the visual outcomes were excellent in eyes of patients with a history of tamsulosin use" [3]. I find this conclusion somewhat reassuring. Nevertheless, I think is most important not to be surprised, and, when possible, to withhold alpha-adrenergic receptor blockers as long as possible before cataract surgery.

References

1. Neff KD, Sandoval HP, Fernandez de Castro LE, Nowacki AS, Vroman DT, Solomon KD. Factors associated with intraoperative floppy iris syndrome. Ophthalmology. 2009;116(4): 658–663.
2. Bell CM, Hatch WV, Fischer HD, et al. Association between tamsulosin and serious ophthalmic adverse events in older men following cataract surgery. JAMA. 2009;301(19):1991–1996.
3. Chang DF, Osher RH, Wang L, Koch DD. Prospective multicenter evaluation of cataract surgery in patients taking tamsulosin (Flomax). Ophthalmology. 2007;114(5):957–964.

###

A Child with a Croupy Cough Whose Symptoms Do Not Respond Promptly to the Home Remedy of Sitting in a Steamy Bathroom Has a Life-Threatening Disease

Croup, aka laryngotracheitis, is a disease of older infants and younger children, typically ages 3 months to 3 years. The distinctive sign is a barking cough – like that of the seal at a zoo. For parents, this can be terrifying, even if they are veterans of previous episodes.

Subcostal and intercostal retraction indicate airway obstruction. Hypoxia, cyanosis and death can occur [1, 2].

Here are some personal observations about croup. Sitting in the hot, steamy bathroom at home is often effective, but sooner or later, the home hot water tank runs dry. Also, after leaving the bathroom "sauna," symptoms can return. As a small town family doctor, I saw a few instances in which riding to the office in the cold night air (These problems always seemed to happen at night) seemed to bring some relief, but this favorable effect cannot be counted upon.

References

1. Cherry JD. Clinical practice: croup. N Engl J Med. 2008;358(4):384–391.
2. Orr ST, Caplan SE. Laryngotracheitis and croup. Am J Dis Child. 1984;138(10):991–992.

###

Most Headache Patients Do Not Require Imaging, but Some Do

A headache accompanied by one of several danger signs – paralysis; papilledema; or drowsiness, confusion, memory impairment and unconsciousness – has been found by Lamont et al. to suggest intracranial pathology. The authors found that the presence of three or more of these manifestations were especially predictive of abnormal imaging [1].

> Some headache patients should have prompt diagnostic imaging. This study describes some key indications. Others include recent onset headaches, seizures and the "worst headache ever."

Reference

1. Lamont MS, Alias NA, Win MN. Red flags in patients presenting with headache: clinical indications for neuroimaging. Br J Radiol. 2003;76(908):532–535.

###

The Combination of Headache, Palpitations and Sweating Suggests the Possibility of Pheochromocytoma

Other possible manifestations of this catecholamine-secreting tumor of the adrenal gland include ST-changes that would seem to suggest myocardial infarction, heart failure, and, rarely, ventricular tachycardia [1].

> If suspicious of pheochromocytoma, laboratory testing may include plasma metanephrine testing or a 24-h urinary collection for catecholamines and metanephrines. Caution: In a study of 26 healthy adults, de Jong et al. found that consumption of catecholamine-rich nuts and fruits can affect test results [2]. Some drugs that can yield falsely high values are listed in Chap. 7.

References

1. Leite LR, Macedo PG, Santos SN, Quaglia L, Mesas CE, De Peola A. Life-threatening cardiac manifestations of pheochromocytoma. Case Report Med. 2010;2010:976120. Epub 2010 Feb 10.
2. de Jong WH, Eisenhofer G, Post WJ, et al. Dietary influences on plasma and urinary metanephrines: implications for diagnosis of catecholamine-producing tumors. J Clin Endocrinol Metab. 2009;94(8):2841–2849.

###

A Diagnosis of "Non-specific Chest Pain" Carries a Significant Mortality Risk over the Next 5 Years

An adult with acute chest pain, evaluated, found to have no evidence of acute coronary artery disease and sent home is at increased risk of dying. A British study of 786 patients with nontraumatic chest pain who were discharged without being admitted to the hospital were found to have a significantly reduced 5-year survival. Half of the deaths in males were caused by ischemic heart disease [1].

This finding was consistent with the conclusion of an earlier study from Sweden that included 6,488 men ages 51–59 who were considered to have "non-specific chest pain." The authors report, "We found a high cardiovascular as well as noncardiovascular mortality among patients with chest pain who had not been considered to have angina pectoris at a three-step procedure. It is important to be suspicious of early coronary heart disease symptoms in men (and women?) with "nonspecific" chest symptoms and to analyze their cardiovascular risk factor pattern further because they are at considerably higher risk for future events than those in whom coronary heart disease is not suspected" [2].

> Robinson et al. looked at nonspecific chest pain in women with the largest sample of all: 83,622 women ages 50–79 years. To no one's surprise, the authors report similar findings: "Older women discharged with a diagnosis of nonspecific chest pain may be at increased risk of coronary heart disease mortality" [3].

References

1. Geraldine McMahon C, Yates DW, Hollis S. Unexpected mortality in patients discharged from the emergency department following an episode of nontraumatic chest pain. Eur J Emerg Med. 2008;15(1):3–8.
2. Wilhelmsen L, Rosengren A, Hagman M, Lappas G. "Nonspecific" chest pain associated with long-term mortality: results from the primary prevention study in Goteborg, Sweden. Clin Cardiol. 1998;21(7):477–482.
3. Robinson JG, Wallace R, Limacher M, et al. Elderly women diagnosed with non-specific chest pain may be at increased cardiovascular risk. J Women's Health (Larchmt). 2006;15(10):1151–1160.

###

Sudden Chest or Abdominal Pain Described as "Tearing" or "Ripping" Is a Red Flag for the Possibility of Aortic Dissection

The adjectives used in the medical history can be the tip-off to a dissecting aortic aneurysm; according to Osler, there is no disease more conducive to clinical humility. Clinical signs pointing to the diagnosis are mediastinal or aortic widening on chest x-ray and pulse or blood pressure differentials.

Note that these signs and symptoms can be ascertained rapidly, important in a situation when prompt diagnosis can be life-saving.

Reference

1. von Kodolitsch Y, Schwartz AG, Nienaber GA. Clinical prediction of acute aortic dissection. Arch Intern Med. 2000;160(19):2977–2982.

###

The Sudden Onset of Fever and Dyspnea in a Nursing Home Patient Is Aspiration Pneumonitis until an Alternative Diagnosis Is Confirmed

There may be cyanosis and abnormal sounds on chest auscultation. On chest x-ray, look for consolidation in the lower lobes (I think of inhaled food dropping by gravity). Marik distinguishes between aspiration pneumonitis (a chemical injury) and aspiration pneumonia (colonization by pathogenic bacteria) [1].

Not all aspiration pneumonitis patients are in nursing homes. Some specific predisposing factors include: neurologic diseases causing dysphagia, an impaired cough reflex, mechanical impairment of the glottic closure owing to tracheostomy, endotracheal intubation, or nasogastric tube feedings.

Reference

1. Marik PE. Aspiration pneumonitis and aspiration pneumonia. N Engl J Med. 2001;344(9): 665–671.

###

The Sudden Onset of Labored and Rapid Breathing in an Otherwise Healthy Person May Be Alarm Symptoms of Pulmonary Embolism (PE)

These two findings – dyspnea and tachypnea – were found by Stein et al. to occur in 90% of 117 PE patients studied. Only about half of the PE patients studied had evidence suggesting deep vein thrombosis of the lower extremity [1]. The telltale dyspnea may be present only upon exertion [2].

The diagnosis of pulmonary embolism is often missed, because the patient with vague shortness of breath and rapid breathing seems otherwise healthy, and because we fail to think of PE. Be especially suspicious of the patient who has recently engaged in prolonged sedentary activity, such as a long airplane trip.

References

1. Stein PD, Terrin ML, Hales CA, et al. Clinical, laboratory, roentgenographic, and electrocardiographic findings in patients with acute pulmonary embolism and no pre-existing cardiac or pulmonary disease. Chest. 1991;100(3);598–603.
2. Stein PD, Beemath A, Matta F, et al. Clinical characteristics of patients with acute pulmonary embolism: data from PIOPED II. Am J Med. 2007;120(10):871–879.

Be Concerned When Presented with the Very Obese Patient with Sleep Disordered Breathing; He or She Might Have the Obesity Hypoventilation (Pickwickian) Syndrome

The clincher in making this diagnosis is finding chronic hypercapnia during wakefulness in the absence of other known causes of hypercapnia. Littleton estimates that this syndrome is present in 10–20% of all obstructive sleep apnea patients [1].

The syndrome is named for the "fat boy" named Joe in Charles Dickens' The Posthumous Papers of the Pickwick Club. Joe would fall asleep while performing his duties or even while eating [2]. Making the diagnosis and initiating treatment of the obesity hypoventilation (Pickwickian) syndrome is important because the disease is associated with a high burden of morbidity and mortality [3].

References

1. Littleton SW, Mokhlesi B. The pickwickian-obesity hypoventilation syndrome. Clin Chest Med. 2009;30(3):467–478.
2. Dickens C. The Posthumous Papers of the Pickwick Club. London: Chapman & Hall. 1837.
3. Mokhlesi B, Tulaimat A. Recent advances in the obesity hypoventilation syndrome. Chest. 2007;132(4):1322–1336.

###

New Onset Diabetes Mellitus in an Older Adult May Herald a Later Diagnosis of Pancreatic Cancer

Chari et al. studied 2,122 newly diagnosed diabetics age 50 years and older. Of these persons, 18 (0.85%) developed pancreatic cancer within 3 years. There may have been a greater risk of pancreatic cancer in ever-smokers, but the numbers did not reach statistical significance [1].

> *In a newly diagnosed older diabetic, be alert for the manifestations of pancreatic cancer: abdominal pain, especially if it radiates through to the back; jaundice; and weight loss.*

Reference

1. Chari ST, Leibson CL, Rabe KG, Ransom J, de Andrade M, Peterson GM. Probability of pancreatic cancer following diabetes: a population-based study. Gastroenterology. 2005;129(2):504–511.

###

In Any Patient with Acute or Chronic Diarrhea Accompanied by Abdominal Distension, the Possibility of Toxic Megacolon Should Be Considered

First recognized as a clinical entity as recently as 1950, toxic megacolon is a segmental or total nonobstructive colonic dilation involving 6 cm or more accompanied by evidence of systemic toxicity [1]. To confirm the diagnosis, look for radiographic evidence of colonic distension accompanied by fever, tachycardia, neutrophilic leukocytosis and anemia. Other manifestations may include altered consciousness, hypotension, dehydration, and electrolyte disturbances. Toxic megacolon is a potentially lethal condition.

> *Levine reminds us that risk factors include barium enema, colonoscopy, and antimotility medications [2].*

References

1. Sheth SG, LaMont JT. Toxic megacolon. The Lancet. 1998;351:509–513.
2. Levine CD. Toxic megacolon. AACN Clin Issues. 1999;10(4):492–499.

###

Low Back Pain Plus Bladder or Bowel Dysfunction Signal a Surgical Emergency

Back pain accompanied by difficulty urinating, fecal incontinence, or saddle anesthesia signals the possibility of a cauda equina syndrome [1]. There may also be bilateral sciatic pain or leg weakness [2]. The patient may present with urinary retention with overflow incontinence.

> *More than 1 in 20 adult Americans experience low back pain each day, and some 60–70% will have low back pain during their lifetimes [1]. In among these throngs of backache sufferers, however, are a few with nerve compression that can lead to permanent sensory or motor loss. In such an instance, prompt surgical referral is mandatory.*

References

1. Kinkade S. Evaluation and treatment of acute low back pain. Am Fam Physician 2007;75: 1181–1188, 1190–1192.
2. Ma B, Wu H, Jia LS, Yuan W, Shi GD, Shi JG. Cauda equina syndrome: a review of clinical progress. Chin Med J. 2009;122(10):1214–1222.

###

When Evaluating a Low Back Pain Patient for Fracture, There Are Three Red Flags to Consider: Prolonged Use of Corticosteroids, Age Greater than 70 Years, and Significant Trauma

These three red flags were identified following a study conducted in Australia of 1,172 consecutive patients receiving primary care for low back pain. Of these subjects, 11 cases of previously undetected spinal pathology were discovered. The most common serious pathology observed was vertebral fracture, found in 8 cases. The authors of the study report studying 25 red flag questions, many of which were found to have very high false-positive rates. Only the three red flags noted above were found to be informative in detecting vertebral fracture [1].

> *In the Australian study, 1 of the 11 patients with serious spinal pathology had cauda equina syndrome. Herniated lumbar discs with nerve root impingement and sciatic pain were not identified as "serious spinal pathology" [1]. The patients with symptomatic lumbar diskopathy might disagree.*

Reference

1. Henschke N, Maher CG, Refshauge KM. Prevalence of and screening for serious spinal pathology in patients presenting to primary care settings with acute low back pain. Arthritis Rheum. 2009;60(10):3072–3080.

###

An Injury Such as a Fall Followed by Bilateral Upper Extremity Weakness Is an Alarm Scenario that May Indicate the Presence of Central Cord Syndrome

There may also be some weakness in the lower extremities, but upper extremity paresis is typically more profound. Some sensory deficit may be noted, but is overshadowed by the patient's difficulty moving the involved extremities [1, 2]. The prognosis can be favorable. Yamazaki et al. recommend timely surgery, preferably within 2 weeks of injury, in selected patients [2].

> *Elderly persons and athletes in contact sports do not share much, but this disease occurs in these two groups of persons. Elderly persons often have predisposing degenerative disease of the spine and occasional cervical spondylosis. Athletes, especially those in impact sports such as football, may suffer causative hyperextension injuries.*

References

1. Nakajima M, Hirayama K. Midcervical central cord syndrome: numb and clumsy hands due to midline cervical disc protrusion as the C3–4 intervertebral level. Neurol Neurosurg Psychiatry. 1995;58:607–613.
2. Yamazaki T, Yanaka K, Fujita K, et al. Traumatic central cord syndrome: analysis of factors affecting the outcome. Surg Neurol. 2005;63(2):95–99.

###

Symmetrical Limb Weakness Following a Respiratory Infection or Gastroenteritis Describes the Classic Onset of Guillain–Barré Syndrome

Weakness generally starts in the lower extremities and moves proximally. Half of all patients show facial weakness [1]. The life-threatening manifestation is weakness of the respiratory muscles, occurring in some 10–30% of cases, requiring ventilatory support [2]. Current therapeutic options include the use of intravenous immunoglobulin [3].

While the motor weakness feature of the disease are well known, Seneviratne et al. remind us that 80% of patients have sensory symptoms, and 90% have pain, which is often severe [1].

References

1. Seneviratne U. Guillain-Barré syndrome. Postgrad Med. 2000;76(902):774–782.
2. Alshekhlee A, Hussain Z, Sultan B, Katirji B. Guillain-Barré syndrome: incidence and mortality rates in U.S. hospitals. Neurology. 2008;70(18):1608–1613.
3. Hughes RA, Dalakas MC, Cornblath DR, Latov N, Weksler ME, Relkin N. Clinical applications of intravenous immunoglobulins in neurology. Clin Exp Immunol. 2009;158 (Suppl 1):34–42.

Patient Distress during Pelvic Examinations May Signal Past Sexual Violence

Weitlauf et al. surveyed female veterans for a history of sexual violence and distress and pain associated with the pelvic examination. A subset of the group were assessed for posttraumatic stress disorder (PSTD). Those women most likely to report distress with the pelvic examination had both a history of sexual violence and PTSD. Next most likely to report pelvic examination pain were those with a history of sexual violence only. Least likely to describe pelvic examination pain were those women with neither a sexual violence history or PTSD [1].

While the subjects in the Weitlauf study were female veterans, Luce et al. remind us that there are other groups at special risk for sexual violence: adolescents, disabled persons, persons with substance abuse problems, homeless persons, survivors of childhood physical or sexual abuse, prison inmates, and sex workers [2].

References

1. Weitlaulf JC, Finney JW, Ruzek JL, et al. Distress and pain during pelvic examinations: effect of sexual violence. Obstet Gynecol. 2008;112(6):1343–1350.
2. Luce H, Schrager S, Gilchrist V. Sexual assault of women. Am Fam Phys. 2010;81(4): 489–495, 496.

###

Be Alarmed and Suspect Ectopic Pregnancy (EP) When a Woman of Childbearing Age Reports Lower Abdominal or Pelvic Pain, Especially Pain that Is Lateral or Described as "Sharp," Occurring 6–8 Weeks Following the Last Menstrual Period

Following a study by Dart et al. of 441 patients with suggestive symptoms, 57 (13%) were found to have an ectopic pregnancy [1]. This study and another by Ankum et al. have identified some factors that make the diagnosis of ectopic pregnancy more likely [1, 2].

Factors Making Ectopic Pregnancy Diagnosis More Likely

Previous ectopic pregnancy
Pain described as sharp or lateral
Pain described as moderate to severe
History of intrauterine device use
History of infertility
History of intrauterine diethylstilbestrol (DES) exposure
Prior pelvic surgery or tubal ligation
Peritoneal signs on physical exam
Cervical motion tenderness
Lateral or bilateral abdominal or pelvic tenderness

The diagnosis of EP was less likely if pelvic examination revealed a uterus larger than 8 week size [1].

> *Happily, a study of 849 tubal pregnancies led authors Job-Spira et al. to conclude, "Although tubal rupture seriously affects the immediate health of the women concerned, it seems to have no independent effect on subsequent fertility" [3].*

References

1. Dart RG, Kaplan B, Varaklis K. Predictive value of history and physical examination in patients with suspected ectopic pregnancy. Ann Emerg Med. 1999;33(3):283–290.
2. Ankum WM, Mol BW, Van der Veen F, Bossuyt PM. Risk factors for ectopic pregnancy: a meta-analysis. Fertil Steril. 1996;65(6):1093–1099.
3. Job-Spira N, Fernandez H, Bouyer J, Pouly JL, Germaine E, Coste J. Ruptured tubal ectopic pregnancy: risk factors and reproductive outcome: results of a population-based study in France. Am J Obstet Gynecol. 1999;180(4):938–944.

###

Gynecomastia Can Be an Early Clue to Testicular Cancer

Gynecomastia, usually but not always associated with elevated levels of human chorionic gonadotropin (hCG) produced by tumor cells, may be present in up to 10% of testicular cancer patients [1].

The finding of gynecomastia developing in a young man calls for careful examination of the scrotum, looking for a firm nodule or painless swelling of one testicle.

Reference

1. Tseng A Jr, Horning SJ, Freiha FS, Resser KJ, Hannigan JF, Torti FM. Gynecomastia in testicular cancer patients. Prognostic and therapeutic implications. Cancer. 1985;56(10):2534–2538.

###

Here Is the Red Flag Scenario for Stevens–Johnson Syndrome (SJS): a Child Or Young Person with an Infectious Disease, Perhaps Treated with an Antibiotic Who, About 2 Weeks Later, Develops Fever and Flu-Like Symptoms Followed by Rash

The rash is typically erythematous macules, often pruritic. Target lesions and bullae may be noted. The inciting event in adults is often antibiotic use; in children it is more likely to be an infection, most commonly *Mycoplasma pneumoniae* [1]. When an infection has been treated with one of the commonly implicated drugs – sulfonamides, penicillin, or cephalosporins – the etiologic picture is a little clouded.

Consider the possibility of malignancy in the elderly patient with SJS. And here is another fact to remember about SJS: Patients with human immunodeficiency virus infections have a 40-fold increased risk of developing SJS or toxic epidermal necrolysis when taking trimethoprim-sulfamethoxazole, when compared with the risk in the general population [2].

References

1. Leaute-Labreze C, Lamireau T, Chawki D, Maleville J, Taieb A. Diagnosis, classification, and management of erythema multiforme and Stevens-Johnson syndrome. Arch Dis Child. 2000;83(4):347–352.
2. Rotunda A, Hirsch RJ, Scheinfeld N, Weinberg JM. Stevens-Johnson syndrome and toxic epidermal necrolysis. Acta Derm Venereol. 2003;83(1):1–9.

###

A Patient with Intermittent Abdominal Pain Who Mentions that His or Her Urine Turns Red upon Standing (In a Glass Container) May Have Acute Intermittent Porphyria (AIP)

Abdominal pain is the most common presenting symptom of this autosomal disorder [1, 2]. Other manifestations may include anxiety, hysteria, phobias, psychoses, seizures, neuropathy of various types, and altered consciousness.

Recall that this disease may have muddled the thinking of King George III during the American Revolutionary War [3]. We are reminded that psychiatric hospitals have a disproportionate number of acute intermittent porphyria patients [4].

References

1. Herrick AL, McColl KEL. Acute intermittent porphyria. Clin Gastroent. 2005;19(2):235–249.
2. Grandchamp B. Acute intermittent porphyria. Semin Liver Dis. 1998;18(1):17–24.
3. Macaline I, Hunter R. The "insanity" of King George 3rd: a classic case of porphyria. BMJ. 1966;1(5479):65–71.
4. Burgovne K, Swartz R, Ananth J. Porphyria: reexamination of the psychiatric implications. Psychother Psychosom. 1995;64(3):121–130.

###

The Diabetic Patient Who also Has Hyperpigmentation of the Skin Might Have Hemochromatosis ("Bronze Diabetes")

The skin hyperpigmentation is due to both melanin and iron deposition. The finding of liver disease, along with diabetes and hyperpigmentation, completes the classic triad of hemochromatosis [1]. Other possible manifestations include lethargy, joint pains, impotence in men, and electrocardiographic abnormalities [2].

Bacon reports that hemochromatosis affects 1 in every 200–400 persons of Northern European descent, making this a not-altogether-rare disease [1].

References

1. Bacon BR. Hemochromatosis: diagnosis and management. Gastroenter. 2001;120(4):718–725.
2. Niederau C, Strohmeyer G, Stremmel W. Epidemiology, clinical spectrum and prognosis of hemochromatosis. Adv Exp Med Biol. 1994;356(3):293–302.

###

Reporting Late to Establish Prenatal Care During a Pregnancy May Be an Alarm Signal Indicating the Presence of Domestic Violence

In a study involving 548 pregnant women who were surveyed regarding physical abuse, 36 (6.6%) described physical abuse during the current pregnancy and 60 (10.9%) before it. Of those abused during the pregnancy, 64% of women reported increased abuse during the pregnancy [1].

In the setting of delayed establishment of prenatal care, look for other markers of spousal abuse: low income, poor education, unmarried status, unemployment, or a history of being abused as a child [2].

References

1. Stewart DE, Cecutti A. Physical abuse in pregnancy. Can Med Assoc J. 1993;149(9):1257–1266.
2. Hegarty K, Gunn J, Chondros P, Small P. Association between depression and abuse by partners of women attending general practice: descriptive, cross sectional survey. BMJ. 2004;328(7440): 621–624.

###

Of All Disease Entities, Cancer Is Especially Likely to Reveal Itself, to Borrow Dr. Trotter's Words, in Casual Parentheses

The list of subtle clues to cancer are many [1]. Here are some of them, all to be considered cancer until proven otherwise, especially in adults and elderly individuals:

- Bright red rectal bleeding
- Hemoptysis in a smoker
- Post-menopausal bleeding
- An upper lobe infiltrate on chest x-ray
- An ulcerated skin lesion that does not heal
- Hematuria found on routine urinalysis
- Sudden gross hematuria
- Unexplained weight loss
- Any breast mass
- Unilateral nipple discharge from the breast
- An enlarged supraclavicular lymph node

Note how often bleeding shows up on this list. Cancer is one of the must-never-miss diagnoses, and we must stay alert to its early hints, often involving the leakage of a few erythrocytes.

Reference

1. Taylor RB. Medical wisdom and doctoring: the art of 21st century practice. New York: Springer. 2010, Chapter 4.

###

Patients Who State that they Are Going to Die Soon Often Do So

This is one of Meador's rules, a collection of wise sayings by experienced physicians [1]. I have been unable to find supporting evidence for the assertion. There have been no long-term clinical trials.

As a family physician with decades of career experience, I have seen this happen. I think we will all witness the self-fulling prophecy of death if we are in practice long enough.

Reference

1. Meador CK. A little book of doctors' rules II. Philadelphia: Hanley & Belfus. 1999;Page 7.

#####

Chapter 9
Therapeutic Insights

There are some patients whom we cannot help;
There are none whom we cannot harm.

American physician Arthur L. Bloomfield (1888–1962) [1]

To introduce this chapter, I selected a case in which we actually helped the patient. Despite all the perils of twenty-first century therapy, we sometimes get things right. Here is one such story.

> Not long ago, following a series of heart attacks, Harvey N, age 75, developed severe heart failure. His symptoms of dyspnea, orthopnea and cough progressed to pretibial edema and liver engorgement. Things became worse following another episode of chest pain, placing him in the coronary care unit of his local community hospital. His doctor was doing her best, including the use of diuretics, ACE inhibitors, vasodilators, as well as salt restriction and oxygen. With what seemed another insult to his myocardium, symptoms became worse. The outlook was grim.
>
> A visiting medical student had an idea, something he had heard about in a lecture. Why not try him on an aldosterone antagonist? Why not?
>
> Harvey's doctor prescribed the drug, and by the next morning there was some improvement. Over the next few days, his edema began to recede and breathing seemed easier. By the end of the week he was ready to go home, supported by his new medication regimen.

In 2009, a group from the Cleveland Clinic reported an observational analysis of 43,625 patients with heart failure admitted to 241 hospitals. They found that of 12,565 patients eligible for aldosterone antagonist therapy, only 4,087 (32.5%) received an aldosterone antagonist at discharge. The use of aldosterone antagonists in hospitals ranges from no use at all to 90.6% use in appropriate cases [2]. What is impressive about less than one-third of eligible patients receiving this useful drug is that all of these patients were enrolled in a guideline-based quality improvement registry.

Knowing the key fact – a novel intervention on the plus side or a little known quirk of therapy that might lead to problems – can make all the difference in treating the next patient you see. In this chapter I tell some insights and warnings in the realm of clinical disease management. I'll begin with some of our more common problems – diabetes, depression and other mental health problems, hypertension, cardiovascular disease, and headache – followed by a selection of situations, such as the sequence in which to administer childhood immunizations, an innovative treatment of lower

R.B. Taylor, *Essential Medical Facts Every Clinician Should Know: To Prevent Medical Errors, Pass Board Examinations and Provide Informed Patient Care*,
DOI 10.1007/978-1-4419-7874-5_9, © Springer Science+Business Media, LLC 2011

urinary tract symptoms, and an little-known risk of primaquine use in malaria prophylaxis, that may improve patient care and prevent clinical missteps.

References

1. Bloomfield AL. Quoted in: Strauss MB. Familiar medical quotations. Boston: Little, Brown; 1968. Page 637.
2. Albert NM, Yancy CW, Liang L, et al. Use of aldosterone antagonists in heart failure. JAMA. 2009;302(15):1658–1685.

###

In the Intensive Care Unit (ICU) Setting, a Target Glucose of 180 mg/dL or Less Yields a Lower Mortality than a Target of 81–108 mg/dL

This is the finding of investigators in the NICE-SUGAR study of 6,104 diabetic patients admitted to the ICU, who were randomized to receive conventional (n = 3,050) versus intensive (n = 3,054) control. In the end, 24.9% of the conventional therapy patients died, compared with 27.5% of the intensive control patients. It is noteworthy that there were 206 instances of severe hypoglycemia (blood glucose of 40 mg/dL or less) in the intensive therapy cohort compared with only 15 such instances in the conventional therapy group [1].

> The findings described above were more-or-less corroborated by a meta-analysis by Griesdale et al., who reviewed 26 trials involving 13,567 patients treated in ICU settings with various targets of insulin therapy. They concluded: "Intensive insulin therapy significantly increased the risk of hypoglycemia and conferred no overall mortality benefit among critically ill patients." They go on, however, to distinguish between medical and surgical ICUs: "However, this therapy may be beneficial to patients admitted to a surgical ICM." Note from the citation below that the Griesdale et al. meta-analysis included the Nice-sugar study with its 6,104 subjects [2].
>
> On a lighter note, I hereby present the Academy Award for the Year's Most Inventive Acronym to the NICE-SUGAR study group. NICE-SUGAR stands for the Normoglycemia in Intensive Care Evaluation (NICE) and Survival Using Glucose Algorithm Regulation (SUGAR) Study. Might this acronym have evolved over a bottle of good wine?
>
> Next I am going to present some other facts about drug therapy of diabetes. As with some other items in this chapter, I might have placed them in Chap. 10 on Drug Effects, but I thought it most helpful to cluster them here.

References

1. Finfer S, Chittock DR, Su SY, et al. Intensive versus conventional glucose control in critically ill patients. N Engl J Med. 2009;360(13):1283–1297.
2. Griesdale DE, de Souza RJ, van Dam RM, et al. Intensive insulin therapy and mortality among critically ill patients: a meta-analysis including the NICE-SUGAR study data. CMAJ. 2009;180(8):821–827.

###

Insulin Use Seems to Increase Mortality Risk

A cohort study of 12,272 type 2 diabetic patients was followed for a mean duration of 5.1 years. During this time, 1,443 (12%) began insulin use and there were 2,681 deaths, with the highest death rate in those with the highest exposure to insulin. The adjusted hazard ratio in the high exposure cohort was 2.79 and in the low exposure group it was 1.75. The investigators reported "a significant and graded association between mortality risk and insulin exposure level."

> Now we clinicians are faced with a dilemma: Given that the risk of death with insulin use is low, shall we share this information with type 2 diabetic patients for whom we are recommending a switch from oral medication to insulin, patients already reluctant to undertake a new regimen involving injections?

Reference

1. Gamble JM, Simpson SH, Eurich DT, et al. Insulin use and increased risk of mortality in type 2 diabetes: a cohort study. Diabetes Obes Metab. 2010;12(1):47–53.

There Are Risks Associated with the Use of Various Oral Antidiabetic Agents

A study of 91,521 diabetic persons in the United Kingdom General Practice Research Database revealed that, when compared to metformin (Glucophage), monotherapy with first or second generation sulfonylureas was associated with a 24–61% excess risk for all cause mortality. In addition, use of second generation sulfonylureas carried an 18–30% excess risk of developing congestive heart failure [1].

Metformin has been used for more than four decades; the drug, however, is not without issues.

Best known is lactic acidosis, occurring in 0.3 instances per 1,000 patient-years of use, and chiefly occurring in persons with decreased renal function. Howlett and Bailey state: "Serious adverse events with metformin are predictable rather than spontaneous and are potentially preventable if the prescribing guidelines are respected." These guidelines include contraindications to use of metformin in heart failure, hypoxic states, and advanced liver disease [2].

One curious effect of metformin use in type 2 diabetic patients is lowering of thyrotropin (TSH) in those who also have hypothyroidism. Capelli et al. studied diabetic patients with hypothyroidism and compared them to euthyroid diabetic patients. All were treated with metformin. One year later a significant drop in TSH was noted in hypothyroid patients, whether of not they were receiving treatment with levothyroxine. There was no TSH change in the euthyroid group, and no significant alteration in free T4 was observed in any group [3].

Then there is exenatide (Byetta), originally isolated from the salivary secretions of the lizard *Heloderma suspectum* (Gila monster). A U.S. Food and Drug Administration (FDA) Alert cautions that an association between the drug and acute pancreatitis is suspected and "Healthcare professionals should instruct patients taking Byetta to seek prompt medical care if they experience unexplained persistent severe abdominal pain which may or may not be accompanied by vomiting" [4].

When added to glucose-lowering monotherapy with metformin or a sulfonylurea in persons with type 2 diabetes, rosiglitazone increased the risk of heart failure and also of upper and distal lower limb fractures, especially in women [5].

On the plus side, Tzoulaki et al. found that, compared with metformin, pioglitazone was associated with a significant 31–39% lower risk of all cause mortality [1].

References

1. Tzoulaki I, Molokhia M, Curcin V, et al. Risk of cardiovascular disease and all cause mortality among patients with type 2 diabetes prescribed oral antidiabetic drugs: retrospective cohort study using UK general practice research base. BMJ. 2009;339:b4731.
2. Howlett HCS, Bailey CJ. A risk-benefit assessment of metformin in type 2 diabetes mellitus. Drug Saf. 1999;20(6):489–503.
3. Capelli C, Rotondi M, Pirola I, et al. TSH-lowering effect of metformin in type 2 diabetic patients: difference between euthyroid, untreated hypothyroid, and euthyroid on L-T4 therapy patients. Diabetes Care. 2009;32(9):1589–1590.
4. FDA Alert: Exenatide (marketed as Byetta). Available at: http://www.fda.gov/Drugs/DrugSafety/PostmarketDrugSafetyInformationforPatientsandProviders/ucm111085.htm. Accessed August 26, 2009.
5. Home PD, Pocock SJ, Beck-Nielsen H, et al. Rosiglitazone evaluated for cardiovascular outcomes in oral agent combination therapy for type 2 diabetes (RECORD): a multicenter, randomized, open-label trial. Lancet. 2009;373(9681):2125–2135.

###

In China, Metformin Has Been Prescribed for Antipsychotic-Induced Weight Gain

Metformin has been prescribed, along with lifestyle modifications, to promote weight loss in patients who gain more than 10% of their pretreatment body weight while taking antipsychotic medications [1].

This innovative use of metformin is intriguing, but are we ready for the chain reaction that could occur as we use one drug to treat the side effects of another?

Reference

1. Wu RR, Zhao JP, Jin H et al. Lifestyle intervention and metformin for treatment of antipsychotic-induced weight gain: a randomized controlled trial. JAMA 2008;299:185–193.

###

Treating Periodontal Disease Can Improve Glycemic Control in Type 2 Diabetic Patients

The evidence for this statement comes from a systematic review and meta-analysis of 5 studies involving 371 patients. The improvement in diabetic control following periodontal treatment lasted for 3 months or more [1].

Although not necessarily inexpensive, treating periodontal disease in diabetic patients contributes both to oral health and improved glycemic control, without the risk of drug side effects.

Reference

1. Teeuw WJ, Gerdes VI, Loos BG. Effect of periodontal treatment on glycemic control of diabetic patients: a systematic review and meta-analysis. Diabetes Care. 2010;33(2):421–427.

###

When Initiating Treatment for the Acute Phase of Major Depression, Sertraline (Zoloft) May Be the Best Choice

To assess the relative efficacy of a variety of antidepressant medications used to treat the acute phase of major depression, Cipriani et al. reviewed 59 studies involving multiple treatment comparisons between sertraline and other antidepressant agents. These authors found "a trend in favor of sertraline over other antidepressive agents both in terms of efficacy and acceptability, using 95% confidence intervals and a conservative approach, with a random effects analysis" [1].

*Recall from Chap. 2 that in the case of mild to moderate depression, the effect of antidepressant medication may minimal or non-existent. This is in contrast to very severe depression, a condition in which, according to Fournier et al., "... the benefit of medication over placebo is substantial" [2]. In this latter setting, sertraline may be the preferred agent. The drug has another advantage in being available in generic form. Could this be a **practice changer?***

References

1. Cipriani A, La Ferla T, Furukawa TA, et al. Sertraline versus other antidepressive agents for depression. Cochrane Database Syst Rev. 2010;Jan 20(1):CD006117.
2. Fournier JC, DeRubeis RJ, Hollon SD, et al. Antidepressant drug effects and depression severity. JAMA. 2010;303(1):47–53.

###

Selective Serotonin Reuptake Inhibitor (SSRI) Use Can Be Associated with Upper Gastrointestinal Bleeding (UGB)

A study conducted in Denmark involving 3,652 persons with UGB over an 11 year period revealed that the adjusted odds ratio of UGB among current, recent and past users of SSRI drugs was 1.67, 1.88, and 1.22, respectively. The occurrence of upper gastrointestinal bleeding was described as consistent with the antiplatelet effects of SSRIs [1].

> *The clinical implication is that these drugs may not be ideal choices in persons at risk of gastrointestinal bleeding. Yet, is there the possibility of some clinical utility for some patients in their antiplatelet effects?*

Reference

1. Dall M, Schaffalitzky de Muckadell OB, Lassen AT, Hansen JM, Hallas J. An association between selective serotonin reuptake inhibitor use and serious upper gastrointestinal bleeding. Clin Gastroenterol Hepatol. 2009;7(12):1314–1321.

The Use of SSRIs in Pregnancy May Adversely Affect Pregnancy Outcomes

A Danish study compared the pregnancy outcomes of 329 pregnant women treated with SSRIs with the outcomes of much larger numbers of women who had a history of psychiatric illness but took no SSRIs and another group with no history of psychiatric illness. The found that the use of SSRIs during pregnancy was associated with a greater risk of preterm delivery, a lower 5-min Apgar scores, and an increased likelihood of admission to the neonatal intensive care unit, which was not explained by lower Apgar scores or gestational age [1].

> *Add SSRIs to the list of drugs to be used with caution in women of child-bearing age.*

Reference

1. Lund N, Pedersen LH, Henriksen TB. Selective serotonin reuptake inhibitor exposure in utero and pregnancy outcomes. Arch Pediatr Adolesc Med. 2009;163(10):949–954.

###

SSRIs Increase the Risk of Hemorrhagic and Fatal Stoke in Postmenopausal Women

But the absolute event risks are low. A study of 136,293 community-dwelling, postmenopausal women in the Women's Health Initiative revealed that SSRI use was associated with incident hemorrhagic stroke (hazard ratio, 2.12) and fatal stroke (hazard ratio, 2.10) [1].

These are not great risks when considered in aggregate, but the incidence is 100% in the woman who suffers a cerebrovascular accident.

Reference

1. Smoller JW, Allison M, Cochrane BB, et al. Antidepressant use and risk of incident cardiovascular morbidity and mortality among postmenopausal women in the Women's Health Initiative study. Arch Intern Med. 2009;169(22):2128–2139.

###

The Risk of Suicidality in Patients Taking Antidepressants Varies with Age

The study was a meta-analysis of data involving 99,231 adults enrolled in 372 randomized clinical trials submitted to the U.S. Food and Drug Administration. In patients for whom antidepressants were prescribed for psychiatric reasons – major depression, other depression, or other psychiatric disorders – the risk of suicidality declined with age. "When age was modeled as a continuous variable, the odds ratio for suicidal behavior or ideation declined at a rate of 2.6% per year of age and the odds ratio for suicidal behaviour declined at a rate of 4.6% per year of age." The authors propose that the use of antidepressants in the patient groups described is neutral for suicidal behavior and possibly protective for suicidal ideation in adults age 25–64 years of age, and that the drugs reduce the risk of suicidality and suicide behavior in patients age 65 and older [1].

The U.S. Food and Drug Administration has issued a boxed warning concerning increased suicidal ideation and behavior associated with antidepressant drug treatment in children and adolescents [2]. The Stone et al. study described here helps clarify the effect of these drugs when used in depressed adults.

References

1. Stone M, Laughren T, Jones ML, et al. Risk of suicidality in clinical trials of antidepressants in adults: analysis of proprietary data submitted to U.S. Food and Drug Administration. BMJ. 2009;339:b3066.
2. Olfson M, Marcus SC, Shaffer D. Antidepressant drug therapy and suicide in severely depressed children and adults. Arch Gen Psychiatry. 2006;63(8):865–872.

###

Testosterone Therapy May Help Relieve Depression in Hypogonadal Older Men with Subthreshold Depression

This report describes a randomized, double-blind, placebo-controlled trial involving 33 older men with low testosterone levels and dysthymia or minor depression. Subjects received 7.5 g of testosterone gel or placebo gel daily for 12 weeks. Then for the next 12 weeks both groups received the testosterone gel. Outcome measures were scores on the Hamilton Rating Scale for Depression and remission of subthreshold depression. At the end of the first 12 weeks, the testosterone gel patients had a greater reduction in the Hamilton Rating Scale score and a higher remission rate of subthreshold depression. At the end of the second phase, in which all received the testosterone gel, the testosterone group had sustained improvement and the control group improved [1].

> *If testosterone were to be used for long-term therapy of mild depression, the risks must be considered. An Endocrine Society Clinical Practice Guideline recommends against starting testosterone therapy in patients with breast or prostate cancer, a palpable prostate nodule or induration or prostate-specific antigen greater than 3 ng/mL without further urological evaluation, erythrocytosis (hematocrit >50%), hyperviscosity, untreated obstructive sleep apnea, severe lower urinary tract symptoms with International Prostate Symptom Score (IPSS) greater than 19, or class III or IV heart failure [2].*

References

1. Shores MM, Kivlahan DR, Sadak TI, Li EJ, Matsumoto AM. A randomized, double-blind, placebo-controlled study of testosterone treatment of hypogonadal older men with subthreshold depression (dysthymia or minor depression). Clin Psychiatry. 2009;70(7):1009–1016.
2. Bhasin S, Cunningham GR. Hayes FJ, et al. Testosterone therapy in adult men with androgen deficiency syndromes: an endocrine society clinical practice guideline. J Clin Endocrinol Metab. 2006; 91(6):1995–2010.

###

The Initiation of Antipsychotic Drug Treatment in Older Diabetic Persons Is Associated with an Increased Risk of Hospitalization for Hyperglycemia

The above statement is the conclusion of a study of 13,817 diabetic persons age 66 or older who began use of antipsychotic medication. Of these patients, 1,515 (11%) were admitted to the hospital for hyperglycemia. It made no difference whether the diabetes was treated with insulin, oral agent or no pharmacologic therapy [1]. The risk of hyperglycemia was noted with both typical and atypical antipsychotic agents, and was especially high with the initial course of treatment.

Here I wonder if we are seeing some sort of metabolic effect, or if the high incidence of hyperglycemia with initial/current antipsychotic use is somehow related to a mood change induced by the drug.

Reference

1. Lipscombe LL, Levesque L, Gruneir A, et al. Antipsychotic drugs and hyperglycemia in older patients with diabetes. Arch Intern Med. 2009;169(14):1282–1289.

###

Initial Treatment of Children and Adolescents with Second Generation Antipsychotic Medications Is Associated with Weight Gain

Correll et al. studied 205 patients age 4–19 years who received one of four second generation antipsychotic drugs (aripiprazole, olanzapine, quetiapine, or risperidone) for a variety of mental health problems. At the end of a median of 10.8 weeks, patients in all four drug groups gained weight. The greatest was in the olanzapine group, 8.5 kg. The least was in the aripiprazole group, 4.4 kg. The control group taking no antipsychotic drugs gained a meagre 0.2 kg [1].

Are we seeing a metabolic drug effect or an increased appetite owing to a mood change?

Reference

1. Correll CU, Manu P, Olshanskiy V, Napolitano B, Kane JM, Malhotra AK. Cardiometabolic risk of second-generation antipsychotic medications during first-time use in children and adolescents. JAMA. 2009;302(16):1765–1773.

###

Patients with Alzheimer Disease Taking Antipsychotic Medications Are at Increased Risk of Death

The evidence is a randomized, placebo-controlled, parallel, two-group treatment discontinuation trial involving 165 Alzheimer disease patients taking antipsychotic medication. Half continued to take their medication; half were changed to oral placebo use. Over the following 12 months, the cumulative probability of survival in the treatment group was 70% compared with 77% in the placebo group [1].

> *This is an unusual study design – subtracting rather that adding a variable (the drug). All subjects were taking antipsychotics at the beginning of the study, and then half were switched to placebo. I find the study to be very well designed.*

Reference

1. Ballard C, Hanney ML, Theodoulou M, et al. The dementia antipsychotic withdrawal trial (DART-AD): long-term follow-up of a randomized placebo-controlled trial. Lancet Neurol. 2009;8(2):151–157.

###

Long-Chain Omega-3 Fatty Acids May Help Prevent the Onset of Psychotic Disorders

Amminger et al. describe a study involving adolescent and young patients in a large public hospital in Vienna. Subjects received omega-3 polyunsaturated fatty acids or placebo for 12 weeks and were followed for 40 weeks. Of 81 enrollees, 76 (93.8%) completed the trial. Of these subjects, 2 of 41 in the omega-3 group progressed to psychosis, compared with 11 of 40 in the placebo group.

> *Given the benign nature of omega-3 fatty acid use, the addition of these products to whatever other therapy is employed in young persons at high risk of transition to psychosis seems reasonable.*

Reference

1. Amminger GP, Schafer MR, Papageorgiou K, et al. Long-chain omega-3 fatty acids for indicated prevention of psychotic disorders: a randomized, placebo-controlled trial. Arch Gen Psychiatry. 2010;67(2):146–154.

###

When It Comes to Preventing Coronary Heart Disease (CHD) Events and Stroke, There Is Little Difference Among the Various Classes of Blood Pressure (BP) Lowering Drugs

Yes, there is the extra protective effect of beta blockers when given following a myocardial infarction, and calcium channel blockers may have a slight edge in stroke prevention. Otherwise, according to the conclusions of a meta-analysis of 147 randomized clinical trials, all the classes of antihypertensive medicines have a similar effect in reducing CHD events and stroke for a given reduction in blood pressure [1].

Nor does age seem to matter much. A meta-analysis by Turnbull et al. looked at relative risk reduction by age afforded by various categories of antihypertensive agents. After reviewing 31 trials involving 190,606 subjects, they reported, "The meta-analysis showed no clear difference between age groups in the effects of lowering blood pressure or any difference between the effects of the drug classes on major cardiovascular events" [2].

It seems that although there are benefits, at all ages, from lowering high blood pressure levels, no single class of drugs can claim clear superiority. Read on to see what might just be a good choice, and what might not, and also to read about a study that is not so sure about the benefits of one of the drug classes.

References

1. Law MR, Morris JK, Wald NJ. Use of blood pressure lowering drugs in the prevention of cardiovascular disease: meta-analysis of 147 randomized trials in the context of expectations from prospective epidemiologic studies. BMJ. 2009;338:b1665.
2. Turnbull F, Neal B, Ninomiya T, et al. Effects of different regimens to lower blood pressure on major cardiovascular events in older and younger adults: meta-analysis of randomized trials. BMJ. 2008;336(7653):1121–1123.

In the Initial Treatment of High Blood Pressure, Low Dose Thiazides Seem to Be a Good Default Choice

A Cochrane Database review of 24 trials including 58,040 patients led to the following conclusion: "First-line low-dose thiazides reduce all morbidity and mortality outcomes. First-line ACE inhibitors and calcium channel blockers may be similarly effective but the evidence is less robust. First-line high-dose thiazides and first-line beta blockers are inferior to first-line low-dose thiazides" [1].

Going ever further as far as beta-blockers are concerned, and challenging the belief that all antihypertensive drug classes are of more or less equal benefit, another Cochrane Database review of 13 randomized trials with 91,561 participants failed to support the use of beta-blockers as first-line drugs. Wiysonge et al. cite relatively weak effect of beta-blockers to reduce stroke, their absence of an effect on coronary heart disease when compared to placebo or no treatment and their trend toward worse outcomes when compared with other classes of agents, including thiazide diuretics [2]. In yet another large Cochrane Database review, Kahn and McAlister conclude that while beta-blockers should not be first-line therapy for older patients in the absence of another indication for their use, the drugs offer "a significant reduction in cardiovascular morbidity and mortality" when used by younger patients [3].

Of course, cost is always a factor, and thiazide diuretics are likely to be the least expensive option–among the drugs, at least. This might be a good time to reflect that, as Lindsay wrote in the 1920s, "The treatment of high blood pressure is a regimen, not a drug" [4].

References

1. Wright JM, Musini VM. First-line drugs for hypertension. Cochrane Database Syst Rev. 2009;July 8(3):CD001841.
2. Wiysonge CS, Bradley H, Mayosi BM, et al. Beta-blockers for hypertension. Cochrane Database Syst Rev. 2007;Jan 24(1):CD002003.
3. Kahn N, McAlister FA. Re-examining the efficacy of beta-blockers for the treatment of hypertension: a meta-analysis. CMAJ. 2006;174(12):1737–1742.
4. Lindsay JA. Medical axioms, aphorisms and clinical memoranda. London: H.K. Lewis Co.; 1923. Page 86.

###

Combination Therapy Yields Greater Decrement in Blood Pressure when Compared with Increasing the Dose of a Single Drug Used to Treat Hypertension

In a review of 42 trials involving 10,968 subjects, Wald et al. studied the incremental effects of combining antihypertensive medications from any two drug classes (thiazides, beta-blockers, angiotensin-converting enzyme inhibitors (ACEI), and calcium channel blockers) compared with doubling the dose of a single drug. They conclude, "The extra blood pressure reduction from combining drugs from 2 different classes is approximately 5 times greater than doubling the dose of 1 drug" [1].

*Granted, adding a second antihypertensive medication increases complexity, brings a second panorama of side effects, and will probably increase treatment cost. Nevertheless, based on this study, the additional drug may often be the best answer. For some, this will be a **practice changer**.*

Reference

1. Wald DS, Law M, Morris JK, Bestwick JP, Wald NJ. Combination therapy versus monother-apy in reducing blood pressure: meta-analysis on 11,000 participants from 42 trials. Am J Med. 2009;122(3):290–300.

###

Treating Patients to Lower than Standard Blood Pressure Targets, ≤140–160/90–100 mmHg, Does Not Reduce Mortality or Morbidity

The above is a direct quotation from the Authors' Conclusions of a review of 7 trials involving 22,089 participants [1]. A report in Lancet, however, described a randomized open-label trial of 1,111 non-diabetic patients assigned to target systolic BP control of 140 mmHg (n = 553) or 130 mmHg (n = 558). The primary end point was the rate of electrocardiographic left ventricular hypertrophy at the end of 2 years. The primary end point occurred in 17.0% of patients in the 140 mmHg target group compared with only 11.4% of those in the 130 mmHg target cohort. A composite cardiovascular endpoint also favored the tighter control group. The authors believe, "Our findings lend support to a lower blood pressure goal than is recommended at present in non-diabetic patients with hypertension" [2].

Let's think. The study finding that lower BP targets do not afford desired morbidity and mortality outcomes is a Cochrane Database review involving more than 22,000 patients. The other study, published in Lancet, advocating a lower BP target includes 1,111 subjects, and is funded by three pharmaceutical companies that market antihypertensive medications. Which study should I rely upon to make practice decisions?

References

1. Arguedas JA, Perez MI, Wright JM. Treatment blood pressure targets for hypertension. Cochrane Database Syst Rev. 2009;Jul 8(3):CD004349.
2. Verdecchia P, Staessen JA, Anteli F, et al. Usual versus tight control of systolic blood pressure in non-diabetic patients with hypertension (Cardio-Sis): an open-label randomized trial. Lancet. 2009;374(9689):525–533.

###

The Patient with Severe but Asymptomatic Hypertension May Not Need Rapid Lowering of Blood Pressure

Severely elevated blood pressure (systolic BP of 180 mm Hg or greater or diastolic BP of 110 mm Hg or greater) usually develops gradually over days to weeks [1]. In the absence of manifestations of end-organ damage, such patients generally do not require urgent blood pressure reduction. Such efforts can be dangerous, resulting in hypotension and hypoperfusion of vital organs, including the brain [2].

Part of the approach will depend on the cardiovascular risk profile. Even in that absence of demonstrable end-organ damage, severe asymptomatic hypertension combined with an alarming cardiovascular risk profile calls for more aggressive therapy than would be indicated in a person without noteworthy cardiovascular risk factors.

References

1. Kessler C, Youdeh Y. Evaluation and treatment of severe asymptomatic hypertension. Am Fam Physician. 2010;81(4):470–476.
2. Decker WW, Godwin SA, Hess EP, Lenamond CC, Jagoda AS, for the American College of Emergency Physicians Clinical Policies Subcommittee (Writing Committee) on Asymptomatic Hypertension in the ED. Clinical policy: critical issues in the evaluation and management of adult patients with asymptomatic hypertension in the emergency department. Ann Emerg Med. 2006;47(3):237–249.

###

Beta-Blocked Patients Tolerate Surgical Anemia Less Well Than Those Who Have Not Received Beta Blockers

In a study of 1,153 patients who received beta blockers within the first 24 h post-operatively matched with beta-blocker naïve patients, major adverse cardiac events occurred in 6.5% of beta blocked patients but in only 0.3% of those not given beta blockers. The key is that this difference was noted only in patients whose hemoglobin decrease exceeded 35% of baseline value [1].

It seems that severe, surgically-induced anemia trumps the cardioprotective effects of beta-blockade.

Reference

1. Beattie WS, Wijeysundera DN, Karkouti K, et al. Acute surgical anemia influences the cardioprotective effects of beta-blockade: a single-center, propensity-matched cohort study. Anesthesiology. 2010;112(1):25–33.

###

In Patients with Atrial Fibrillation (AF) and Heart Failure (HF), Rhythm Control Is Not Superior to Rate Control

In treating patients with atrial fibrillation and congestive heart failure, controlling rhythm (to maintain sinus rhythm) does not yield better clinical outcomes than rate control, making the simpler rate control the treatment of choice in these patients [1]. This is the outcome of a study of 1,376 patients with a left ventricular ejection fraction of 35% or less, heart failure symptoms and a history of AF. Patients were randomized to two more or less equal groups. One group received therapy aimed at rhythm control; the other group was treated with drugs aimed to control heart rate. After 37 months the deaths due to CV disease were as follows: 27% in the rhythm control group and 25% in the rate control group.

> There was no advantage demonstrated for attempts at rhythm control. This is a clinically relevant study, given that patients with heart failure are at increased risk for atrial fibrillation, and that AF is considered a predictor of death in HF patients [1].

Reference

1. Roy D, Talajic M, Nattel S, et al. Rhythm control versus rate control for atrial fibrillation and heart failure. N Engl J Med 2008; 358:2667–2777.

###

Lenient Rate Control in Patients with Atrial Fibrillation Is as Effective as Strict Rate Control

In a study of patients with atrial fibrillation randomly assigned to receive lenient rate control (resting heart rate < 110 beats per minute) versus strict rate control (resting heart rate < 80 beats per minute and heart rate during moderate exercise < 110 beats per minute), the authors followed patients for 2–3 years, looking for death from cardiovascular causes, hospitalization for heart failure, and stroke, systemic embolism, bleeding and life-threatening arrhythmic events. They conclude: "In patients with permanent atrial fibrillation, lenient heart rate control is as effective as strict rate control and is easier to achieve" [1].

> Lenient rate control would also seem to be less fraught with unwanted drug effects. Yet the authors report, "The frequencies of symptoms and adverse events were similar in the two groups" [1].

Reference

1. Van Gelder I, Groenveld HF, Crijns HJG, et al. Lenient versus strict rate control in patients with atrial fibrillation. N Engl J Med. 2010;362(15):1363–1373.

###

In a Patient with Acute Cardioembolic Stroke, Anticoagulation Therapy May Not Be the Best Choice

A meta-analysis of 7 studies, involving 4,624 patients with acute cardioembolic stroke led the authors to conclude: "Our findings indicate that in patients with acute cardioembolic stroke, early anticoagulation is associated with a nonsignificant reduction in recurrence of ischemic stroke, no substantial reduction in death and disability, and an increased intracranial bleeding" [1].

> *As we consider this finding in the context of the previous fact about AF and HF, it is interesting to note that in the study by Paciaroni et al., 82% (n = 3,797) of patients had atrial fibrillation [1].*

Reference

1. Paciaroni M, Agnelli G, Micheli S, Caso V. Efficacy and safety of anticoagulant treatment in acute cardioembolic stroke: a meta-analysis of randomized controlled trials. Stroke. 2007;38(2):423–430.

###

The HMG-CoA Reductase Inhibitors (Statins) Have Diverse and Generally Beneficial Effects, Actions That Involve More than Reduction in Lipid Levels

In patients with heart failure, statin drugs improve left ventricular ejection fraction (LVEF) and decrease hospitalization for worsening HF. This is the conclusion of a meta-analysis of 10 studies, with 10,192 participants taking a variety of statin drugs versus placebo. There were some differences among the statins; for example simvastatin (Zocor) was more likely than rosuvastatin (Crestor) to cause improvement in LVEF [1].

A case-control analysis using the UK-based General Practice Research Database reviewed the records of 27,035 patients who had had cholecystectomy, including 2,396 who had used statin drugs. These were matched with 106,531controls of whom 8,868 had used statins. The authors of the report found, "Longterm use of statins was associated with a decreased risk of gallstones followed by cholecystectomy" [2].

A report of a meta-analysis published in the American Journal of Medicine describes a review of 65 trials with 200,607 patients. The investigators state: "This meta-analysis suggests that statins reduce the incidence of stroke in patients with and without coronary heart disease" [3].

From my own institution here in Portland, Oregon comes a case-control study of 100 prostate cancer patients compared with age-matched prostate-specific antigen-normal controls. The investigators found that statin use was associated with a significant reduction in prostate cancer risk (odds ratio = 0.38). Curiously, the inverse relationship to statin use was seen only in men with more aggressive cancers, that is, with Gleason scores of 7 or greater. The authors suggest that "statins may reduce the risk of total prostate cancer and, specifically, more aggressive prostate cancer" [4].

A major cause of perioperative morbidity and mortality is cardiovascular complications. According to Durazzo et al., statin therapy given perioperatively, whether or not the patient has hypercholesterolemia, may help reduce cardiac events. The mechanism seems to be through stabilization of coronary artery plaques [5]. Schouten et al. report similar favorable results with fluvastatin in patients undergoing vascular surgery [6]. Studies such as this lead Brookes et al. to wonder if statins should not become routine preoperative medications for all. They cite statins' "beneficial effects beyond those of lipid-lowering, including reducing the perioperative risk of cardiac complications and sepsis" [7].

At this point, one might wonder: Why stop at prescribing statins just for surgery patients? Why not statins for all adults? Why not statins for children? Why not just put them in the drinking water, like we do fluoride? Well, there are some adverse effects to consider. Read on.

References

1. Lipinski MJ, Cauthren CA, Biondi-Zoccai GG, et al. Meta-analysis of randomized controlled trials versus placebo in patients with heart failure. Am J Cardiol. 2009; 104(12):1708–1716.
2. Bodmer M, Brauchli YB, Krähenbühl S, Jick SS, Meier CR. Statin use and risk of gallstone disease followed by cholecystectomy. JAMA. 2009;302(18):2001–2007.
3. Briel M, Studer M, Glass TR, Bucher HC. Effects of statins on stroke prevention in patients with and without coronary heart disease: a meta-analysis of randomized controlled trials. Am J Med. 2004;117(8):596–606.
4. Shannon J, Tewoderos S, Garzotto M, et al. Statins and prostate cancer risk: a case-control study. Am J Epidemiol. 2005;162(4):318–325.
5. Durazzo AE, Machado FS, Ikeoka DT, et al. Reduction in cardiovascular events after vascular surgery with atorvastatin: a randomized trial. J Vasc Surg. 2004;39(5):967–976.
6. Schouten O, Boersma E, Hoeks SE, et al. Fluvastatin and perioperative events in patients undergoing vascular surgery. N Engl J Med. 2009;361(10):980–989.
7. Brookes ZL, McGown CC, Reilly CS. Statins for all: the new premed? Br J Anaesth. 2009;103(1):99–107.

###

There Are Some Adverse Effects That Can Occur with Use of Statins

Granted, the spectre of liver toxicity once feared during the early years of statin use has not turned out to be much of a problem. Low to moderate dose statin use is not associated with a significant risk of liver function test abnormalities [1]. Furthermore, a study of patients with elevated baseline liver enzymes suggested that these individuals do not have a higher risk of hepatotoxicity from statins [2].

Rhabdomyolysis, however, continues to be a life-threatening but mercifully uncommon adverse effect [3]. Lenz suggests that physically active persons taking statins might be at increased risk for myopathy, citing a study of professional athletes with familial hypercholesterolemia in which 16 of 22 persons could not tolerate statin drugs [4].

A possibility to be watched is documented in a report from Duke University Medical Center, reporting 60 instances of memory loss associated with statin use. Various statin drugs were identified and the adverse cognitive effect began within the first 2 months of therapy in half of all instances [5].

Sattar et al. reviewed 13 randomized statin trials involving 91,140 subjects. They found statin therapy associated with a 9% increased risk of diabetes, with the greatest risk, not unexpectedly, in older subjects. Stated in another way, there will be 1 additional case of diabetes for every 255 patients taking statin drugs for 4 years. The authors consider the risk low when compared with the reduction in coronary events afforded by the use of statin drugs [6].

Persons intolerant to statins have another option. Becker et al. studied the action of red yeast rice on low density lipoprotein (LDL) levels. Patient with dyslipidemia who had discontinued statins were randomized to a group (n = 31) who received 1,800 mg of red yeast rice twice daily or a similar-appearing placebo (n = 31) for 24 weeks. All subjects also participated in a lifestyle change program. LDL levels were significantly lower in the red yeast rice group when measured at 12 and 24 weeks, with no difference in liver enzymes, creatine phosphokinase or pain levels between groups [7].

All things considered, the benefits of statin therapy for appropriate clinical indications seem to outweigh the risks cited. Yet patients should be warned about symptoms of myopathy and perhaps to be alert for the admittedly-rare cognitive effects.

References

1. de Denus S, Spinler SA, Miller K, Peterson AM. Statins and liver toxicity: a meta-analysis. Pharmacotherapy. 2004;24(5):584–591.
2. Chalasani N, Aljadhey H, Kesterson J, Murray MD, Hall SD. Patients with elevated liver enzymes are not at higher risk for statin hepatotoxicity. Gastroenterology. 2004;126(5):1287–1292.
3. Schreiber DH, Anderson TR. Statin-induced rhabdomyolysis. J Emerg Med. 2006;31(2): 177–180.
4. Lenz TL. Are physically active individuals taking statins at increased risk for myopathy? Am J Lifestyle Med. 2009;3(4):287–289.
5. Wagstaff LR, Mitton MW, Arvik BM, Doraiswamy PM. Statin-associated memory loss: analysis of 60 case reports and review of the literature. Pharmacotherapy. 2003;23(7):871–880.

6. Sattar N, Preiss D, Murray HM, et al. Statins and risk of incident diabetes: a collaborative meta-analysis of randomized statin trials. Lancet. 2010;375(9716):735–742.
7. Becker DJ, Gordon RY, Halbert SC, French B, Morris PB, Rader DJ. Red yeast rice for dyslipidemia in statin-intolerant patients. Ann Intern Med. 2009;150(12):830–839.

###

Triptan Medications Should Not Be Used in Complicated Migraine Headaches, Such as Hemiplegic or Basilar Migraine

When introduced in 1991, sumatriptan (Imitrex) was the first of the 5-hydroxytriptamine agonists or triptans. The new drug class represented a giant step forward in the treatment of migraine headaches, which affect some 18% of US women and 6% of men during their lifetimes. Triptan drugs are widely prescribed, reasonably effective, and generally safe. (One safety concern is the risk of serotonin syndrome, described in Chap. 11.) When considering the use of triptans in migraine, however, there is one important caveat. They should not be used in patients with basilar migraine and hemiplegic migraine. Both of these "complicated" migraine syndromes have features consistent with vasospasm (Note my careful use of words), although not all agree, as described shortly. If cerebral vasospasm is present, it seems illogical and risky to give a drug that is fundamentally a vasoconstrictor. Perhaps the best reason for this prohibition is that there is a contraindication warning in bold type against such use in the *Physicians' Desk Reference* (PDR), and hence a prescription in this setting would be dangerously "off-label" [1].

This prohibition is not without its detractors, one of whom cites "the absence of any data convicting basilar-type migraine as a vasospastic condition" [2]. And a group in Finland, based on a series of 76 subjects who each used triptans for one or more familial or sporadic hemiplegic migraine attacks without suffering an ischemic stroke or heart attack, concluded, "Triptans seem to be safe and effective treatment for most hemiplegic migraine patients" [3].

Despite the occasional paper advocating such use, I continue to rely on my reference sources and my own clinical logic in avoiding triptan use in patients with basilar and hemiplegic migraine.

References

1. Physicians' Desk Reference, 2009, page 1476.
2. Kaniecki RG. Basilar-type migraine. Curr Pain Headache Rep 2009; 13(3):217–220.
3. Artto V, Nissilä M, Wessman M, et al. Treatment of hemiplegic migraine with triptans. Eur J Neurol 2007; 14(9):1053–1056.

###

High-Flow Oxygen May Be Useful in Treating Cluster Headache

Cluster headache, an uncommon headache syndrome affecting more men than women, can be very hard to control. Cohen et al. randomized 109 cluster headache patients to receive oxygen (inhaled O2 at 100%, 12 L/min) or high-flow air placebo. The end point was becoming pain free (a remarkable outcome to those of us familiar with cluster headache) or at least to have adequate relief in 15 min. Of the oxygen group, relief was attained by 78%, compared to 20% for the air/placebo group [1].

> *Physiologically, oxygen is a non-specific cerebral vasoconstrictor, which probably explains its effect on the vascular headache. Also significant is the fact that the study intervention – inhaled oxygen – caused no adverse effects [1]. Few drugs can make this claim.*

Reference

1. Cohen AS, Burns B, Goadsby PJ. High-flow oxygen for treatment of cluster headache: a randomized trial. JAMA. 2009;302(22):2451–2457.

###

Varenicline Can Cause Potentially Dangerous Psychiatric Symptoms

Varenicline (Chantrix), widely use for smoking cessation, can cause syncope and psychiatric side effects [1]. In the fourth quarter of 2007, the drug accounted for more reported serious injuries than any other prescription drug, prompting a February, 2008 FDA Public Health Alert about varenicline-induced psychiatric side effects [2].

In May 2008, the Institute for Safe Medical Practices (ISMP) published a Strong Safety Signal that read, "We have immediate safety concerns about the use of varenicline among persons operating aircraft, trains, buses and other vehicles, or in other settings where a lapse in alertness or motor control could lead to massive, serious injury. Other examples include persons operating nuclear power reactors, high-rise construction cranes or life-sustaining medical devices. Based on reports of sudden loss of consciousness, seizures, muscle spasms, vision disturbances, hallucinations, paranoia and psychosis, we believe varenicline may not be safe to use in these settings. The extent to which varenicline has already contributed to accidental death and injury has not yet been investigated because these adverse effects had not been previously reported. The Federal Aviation Administration approved varenicline for use by airline pilots before most of these reports were available" [3]. Following this report, the Federal Aviation Administration issued a statement that actively employed airline pilots and air traffic controllers could no longer receive varenicline therapy [4].

*The psychiatric manifestations seem to go far beyond the effects of nicotine withdrawal. You may consider this a **practice changer** in that full disclosure would seem to mandate that patients for whom we prescribe varenicline be warned of the dangers of driving while taking the drug.*

That said, consider the statistics: The ISMP report describes 227 reports of suicide acts, thoughts or behaviors, 397 cases of possible psychosis, and 525 reports of hostility or aggression; among these, there are 41 mentions of homicidal actions [3]. Now consider that the next time you are in your car, the driver in an approaching vehicle might be a recovering smoker taking varenicline.

There may be one bright spot, however. Patterson et al. conducted a double-blind within-subject crossover study of 67 smokers who received varenicline therapy. While taking varenicline, compared with placebo, subjects described significantly greater positive affect, sustained attention, and working memory [5].

References

1. Pumariega AJ, Nelson R, Rotenberg L. Varenicline-induced mixed mood and psychotic episode in a patient with a past history of depression. CNS Spectr 2008;13(6):511–514.
2. Pharmacology Watch. December, 2008. Page 2.
3. Moore TJ, Cohen MR, Furberg CD. Strong safety signal seen for new varenicline risks. The Institute for Safe Medication Practices. Published May 21, 2008. Available at: http://www.ismp.org/docs/vareniclineStudy.asp/ Accessed March 12, 2010.
4. McIntyre RS. Varenicline and suicidality: a new era in medication safety surveillance. Expert Opin Drug Saf. 2008;7(5):511–514.
5. Patterson F, Jepson C, Strasser A, et al. Varenicline improves mood and cognition during smoking abstinence. Biol Psychiatry. 2009;65(2):144–149.

###

A Mother's Antiepileptic Therapy During Pregnancy Risks Impaired Cognitive Function in the Child

According to a study reported in 2009, there is an increased risk of impaired cognitive function at age 3 years in infants exposed in utero to valproate (Depakote). The degree of impairment was dose related. Similar findings were not documented with other commonly prescribed antiepileptic drugs carbamazepine (Tegretol), lamotrigine (Lamictal) and phenytoin (Dilantin) [1].

Every drug used during pregnancy could possibly affect the fetus. In the case of valproate, we know some of the risks. Note that this drug is also used for prophylaxis headaches, a common symptom in women of child-bearing age.

Reference

1. Meador KJ, Baker GA, Browning N, et al. Cognitive function at 3 years of age after fetal exposure to antiepileptic drugs. N Engl J Med 2009;360(16):1597–1605.

###

Oral Acyclovir (Zovirax) Does Not Seem to Be Helpful in Preventing Postherpetic Neuralgia

In a Cochrane Database review, Li et al. examined 6 randomized controlled trials with 1,211 subjects, and found no significant difference in acyclovir-treated and control groups at 4 and 6 months in the incidence of postherpetic neuralgia following an acute herpetic rash.

> *Still, the use of antivirals in this setting seems intuitive, and the drugs may shorten the duration of acute symptoms. The trials examined did not, in total, have very many subjects. The Li et al. study may be one of those that, instead of providing a definitive answer, show that a large, multi-center, randomized study is needed.*

Reference

1. Li Q, Chen, Yang J, et al. Antiviral treatment for preventing postherpetic neuralgia. Cochrane Database Syst Rev. 2009;April 15(2):CD006866.

Steroids Are Helpful in Treating Bell Palsy; Antiviral Agents May or May Not Be Beneficial

De Almeida et al. reviewed 18 trials involving 2,786 patients with Bell palsy. Regression analysis showed a synergistic effect with the combined use of corticosteroids and antivirals compared with either of these alone. The conclusion: "In Bell palsy, corticosteroids are associated with a reduced risk of unsatisfactory recovery. Antiviral agents, when administered with corticosteroids, may be associated with additional benefit" [1].

This seems fairly clear, at least until we look at the report by Quant et al. published in the same month in another prestigious medical journal. Their meta-analysis involved 6 trials with 1,145 patients in which Bell palsy was treated with steroids alone (n = 574) or steroids plus antivirals (n = 571). These investigators concluded: "Antivirals did not provide an added benefit in achieving at least partial facial muscle recovery compared with steroids alone in patients with Bell palsy" [2].

Then there is the report by Sullivan et al. that describes a randomized clinical trial of 496 patients treated with prednisolone, acyclovir, both drugs, or placebo. The primary outcome was return of facial function. They conclude: "In patients with Bell palsy, early treatment with prednisolone significantly improves the chances of complete recovery at 3 and 9 months. There is no evidence of benefit of acyclovir given alone or and additional benefit of acyclovir in combination with prednisolone" [3].

In these 3 reports, we have support for steroid therapy of Bell palsy, and none for antivirals alone. As for added corticosteroids plus antivirals, score one "may be associated with addition benefit" versus 2 studies showing no additional benefit, including the single randomized controlled trial in the group.

References

1. de Almeida JR, Al Khabori M, Guyatt GH, et al. Combined corticosteroid and antiviral treatment for Bell palsy: a systematic review and meta-analysis. JAMA. 2009;302(9): 1003–1004.
2. Quant EC, Jeste SS, Muni RH, et al. The benefits of steroids versus steroids plus antivirals for treatment of Bell palsy: a meta-analysis. BMJ. 2009;339:b3354.
3. Sullivan FM, Swan IR, Donnan PT, et al. Early treatment with prednisolone or acyclovir in Bell palsy. N Engl J Med. 2007;357(16):1598–1607.

###

Neither Antibiotic nor Topical Steroid Therapy Is Likely to Be Effective in the Treatment of Acute Sinusitis

Williamson et al. conducted a double-blind, randomized, placebo-controlled trial involving 240 adults with acute nonrecurrent sinusitis. Patients were randomized to receive one of four treatments: Antibiotic and nasal steroid; nasal steroid and placebo antibiotic; antibiotic and placebo nasal steroid; and placebo antibiotic and placebo nasal steroid. The drugs used were 500 mg of amoxicillin 3 times daily for 7 days and 200 mg of budesonide in each nostril daily for 10 days. Upon conclusion of therapy, there was not much difference among the groups, leading the authors to conclude, "Neither an antibiotic nor a topical steroid alone or in combination was effective as a treatment for acute sinusitis in the primary care setting" [1].

I have two thoughts here. First of all, these patients did not have trivial disease. The criterion for inclusion in the study was acute sinusitis manifested as 2 or more of the following: purulent rhinorrhea with unilateral predominance; local pain with unilateral predominance; purulent rhinorrhea bilaterally; or presence of pus in the nasal cavity [1].

My second thought is this. The outcome of this study brings to mind an aphorism from Meador: The well-trained physician knows what to do for his or her patients. The especially well-trained physician knows what not to do [2].

References

1. Williamson IG, Rumsby K, Benge S, et al. Antibiotics and topical nasal steroid treatment of acute maxillary sinusitis: a randomized controlled trial. JAMA. 2007;298(21):2487–2496.
2. Meador CK. A little book of doctors' rules. Philadelphia: Hanley & Belfus; 1999. Rule number 25.

###

Steroids May Be Useful Adjuvant Therapy in Acute Pharyngitis

A review of 8 randomized controlled trials of 806 adults and children in whom steroids were used as adjunctive therapy to control pain revealed "statistically significant faster reduction of pain or complete pain relief from steroid use compared with placebo." The relief was reported in all 8 studies. The authors reported no serious adverse effects [1].

The authors wisely caution against over-enthusiasm in employing the results of the study in practice. Issues involve the need to balance pain relief with possible adverse drug effects if steroids come to be widely used in treating pharyngitis. Then there is the issue of antibiotic use. In the study described here, most patients received concomitant antibiotics. If sore throats are managed without antibiotics and with steroids alone, will we begin to see adverse outcomes? This review is not a practice-changer; instead it is a classic case of a report calling for further studies to establish safety to balance the apparent effectiveness of adjuvant steroid use in pharyngitis pain control.

Reference

1. Korb K, Scherer M, Chenot JF. Steroids as adjuvant therapy for acute pharyngitis in ambulatory patients: a systematic review. Ann Fam Med. 2010;8(1):58–63.

###

The Use of Long-Acting Beta Agonists in Asthma May Increase the Risk of Asthma-Related Intubations and Death

This assertion is based on a pooled trial involving 36,588 persons. The authors found a 2-fold increase in asthma-related intubations or death with long-acting beta-agonists compared with placebo [1].

The authors report that the increased risk of catastrophic events with long-acting beta- agonist therapy of asthma was seen even with the concomitant use of inhaled corticosteroids [1].

Reference

1. Salpeter SR, Wall AJ, Buckley NS. Long-acting beta-agonists with and without corticosteroids and catastrophic asthma events. Am J Med. 2010;123(4):322–328.

###

A Selective Serotonin Reuptake Inhibitor (SSRI) May Be Useful in Treating Premature Ejaculation (PE)

From Spain comes a 2009 paper – no meta-analysis, no randomized clinical trial – advocating for the use of an SSRI to treat premature ejaculation, citing these drugs' tendency to cause delayed ejaculation. The author singles out dapoxetine, described as an SSRI that "has been specifically developed for on-demand use in PE." Attributes of this specific drug are "rapid absorption, a short initial half-life of 1.3–1.4 h and rapid elimination" [1].

This article prompted me to search PubMed and, sure enough, there have been randomized clinical trials. Pryor et al. report the integrated analysis of two 12-week randomized, double-blind, placebo-controlled trials of identical design done independently, in parallel, at 121 sites in the USA. There were 870 men with moderate-to-severe premature ejaculation who took dapoxetine 30 or 60 mg on-demand. Both doses were found to be effective on first dose, and the drug was found to be "an effective and generally well tolerated treatment for men with moderate-to-severe premature ejaculation" [2].

As a family physician, I have generally found that patients with a pesky problem are often willing to try something that is not quite in the mainstream, as long as it seems fairly safe. We are all familiar with the side effects of SSRIs. In the appropriate clinical setting, my sense would be to give it a try, following a thorough discussion with the patient regarding such off-label use and documentation of that discussion.

References

1. Owen RT. A novel treatment for premature ejaculation. Drugs Today. 2009;45(9):669–678.
2. Pryor JL, Althof SE, Steidle C, et al. Efficacy and tolerability of dapoxetine in treatment of premature ejaculation: an integrated analysis of two double-blind, randomized controlled trials. Lancet. 2006;368(9539):929–937.

###

Phosphodiaesterase-5 (PDE5) Inhibitors May Be Useful in Treating Lower Urinary Tract Symptoms (LUTS)

McVary et al. conducted a 12-week, double-blind, placebo controlled trial of sildenafil (Viagra) in men age 45 or older with both erectile dysfunction and LUTS. Men in the sildenafil group (n = 189) reported greater improvement in erectile function, in their prostate symptom scores and in their quality of life than those in placebo group (n = 180) [1].

Mouli and McVary suggest that there may be a causal relationship between LUTS and erectile dysfunction [2]. Thus, daily doses of a PDE5 inhibitor may benefit both.

References

1. McVary KT, Monnig W, Camps J Jr, Young J, Tseng L, von den Ende G. Sildenafil citrate improves erectile function and urinary symptoms in men with erectile dysfunction and lower urinary tract symptoms associated with benign prostatic hypertrophy: a randomized, double-blind trial. J Urol. 2007;177(3):1071–1077.
2. Mouli S, McVary KT. PDE5 inhibitors for LUTS. Prostate Cancer Prostatic Dis. 2009;12(4):316–324.

###

Sildenafil Increases Exercise Capacity Under Hypoxic Conditions

Our colleagues in Germany conducted an ambitious study. The subjects were 14 healthy mountaineer and trekkers, who underwent various tests during exercise (cycle ergometry) while breathing a hypoxic gas mixture. Tests were conducted at both low altitude and at high altitude locations. The high altitude site was the Mount Everest base camp! Subjects were studied while taking sildenafil or placebo. At low altitude sildenafil significantly increased arterial oxygen saturation during exercise, although this effect was not seen at high altitude. The authors conclude: "Sildenafil reduces hypoxic pulmonary hypertension at rest and during exercise while maintaining gas exchange and systemic blood pressure" [1].

This report has many implications, and is one that should be read in its entirety by all involved in sports medicine, high altitude medicine and exercise physiology. The authors are careful to state that they did not examine the effects of the drug on normoxic exercise tolerance, but can such a study be far behind? Will we soon see sildenafil listed as a performance-enhancing drug (in sports, that is)? And will we find that the effects described in this report are shared by all PDE5 inhibitors?

Reference

1. Ghofrani HA, Reichenberger F, Kohstall MG, et al. Sildenafil increased exercise capacity during hypoxia at low altitudes and at Mount Everest base camp: a randomized, double-blind, placebo-controlled crossover trial. Ann Intern Med. 2004;141(3):169–177.

###

A Small Dosage Increment of Phenytoin Can Bring a Large Increase in Serum Levels of the Drug

Phenytoin is probably the most cited example of the Michaelis–Menten non-linear pharmacokinetics phenomenon, in which a small dose increase in the middle therapeutic range may lead to disproportionate increase in serum drug levels, potentially leading to overdosage [1].

Recent medical school graduates almost certainly learned about non-linear pharmacokinetics, a favorite topic of academic pharmacologists. But memory sometimes fades, and I thought it might be helpful to include a reminder here.

Reference

1. Winter ME, Tozer TN. Phenytoin. In: Burton ME, Shaw LM, Schentag JJ, Evans WE, eds. Applied pharmacokinetics and pharmacodynamics: Principles of therapeutic drug monitoring. Ed 4. Philadelphia: Lippincott, Williams & Wilkins; 2005. Pages 464–490.

###

Some Drugs We Commonly Prescribe Are Restricted or Banned from Athletic Competition

Physicians treating National Collegiate Athletic Association (NCAA) or potential Olympic class athletes need to be aware of prohibited substances that may be considered performance enhancing. The following are current examples of NCAA Banned Substances [1]:

Class	Examples
Stimulants	Amphetamine (Adderall); methylphenidate (Ritalin)
Anabolic agents	DHEA; testosterone
Alcohol and beta blockers (banned for rifle only)	Alcohol; propranolol
Diuretics	Furosemide; hydrochlorothiazide
Street drugs	Heroin; marijuana
Peptide hormones and analogues	Human growth hormone; erythropoietin (EPO)
Anti-estrogens	Clomiphene; tamoxifen
Beta-2 agonists	Salbutamol; salmeterol

Any substance chemically related to a class of banned drugs, unless otherwise noted, is also banned.

There is a similar, but not identical, list of prohibited substances published by International Olympic Committee/World Anti-Doping Agency [2].

Note two facts about these lists: First, they change often, as competitors find new ways to game the system chemically. Secondly, it is easy to cause a problem innocently. For example, some commonly used diuretics and anti-asthma drugs are on the NCAA Banned Substances List. Therapeutic use exemptions may be possible; for information relative to NCAA and other restrictions, visit www.drugfreesport.com.

References

1. 2009–2010 NCAA Banned Drugs. Available at: http://www.ncaa.org/wps/wcm/connect/53e6f 4804e0b8a129949f91ad6fc8b25/2009–10+Banned+Drug+Classes.pdf?MOD=AJPERES&CA CHEID=53e6f4804e0b8a129949f91ad6fc8b25. Accessed March 15, 2010.
2. The 2010 Prohibited List. World Anti-Doping Agency. Available at: http://www.wada-ama.org/ en/World-Anti-Doping-Program/Sports-and-Anti-Doping-Organizations/International-Standards/Prohibited-List/ Accessed March 15, 2010.

Short Course Treatment of Uncomplicated, Symptomatic Lower Urinary Tract Infections (UTIs) Works as Well as Longer Duration Treatment

A Cochrane Database review of 15 studies involving 1,644 elderly women examined various treatment duration when treating UTIs. Single dose treatment did not fare well when compared with short course treatment (3–6 days) and with longer course treatment (7–10 days) in the 2 weeks post-treatment. In the long term, single dose and long-course treatment showed no significant difference. Perhaps most important is that no significant difference in efficacy was noted when short-duration and long-duration therapy were compared [1].

Of the options studied, short-course therapy – the middle of the three possibilities–seems best.

Reference

1. Lutters M, Vogt-Ferrier NB. Antibiotic duration for treating uncomplicated, symptomatic lower urinary tract infections in elderly women. Cochrane Database Syst Rev. 2008; Jul 16;(3);CD1535.

###

Procalcitonin Testing Can Provide Useful Guidance when Deciding About Antibiotic Use in Lower Respiratory Tract Infections (LRTIs)

A multicenter, randomized clinical trial conducted at 6 tertiary care centers in Switzerland involved 1,359 patients with LRTIs, most of which were described as severe. One randomized group was managed using guidance from levels of procalcitonin, a laboratory determination that reflects the likelihood of bacterial rather than viral infection. The other group received usual care based on the decisions of the physicians involved. Although the two groups had similar rates of adverse outcomes (recurrent infection requiring antibiotic treatment within 30 days, disease-specific complications, intensive care unit admission, or death), the procalcitonin group had less antibiotic use and less antibiotic adverse effects [1].

The cost of a procalcitonin test is about $45 (30 British pounds) [2]. In the current environment of antibiotic parsimony, will use of this test become considered cost-effective?

References .

1. Schuetz P, Chrit-Crain M, Thomann R, et al. Effect of procalcitonin-based guidelines vs standard guidelines on antibiotic use in lower respiratory tract infections: the ProHOSP randomized controlled trial. JAMA. 2009;302(10):1059–1066.
2. Can procalcitonin testing reduce antibiotic prescribing for respiratory infections? Age and Ageing. Available at: http://ageing.oxfordjournals.org/cgi/content/full/35/6/625. Accessed March 15, 2010.

###

C-Reactive Protein (CRP) Point-of-Care Testing Can Be Helpful in Deciding About Antibiotic Prescribing in LRTIs and Rhinosinusitis

Cals et al. randomized 258 patient with LRTI (n = 107) and rhinosinusitis (n = 151) to use CRP assisted or routine care. In the CRP-assisted care group there were fewer antibiotic prescriptions (43.4%) than in the control group and fewer delayed prescriptions filled (23% vs. 72%). The recovery from the illness was the same in both groups, and patients in the CRP-assisted group reported greater satisfaction with care [1].

C-reactive protein, like procalcitonin, may prove helpful in distinguishing bacterial from viral infections. Some day these findings may prove to be practice changers. In the meantime, as with procalcitonin, the overall cost of care will be a key determinant in whether or not these point-of-care decisions become part of everyday clinical practice.

Reference

1. Cals JW, Schot MJ, de Jong SA, Dinant GJ, Hopstaken RM. Point of care C-reactive protein testing and antibiotic prescribing for respiratory tract infections: a randomized controlled trial. Ann Fam Med. 2010;8(2):124–133.

###

Consider the Possibility of Glucose-6-Phosphate Dehydrogenase (G6PD) Deficiency Before Prescribing Primaquine for Malaria Prophylaxis

Primaquine, when ingested by a G6PD deficient person, can cause severe and potentially fatal hemolysis [1].

> G6PD deficiency is a fairly common, but generally asymptomatic, X-linked genetic disorder [2]. Asymptomatic, of course, unless an event-triggering drug or food is ingested. Other drugs considered unsafe in affected persons include the following: dapsone, nalidixic acid, nitrofurantoin, sulfacetamide, and sulfapyridine.

References

1. Primaquine. Centers for Disease Prevention and Control. The Pre-travel consultation. Available at: http://wwwnc.cdc.travel/yellowbook/2010/chapter-2/malaria.aspx. Accessed March 15, 2010.
2. Mason PJ, Bautista JM, Gilsanz F, et al. G6PD deficiency: the genotype-phenotype association. Blood Rev. 2007;21(5):267–283.

###

The Sequence of Infant Vaccine Injections Matters

Ipp et al. conducted a study involving 120 infants receiving two childhood immunizations at the same visit – diphtheria, polio, and tetanus toxoids and acellular pertussis and Haemophilus influenzae type b (DPTaP-Hib) vaccine and the pneumococcal conjugate vaccine (PCV). Half the infant subjects received DPTaP-Hib first; the other half received PCV first. The assessment was by the Modified Behavioral Pain Scale using videotaped recordings, by parental rating using a 1–10 scale, and by the presence or absence of crying. The researchers found significantly less pain ($p < 0.001$) when the DPTaP-HIB is administered first, before the PCV [1].

*I found myself wondering how the authors came up with the idea for this study, but the outcome offers an easy way to reduce infant discomfort when administering routine immunizations. Is this a **practice changer**? Maybe so.*

Reference

1. Ipp M, Parkin PC, Lear N, et al. Order of vaccine injection and infant pain response. Arch Pediatr Adolesc Med. 2009;163(5):469–472.

The Antiemetic Ondansetron (Zofran) Is Useful in Controlling Vomiting in Children with Acute Gastroenteritis and Mild/Moderate Dehydration Who Fail to Tolerate Oral Rehydration

In a randomized controlled trial, 106 patients ages 1–10 years of age received ondansetron or placebo. Of the ondansetron group (n = 51), 11 (21.6%) required intravenous rehydration, compared to the placebo group (n = 55), in which 30 (54.5%) required intravenous rehydration. Admission to the hospital was needed for 5.9% of the ondansetron group compared with 12.7% of the placebo group [1].

Another study, a systematic review and meta-analysis of 6 randomized, double-masked, placebo control trials, led the authors to conclude that ondansetron therapy decreases the risk of persistent vomiting, the use of intravenous fluid, and hospital admission of children with gastroenteritis-induced vomiting [2].

Each year there are approximately 1.5 million doctor visits by children with gastroenteritis and dehydration, and a diagnosis of "diarrhea" is coded in 13% of all childhood hospitalizations [3]. The use of ondansetron, a selective 5-hydroxytryptamine receptor antagonist available as oral solution or orally disintegrating tablets, will be helpful in many of these instances, especially since this drug minimizes the extrapyramidal and sedative problems seen with older drugs used to suppress vomiting, such as prochlorperazine, promethazine, and metoclopramide.

References

1. Roslund G, Hepps TS, McQuillen KK, et al. The role of oral ondansetron in children with vomiting as a result of acute gastritis/gastroenteritis who have failed oral rehydration therapy: a randomized controlled trial. Ann Emerg Med. 2008;52(1):22–29.
2. DeCamp LR, Byerley JS, Doshi N, Steiner MJ. Use of antiemetic agents in acute gastroenteritis: a systematic review and meta-analysis. Arch Pediatr Adolesc Med. 2008;162(9):858–865.
3. Malek MA, Curns AT, Holman RC, et al. Diarrhea-and rotavirus-associated hospitalizations among children less than 5 years of age: United States, 1997 and 2000. Pediatrics. 2006; 117(5):1887–1892.

###

Oral Bisphosphonates Have Not Been Shown to Cause Atypical Subtrochanteric Fractures of the Femur

This is the conclusion stated in an FDA Drug Safety Communication dated March 10, 2010.

A relationship between bisphosphonate use and atypical femur fractures has been raised, and has now been confronted by the FDA, whose "no clear connection" conclusion is supported by the findings of Abrahamsen et al., following a review of two large studies involving 22,318 patients [1]. A subsequent study by Black et al. also found that "there was no significant risk associated with bisphosphonate use" [2].

The initial suggestion of a link between bisphosphonates and atypical femur fractures probably gained some traction owing to the documented association of these drugs with osteonecrosis of the jaw [3]. This assertion seem to have been put to rest, at least for now.

References

1. Abrahamsen B, Eiken P, Eastell R. Subtrochanteric and diaphyseal femur fractures in patients treated with alendronate: a register-based national cohort study. J Bone Miner Res. 2009;24(6):1095–1102.
2. Black DM, Kelly MP, Genant HK, et al. Bisphosphonates and fractures of the subtrochanteric or diaphyseal femur. N Engl J Med. 2010;362(19):1761–1771.
3. Woo SB, Hellstein JW, Kalmar JR. Systematic review: bisphosphonates and osteonecrosis of the jaws. Ann Intern Med. 2006;144(10):753–761.

###

In Older Persons with Memory Problems, Physical Activity May Improve Cognition

The study to support this statement involved 170 persons age 50 and older who reported memory problems. Those involved in the study were randomized to a group who received a home-based physical activity program or to group who received education and usual care. Of those who began the program, 138 were followed for 18 months. Subjects were evaluated using a variety of dementia/Alzheimer disease instruments. The investigators concluded that in the case of adults with subjective memory impairment, a 6-month program of physical activity provided a modest improvement in cognition over an 18-month follow-up period [1].

I am pleased to report that there was not a single adverse drug effect in the study group.

Reference

1. Lautenschlater NT, Cox KL, Flicker L, et al. Effect of physical activity on cognitive function in older adults at risk for Alzheimer disease. JAMA. 2008;300(9):1027–1037.

###

Vitamin D Deficiency May Play a Role in Chronic Tension-Type Headache

A study conducted in India involved 8 patients with tension-type headache and vitamin D deficiency associated osteomalacia. When treated with vitamin D and calcium, both the headache and the osteomalacia of all patients improved.

Ask any group of people if they have chronic tension-type headache and most, if not all, will respond, "Yes." Wouldn't it be interesting if correcting a vitamin D deficiency could control this almost-universal ailment? This might be actually be possible, at least in some instances.

Reference

1. Prakash S, Shah ND. Chronic tension-type headache with vitamin D deficiency: casual or causal association? Headache. 2009;49(8):1214–1222.

###

Vitamin B$_{12}$ Is Worth a Try in Treating the Patient with Recurrent Aphthous Stomatitis (RAS)

In a randomized, double-blind, placebo controlled trial involving 58 patients with RAS, 31 received a daily dose of 1,000 mcg of vitamin B12 as a sublingual tablet. A control group of 27 patients received placebo therapy. At 5 and 6 months, the duration of outbreaks, the number of ulcers, and the level of pain were all significantly reduced in the treatment group when compared to the placebo group. During the last month of therapy, 74.1% of B12 users reported no aphthous ulcers, compared with only 32.0% of the control group [1].

This treatment seems safe, cheap and reasonably effective, all attributes I look for in a medication.

Reference

1. Volkov I, Rudoy I, Freud T, et al. Effectiveness of vitamin B12 in treating recurrent aphthous stomatitis: a randomized, double-blind, placebo-controlled trial. J Am Board Fam Med. 2009;22:9–16.

###

Supplementary Antioxidant Vitamin Use Does Not Reduce the Incidence of Heart Attacks or Other Vascular Events, Cancer, or Other Major Outcome

In the United Kingdom, researchers studied 20,536 adults randomized to a study group who received antioxidant vitamin supplements (250 mg vitamin C, 600 mg vitamin E, and 20 mg beta-carotene) daily or to a control group who received a matching placebo. An average of 83% of participants in both groups completed the 5-year study. When data were analyzed, researchers found no significant differences in all-cause mortality, or in deaths due to vascular or non-vascular causes. There were also no significant differences in the incidence of myocardial infarction, stroke, or death from either of these causes. Although the use of vitamin supplementation increased the blood levels of the vitamins involved, and did so without safety issues, the bottom line seems to be that antioxidant supplementation "did not produce any significant reduction in the 5-year mortality from, or the incidence of, any type of vascular disease, cancer, or other major outcome" [1].

> *The expensive drug is the one that doesn't work. I think that truism also applies to vitamin supplementation.*

Reference

1. Heart Protection Study Collaborative Group. MRC/BHF Heart Protection Study of antioxidant vitamin supplementation in 20,536 high-risk individuals: a randomized placebo-controlled trial. Lancet. 2002;360(9326):23–33.

#####

Chapter 10
Idiosyncratic and Uncommon Drug Effects

A desire to take medicines is, perhaps, the great feature which distinguishes man from other animals.

Sir William Osler, Quoted in Bean and Bean [1].

Humans seems to the only species to use tools to make tools. Here Sir William offers one more distinguishing characteristic of *homo sapiens*. We certainly take a lot of drugs and, which should be no surprise, we suffer a lot of side effects.

Terri K, a 26 year-old first grade teacher, received word that one of her students, one whom she had comforted when he developed a fever while at school, had been admitted to the hospital with meningococcal meningitis. She telephoned her physician, who recommended prophylaxis with rifampin.

The day after beginning her prophylactic medication, she was horrified to find her urine and tears to be a bright orange-red hue. Later that afternoon, during a workout at the gym, she noted that the beads of sweat on her body were red. This prompted a call to the physician, who reassured her that she was just experiencing a harmless side effect sometimes seen with rifampin. "I guess I should have warned you that this might happen," said the physician.

The fact that rifampin can cause red urine and other body fluids has been known for three decades [2]. In fact the discoloration may be seen in not only urine, tears, and sweat. It may also be noted in sputum, saliva, and feces. It can permanently stain soft contact lenses. The red urine can stain clothing, which may cause Terri to consider the side effect not totally harmless after all. Rifampin use is part of the differential diagnosis of red urine.

Countless drugs cause fatigue, nausea, headache, and so forth. This chapter tells about the odd, unexpected, and sometimes serious side effects of the medications we use each day. Although only serious to clothing and soft contact lenses, the red discoloration of body fluids with rifampin is a good example of a curious and idiosyncratic drug effect.

In considering unexpected side effects of drugs, I should point out that not all are harmful. In fact, some unanticipated outcomes are helpful, and I will describe a few of these.

R.B. Taylor, *Essential Medical Facts Every Clinician Should Know: To Prevent Medical Errors, Pass Board Examinations and Provide Informed Patient Care*, DOI 10.1007/978-1-4419-7874-5_10, © Springer Science+Business Media, LLC 2011

In a study by Tam et al. in Hong Kong, a chart review revealed a 2.03% rate of medication misadventures, four times the rate detected using voluntary reporting [3]. In this study, the leading offenders, causing 82% of all adverse drug reactions, were beta blockers, diuretics, angiotensin-converting enzyme (ACE) inhibitors, aspirin, and non-steroidal anti-inflammatory drugs. I will begin with these.

References

1. Bean RB, Bean WB. Aphorisms by Sir William Osler: New York: Henry Schuman; 1950. Chapter 3.
2. Snider DE, Farer SL. Rifampin and red urine. JAMA. 1977; 238(15):1628.
3. Tam KW, Kwok HK, Fan YM, et al. Detection and prevention of medication misadventures in general practice. Int J Qual Health Care. 2008; 20(3):192–199.

###

Beta Blockers Can Cause or Aggravate Psoriasis

Yilmaz et al. report a case of beta-blocker-induced psoriasis, suggesting an action at the cellular level [1].

> *Because beta blockers are generally taken for a prolonged period of time, as in the treatment of chronic hypertension, when psoriasis begins weeks or months later, I can see why a physician might fail to relate this rare effect to the offending drug.*

Reference

1. Yilmaz MB, Turhan H, Akin Y, Kisacik HL, Korkmaz S. Beta-blocker-induced psoriasis: a rare side effect – a case report. Angiology. 2002; 53(6):737–739.

###

Spironolactone Causes Changes in the Ratio of Testosterone to Estradiol, Contributing to the Likelihood of Gynecomastia as a Side Effect

Gynecomastia is a well-recognized effect of spironolactone use. But why does this occur?

Rose et al. measured hormone levels in 16 hypertensive patients. Six were treated with spironolactone and developed gynecomastia; the other 10 patients were considered control subjects. Following therapy, the spironolactone-treated group had lower blood testosterone levels and higher estradiol levels than the control group [1].

Reference

1. Rose LI, Underwood RH, Newmark SR, Kisch ES, Williams GH. Pathophysiology of spironolactone-induced gynecomastia. Ann Intern Med. 1977;87(4):398–403.

###

Acetazolamide Has Two Curious Side Effects: It Can Cause Tingling of the Fingertips and Can Make Carbonated Beverages Seem to Have an Unpleasant Taste

Carbonic anhydrase inhibitors, useful in preventing and treating altitude sickness, tend to produce an acidotic state, which prompt increased ventilation and improved oxygenation [1].

As one who does some adventure travel to high altitudes, I have experienced both of these effects. The tingling of the fingertips, which I first thought was caused by the straps of my backpack, is the result of increased ventilation, and can be caused by any state that causes "overbreathing." The bad taste of carbonated beverages, including beer and champagne, I cannot explain as readily, but I can attest that it occurs. Graber and Kelleher named it "the champagne blues" [2].

References

1. Burki NK, Khan SA, Hameed MA. The effects of acetazolamide on the ventilatory response to high altitude hypoxia. Chest. 1992;101(3);736–741.
2. Graber M, Kelleher S. Side effects of acetazolamide: the champagne blues. Am J Med. 1988;84(5):978–980.

###

ACE Inhibitors and Angiotensin Receptor Blockers (ARBs) Help Prevent the Development of Diabetes Mellitus

Andraws and Brown reviewed 13 prospective, randomized, controlled clinical trials involving 93,451 patients taking a renin-angiotensin system inhibitor. They found that both drugs helped protect against diabetes. In the ACE inhibitor group, the odds of developing diabetes were reduced by 28%, while in the ARB group the reduction was 27%.

This study is included just to show that not all unexpected drug effects are deleterious. To learn of more happy news about drugs, read on.

Reference

1. Andraws R, Brown DL. Effect of inhibition of the renin-angiotensin system on development of type 2 diabetes mellitus (meta-analysis of randomized trials). Am J Cardiol. 2007;99(7): 1006–1012.

###

Valsartan Use in Hypertension May Help Prevent Cardiovascular Events

A study of 3031 Japanese patients with uncontrolled hypertension randomized to valsartan add-on treatment or non-ARB treatment, followed for 3.7 years, showed less cardiovascular events – such as stroke, transient ischemic attack (TIA) or angina pectoris – in the valsartan-treated group [1].

This study also showed decrease in diabetes in the valsartan-treated group [1].

Reference

1. Sawada T, Yamada H, Dahlof B, et al. Effects of valsartan on morbidity and mortality in uncontrolled hypertensive patients with high cardiovascular risks: KYOTO HEART Study. Eur Heart J. 2009;30(20):2461–2469.

###

Angiotensin Receptor Blockers May Reduce the Development or Progression of Alzheimer Disease and Dementia

The study leading to this conclusion involved 819,491 U.S. veterans with cardiovascular disease followed over a 4 year period. ARBs were compared with lisinopril and other cardiovascular drugs. Although there were only minor differences in blood pressure among the groups, there was a difference in regard to Alzheimer disease and dementia incidence and progression. The authors of the study conclude: "Angiotensin receptor blockers are associated with a significant reduction in the incidence and progression of Alzheimer's disease and dementia compared with angiotensin converting enzyme inhibitors or other cardiovascular drugs in a predominantly white population" [1].

I am beginning to like the side effect profile of the ARBs.

Reference

1. Li NC, Lee A, Whitmer RA, et al. Use of angiotensin receptor blockers and risk of dementia in a predominantly male population: prospective cohort analysis. BMJ. 2010 Jan 12; 340: b5465. Doi: 10.1136bmj.b5465.

###

Regular Analgesic Use Can Lead to Hearing Loss

In a study involving 26,917 men ages 40–74 who completed questionnaires every 2 years, there were 3,488 incident cases of hearing loss in 369,079 person-years of follow-up. Analgesics studied were aspirin, acetaminophen and non-steroidal anti-inflammatory drugs (NSAIDs). With regular use of the drugs compared with those not using the drugs regularly, the hazard ratio for hearing loss with aspirin use was 1.12; with acetaminophen use, 1.22; and with NSAID use, 1.21. Not surprisingly, for acetaminophen and NSAIDs, the incidence of hearing loss increased with longer duration of regular use. The impact was greater on younger men [1].

I think that an important key to this study is the definition of "regular use," that is, use of the drug 2 or more times per week, which I do not consider to be very frequent use. Also, note that the study cited included only male subjects.

Reference

1. Curhan SG, Eavey R, Shargorodshy J, Curhan CC. Analgesic use and the risk of hearing loss in men. Am J Med. 2010;123(3):231–237.

###

Non-Steroidal Anti-Inflammatory Drugs Can Cause a Wide Variety of Skin Rashes

Most commonly reported are morbilliform rashes, urticaria and angioedema, but the spectrum includes a wide range of dermatologic manifestations [1]. One example is a fixed drug eruption, which recurs at the same site when a course of NSAID use is repeated. Other possibilities include Stevens-Johnson syndrome, vasculitis, photosensitivity, livedo-like dermatitis, lichenoid eruption, exanthematous eruption, and pemphigoid [1].

We are all familiar with the tendency of NSAIDs to cause gastrointestinal distress, but we sometimes forget about the other adverse effects of these very commonly used and readily available medications.

Reference

1. Sanches-Borges M, Cariles-Hulett A, Caballero-Fonseca F. Risk of skin reactions when using ibuprofen-based medicines. Expert Opin Drug Saf. 2005;4(5):837–848.

###

Salicylates Carry a Significant Risk of Toxicity

To support this fact I offer two reports, both concerning methyl salicylate, found in oil of wintergreen (98% methyl salicylates) and various creams used for sore muscles. Davis tells of several "well-documented deaths" of children less than 6 years of age who had taken a teaspoonful (5 ml) or less of oil of wintergreen [1]. *Scienceline* reports that a teaspoon of oil of wintergreen is the equivalent of 22 adult aspirin tablets [2].

A chilling story describes the death of high school cross-country runner Arielle Newman, who died of acute salicylate toxicity after extensive application of methyl salicylate-containing products to her aching muscles [2]. The reports identify BenGay by name, but point out that methyl salicylate can also be found in Bayer Muscle Joint Cream, Tiger Balm, and Icy Hot. Look for it also in herbal remedies, and as flavoring in food, candy, and toothpaste.

> *I became aware of the toxic effects of salicylates when I was a young small-town physician, called to the home of a 14-year-old girl. Her mother described how the child had had a fever – persistent, but not excessively high – over the past two days. The mother had dutifully treated her daughter's fever with aspirin every 4–6 h but to no avail. Then on the morning of my visit, the daughter had awakened, still febrile, but now also agitated and confused. My diagnosis: salicylate toxicity, caused by too much aspirin for body weight, given too often. I decided not to sedate her, and advised the mother to do nothing other than apply some cool compresses to her head and chest. I called later in the day, and the mother reported that her daughter was sleeping peacefully and the fever seemed to have subsided.*

References

1. Davis JE. Are one or two dangerous? Methyl salicylate exposure in toddlers. J Emerg Med. 2007;32(1):63–69.
2. How can you overdose on BenGay? Available at: http://scienceline.org/2007/08/13/ask-cooper-bengaydeath/ Accessed February 4, 2009.

###

Antibacterial Agents Can Cause a Panoply of Neurotoxic Manifestations

In contradistinction to the findings of Tam et al., cited above, I believe that antimicrobial agents are the most common causes of adverse drug reactions. (Sanches-Borges et al., also cited above, agree with me.) Granted, most of these reactions are mundane: nausea, diarrhea, skin rashes and so forth. But some are more serious, including a wide variety of neurotoxic reactions.

Here, based on a review by Snavely and Hodges [1], are some of them:

Types of Reaction	Possible Causes
Central nervous system reactions:	Penicillins, cephalosporins, tetracyclines,
Bulging fontanelles, seizures, encephalopathy, and psychiatric manifestations	sulfonamides, chloramphenicol, colistin, aminoglycosides, metronidazole, isoniazid, rifampin, cycloserine, and dapsone
Cranial nerve toxicities:	Erythromycin, sulfonamides, tetracyclines,
Myopia, optic neuritis, deafness, vertigo, and tinnitus	chloramphenicol, colistin, aminoglycosides, vancomycin, isoniazid, and ethambutol
Peripheral nerve symptoms:	Penicillins, sulfonamides, chloramphenicol,
Paresthesias, motor weakness, and sensory impairment	colistin, metronidazole, isoniazid, and dapsone

Wilson et al. provide us with a helpful review of the neurotoxic manifestations that might be seen with cephalosporins: disorientation, confusion, twitching, somnolence, myoclonus, and seizures [2]. All these might occur with what otherwise are considered relatively safe antibiotics.

When we think of the possibility of adverse reactions to antibiotics, we must consider risk factors. The one that is mentioned most often as a contributor to antibiotic neurotoxicity is renal impairment [2, 3].

References

1. Snavely SR, Hodges GR. The neurotoxicity of antibacterial agents. Ann Intern Med. 1984;101(1):92–104.
2. Wilson NS, Duhart B, Self TH. Cephalosporins: how to minimize the risk of neurotoxicity. Consultant. February 2010: 90–91.
3. Chow KM, Szeto CCV, Hui AC, Li PK. Mechanisms of antibiotic neurotoxicity in renal failure. Int J Antimicrob Agents. 2004;23(3):213–217.

###

Tetracycline and Its Derivatives Can Stain Adult Teeth

The potential for tetracycline to cause staining during intrauterine tooth development is widely recognized. Less well known is that this drug and its derivatives can also stain the teeth of adults, a clinically significant fact given that tetracycline drugs are used for a variety of indications, including acne [1, 2].

Sánchez et al. describe the staining which may occur with minocycline, a semisynthetic derivative of tetracycline. The drug can cause darkening of the crowns of permanent teeth and a black or green discoloration of the roots. These authors report a 3–6% prevalence of staining with tetracycline and minocycline.

> *The staining can also involve the conjunctiva, sclera and skin. All these possibilities speak to the need to warn patients for whom we prescribe tetracyclines, especially for long-term use, as in acne therapy.*

References

1. Sánchez AR, Rogers R, Sheridan PJ. Tetracycline and other tetracycline-derivative staining of the teeth and oral cavity. Int J Dermatology. 2004;43(10):709–712.
2. McKenna BE, Lamey PJ, Kennedy JG, Bateson J. Minocycline-induced staining of the adult permanent dentition: a review of the literature and report of a case. Dent Update. 1999;26(4):160–162.

###

Fluoroquinolone Antibiotics Can Cause Tendinitis or Tendon Rupture

The cartilage-damaging effect of quinolones on juvenile experimental animals has been well documented [1]. But are you aware that quinolone antibiotics such as levofloxacin (Levaquin) can also cause tendinitis, sometimes leading to Achilles tendon rupture in adults? The complication is rare, but it happens, and was added as a "black box warning" in 2008 [2].

> *The risk of Achilles tendinitis with possible rupture increases with age, with steroid use, and with renal impairment, and the onset of tendon pain can come soon after beginning quinolone therapy. Patients with the risk factors mentioned and, in fact, probably all patients taking a quinolone should be alerted to stop the drug and call the doctor if tendon pain is noted.*

References

1. Stahlmann R. Cartilage-damaging effect of quinolones. Infection 1991; 19 Suppl 1: S38–46.
2. Fluoroquinolones and tendon injuries. The medical letter. 2008; 50 (1300):93.

###

Some, But Not All, Fluoroquinolones Can Disrupt Glucose Homeostasis, Causing Severe Hypoglycemia or Hyperglycemia

A Veteran's Administration study conducted over 3 years showed a significantly greater incidence of severe hypo- and hyperglycemia with levofloxacin and gatifloxacin, but not with ciprofloxacin, compared with azithromycin [1].

Here are two thoughts about this study: The first is that I consider the risk of perturbed glucose metabolism most worrisome when choosing a fluoroquinolone for a diabetic patient. Secondly, the tendency to cause dysglycemia seems not to be a class effect, in contradistinction to the tendency of these drugs to cause cartilage or tendon damage.

Reference

1. Aspinall SL, Good CB, Jiang R, McCarren M, Dong D, Cunningham FE. Severe dysglycemia with the fluoroquinolones: a class effect? Clin Infect Dis. 2009;49(3):402–408.

###

Fluoroquinolones May Cause Diplopia

Fraunfelder and Fraunfelder rummaged around in the *National Registry of Drug-Induced Ocular Side Effects*, and found 171 case reports of diplopia associated with fluoroquinolone use [1]. The median time from initiation of drug use to onset of symptoms was 9.6 days.

Now here is a curious item in this report: Of the 171 persons with diplopia, 17 had concomitant tendinitis. This seems a very high percentage of tendinitis patients, given that the incidence of fluoroquinolone-induced tendon injury in the general population is estimated to be 0.14 to 0.4% [2]. Granted, the patients with diplopia were older (49 were age 60 or older), one had renal cysts and 4 were taking corticosteroids. I submit that 17 reports of concomitant tendinitis among171 subjects still seems many more than would be expected.

References

1. Fraunfelder FW, Fraunfelder FT. Diplopia and fluoroquinolones. Ophthalmology. 2009;116(9): 1814–1817.
2. Fluoroquinolones and tendon injuries. The Medical Letter. 2008;50(1300):93.

###

Serotonin Selective Reuptake Inhibitors (SSRIs) Can Cause Delayed Ejaculation in Men, Although the Effect Varies Among Specific Agents

Waldinger et al. in the Netherlands have conducted studies of the effect various SSRIs on intravaginal ejaculation latency time (IELT), measured at home using stopwatches. Drugs studied were fluoxetine (Prozac), fluvoxamine (Luvox), paroxetine (Paxil), and sertraline (Zoloft). They found delayed IELT with fluoxetine, sertraline, and paroxetine, with paroxetine causing the greatest prolongation of the latency time. Fluvoxamine caused no significant delay in ejaculation.

If the drugs do not delay ejaculation, use of a stopwatch in the bedroom just might. The differences among various SSRIs described here may be pertinent when selecting the best one to use for a male patient. On a more positive note, SSRIs have been used to treat men suffering from premature ejaculation, as described in Chapter 9.

References

1. Waldinger MD, Hengeveld MW, Zwinderman AH, Olivier B. Effect of SSRI antidepressants on ejaculation: a double-blind, randomized, placebo-controlled study with fluoxetine, fluvoxamine, paroxetine, and sertraline. J Clin Psychopharmacol. 1998; 18(4):274–281.
2. Waldinger MD, Olivier B. Selective serotonin reuptake inhibitor-induced sexual dysfunction: clinical and research considerations. Int Clin Psychopharmacol. 1998; 13 Suppl 6: S27–33.

###

Trazodone (Desyrel) Can Cause Priapism

The adverse effect tends to occur during the first month of therapy and to be noted with doses of 150 mg/d or less. The age of the patient does not seem to matter as a risk factor for the occurrence of priapism [1, 2]. There is even a report of a case of priapism of the female clitoris associated with the use of trazodone [3].

Not long ago I lectured on some of these quirky side effects of drugs at a continuing medical education meeting. One of the attendees, who practices medicine at a substance abuse clinic, told that her patients refer to trazodone as "traz-erect."

References

1. Warner MD, Peabody CA, Whiteford HA, Hollister LE. Trazodone and priapism. J Clin Psychiatry. 1987; 48(6):244–245.
2. Carson CC 3rd, Mino RD. Priapism associated with trazodone therapy. J Urol. 1988; 139(2): 369–370.
3. Pescatori ES, Engelman JC, Davis G, Goldstein I. Priapism of the clitoris: a case report following trazodone use. J Urol. 1993; 149(6):1557–1559.

###

The Nonbenzodiazepine Receptor Agonist (NBRA) Hypnosedatives Can Induce Sleep-Related Complex Behaviors

A review of the literature revealed 10 reports involving 17 patients, all of whom displayed some sort of NBRA-induced complex behaviors. Of these 17 patients, 15 had taken zolpidem (Ambien), one had taken zaleplon (Sonata), and one had taken zopiclone (Rhovane [Canada only]). Various sleep-related complex behaviors described included: sleep eating, sleep conversations, sleepwalking with object manipulation, sleep driving, sleep shopping, and sleep sex [1].

Is zolpidem more likely to cause the adverse effects described, or is it simply prescribed much more often?

Reference

1. Dolder CR, Nelson MH. Hypnosedative-induced complex behaviors: incidence, mechanisms, and management. CNS Drugs. 2008; 22(12):1021–1036.

###

Epilepsy and Other Illnesses for Which Antiepileptic Drugs (AEDs) Are Prescribed Are Associated with an Increased Risk of Suicidal Thoughts or Behavior

This statement is taken directly from a Food and Drug Administration (FDA) update issued May 5, 2009 [1]. Bell et al. report on a meta-analysis of 199 placebo-controlled trials of antiepileptic drugs taken for seizure control, psychiatric or "other" indications. These authors find an odds ratio of 1.8 for suicidal ideation and behavior in patients taking AEDs for epilepsy. They note, "The odds ration was significantly raised for people taking AEDs for epilepsy, but not for the other indications" [2].

Is there some cognitive dissonance here? The FDA tells of an increased suicide risk in patients taking AEDS for epilepsy and other illnesses [1]. Yet Bell et al. state that the increased odds ratio for suicidal ideation and behavior was not found in patients taking the drugs for other indications [2]. The almost two-fold increased risk of suicidal thoughts and behavior in epileptic patients taking AEDs is noteworthy and merits monitoring for behavioral change that could indicate the emergence or worsening of suicidal thoughts or behavior or depression [1]. But what about the tens of thousands of migraine patients using antiseizure drugs for headache prophylaxis? Are they also at risk, and do they merit special monitoring?

Also, the risk is not the same with all anticonvulsant medications. When compared with topiramate, the hazard ratios for other drugs were: gabapentin, 1.42; valproate, 1.65; lamotrigine, 1.84; oxcarbazepine 2.07; and tiagabine, 2.41. Review of data in regard to violent deaths yielded similar findings [3]. Thus topiramate appears to be the safest in regard to suicidality and violent deaths, although the drug is not totally problem-free, as described next.

References

1. Suicidal behavior ideation and antiepileptic drugs: Update 5/5/2009. Available at: http://www. fda.gov/Drugs/DrugSafety/PostmarketDrugSafetyInformationforPatientsandProviders/ ucm111085.htm/ Accessed August 12, 2010.
2. Bell GS, Mula M, Sander JW. Suicidality in people taking antiepileptic drugs: what is the evidence? CNS Drugs. 2009;23(4):281–292.
3. Patorno E, Bohn RL, Wahl PM. Anticonvulsant medications and the risk of suicide, attempted suicide or violent death. JAMA. 2010;303(14):1401–1409.

###

Topiramate (Topamax) Can Cause Impaired Cognitive Function

Several studies have found similar results. Lee et al. describe two studies involving a total of 20 patients tested both on and off topiramate. A variety of cognitive tasks were evaluated, revealing a performance decrement while patients were taking topiramate [1]. In a retrospective study of 18 patients tested before and after beginning topiramate therapy and compared with matched controls, five of the topiramate patients had complaints indicating cognitive decline [2].

> I think of the many patients using topiramate for migraine prophylaxis and wonder if all are aware of the possibility of cognitive decline.
>
> On a more intriguing note comes a report from Italy, with 5 authors and requiring 3 journal pages, telling of a single patient with seizures who experienced intermittent hyperthermia and reduced sweat response while taking topiramate [3]. Aside from the extravagant use of author time and journal pages, this reported phenomenon is one more example of Meador's Rule 31: As yet no drug has been found with a single action and no body with a single reaction [4].

References

1. Lee S, Sziklas V, Andermann F, et al. The effects of adjunctive topiramate on cognitive function in patients with epilepsy. Epilepsia. 2003;44(3):339–347.
2. Thompson PJ, Baxendale SA, Duncan JS, Sander JWAS. Effects of topiramate on cognitive function. J Neurol Neurosurg Psychiatry. 2000;69:636–641.
3. Cerminara C, Seri S, Bombardieri R, Pinnci M, Curatolo P. Hypohidrosis during topiramate treatment: a rare and reversible effect. Pediatr Neurol. 2006;34(5):392–394.
4. Meador CK. A little book of doctors' rules II. Philadelphia: Hanley & Belfus, 1999. Rule 31.

###

Carbamazepine (Tegretol) Can Cause a Shift in Musical Pitch Perception

From Japan comes a report of two instances of carbamazepine-induced pitch perception shifts, which could be especially troublesome to musicians [1].

This chapter is, after all, about some uncommon drug effects, and this one is probably very uncommon.

Reference

1. Kobayashi T, Nisijima K, Ehara Y, Otsuka K, Kato S. Pitch perception shift: a rare side-effect of carbamazepine. Psychiatry Clin Neurosci. 2008;55(4):415–417.

###

Purple Glove Syndrome Is a Rare, But Serious, Complication of Intravenous Phenytoin (Dilantin) Therapy

Physicians are well aware that phenytoin (Dilantin) often causes gum hyperplasia, a side effect that can be especially distressing to young persons with epilepsy. Less well known is the risk that when injected intravenously, the drug can cause purple glove syndrome, a rare complication manifested as pain, swelling and discoloration of the hand distal to the injection site, a condition that may require surgery [1].

If you have ever seen a patient – or a photo of a patient – with purple glove syndrome, you will understand how the condition got its name. Photos are available on Google Images, and on my path through Google I encountered a solicitation by a law firm offering free evaluations to victims of purple glove syndrome.

Reference

1. Chokshi R, Openshaw J, Mehta NN, Mohler E. Purple glove syndrome following intravenous phenytoin administration. Vasc Med. 2007; 12(1):29–31.

###

Sumatriptan (Imitrex) and Related Triptan Drugs Can Cause Ischemic Colitis

There have now been several reports of triptan-induced ischemic colitis and mesenteric ischemia [1, 2, 3]. Hodge and Hodge present the youngest patient reported to date (age 35), who had no risk factors for ischemia, did not smoke, and who had sumatriptan-associated ischemic colitis with no diarrhea or hematochezia [4].

> *It would be grand if sumatriptan and related medications were simply selective constrictors of intracranial arteries [1]. Experience has shown, however, that the drugs' vasopressor response can be manifested elsewhere, causing reports of coronary vasospasm and myocardial infarction. Should we be surprised that the triptans can also cause ischemia in arteries supplying the structures in the abdominal cavity?*

References

1. Knudsen JF, Friedman B, Chen M, Goldwasser JE. Ischemic colitis and sumatriptan use. Arch Intern Med. 1998;158(17):1946–1948.
2. Liu JJ, Ardolf JC. Sumatriptan-associated mesenteric ischemia. Ann Intern Med. 2000;132(7):597.
3. Schwartz DC, Smith DJ. Colonic ischemia associated with naratriptan use. J Clin Gastroenterol. 2004;38(9):790–792.
4. Hodge JA, Hodge KD. Ischemic colitis related to sumatriptan overuse. J Am Board Fam Med. 2010;23(1):124–127.

###

Sumatriptan, in Large Doses, Can Cause Sulfhemoglobinemia

Flexman et al. report a rare case of sulfhemoglobinemia, noted as "dark green blood in the operating theater," found in a 42-year-old man undergoing surgery for a compartment syndrome in both legs. The patient had been taking 200 mg of sumatriptan daily [1].

> *This phenomenon, which is surely a "fascinemia," is not listed as a side effect in the 2010 edition of the Physicians' Desk Reference.*

Reference

1. Flexman AM, Del Vicario G, Schwarz SK. Lancet. 2007 June 9; 369(9577):1972.

###

Digitalis, Even in Modest Doses, Can Cause Yellow Vision

In fact, digitalis can cause a variety of visual symptoms, including blurred vision, "snowy" vision, and a sensation of seeing lights (photopsia). Most characteristic, however, is a disturbance of color vision, notably chromatopsia, described by Butler et al. as a subjective perception that objects possess colors other than their objective colors. Yellow and green are colors likely to be described. The visual phenomena can be seen with therapeutic or even subtherapeutic serum digitalis levels [1].

As an interesting historical aside, Lee speculates that the Dutch postimpressionist painter Vincent van Gogh may have suffered from digitalis-induced visual manifestations. Later in his career, his paintings often had yellow colors and halos. Lee's hypothesis is based on the artist having twice painted his personal physician holding a foxglove plant, a source of digitalis "leaf" [2]. Van Gogh is reported to have been fond of the drink absinthe, which can also cause yellow vision.

References

1. Butler VP, Odel JG, Rath E. et al. Digitalis-induced visual disturbances with therapeutic serum digitalis concentrations. Ann Intern Med. 1995;123(9):676–680.
2. Lee TC. Van Gogh's vision: digitalis intoxication? JAMA. 1981;245(7):727–729.

###

Under Certain Circumstances, Acid-Suppressing Drugs May Be Associated with an Increased Risk of Community Acquired Pneumonia (CAP)

Laheij et al. studied 5551 first occurrences of pneumonia occurring among a population of 364,683 individuals. The found that the incidence rate of pneumonia among acid-suppressive users was 2.45 per 100 person-years, compared with 0.6 for those not taking acid-suppressive drugs. The adjusted relative risk of phenomena among those currently using protein pump inhibitors (PPIs) was 1.89 compared with those who ceased using the drugs. For H2-receptor antagonists, the relative risk of developing pneumonia of those taking the drugs compared to non-users was increased 1.63 [1].

Somewhat similar findings were reported in a study of 248 recurrent pneumonia cases in a population of high-risk elderly persons. The authors found that the association was confined to patients beginning acid-suppressing drug use after hospital discharge [2].

Sarkar et al. examined the issue using a nested case-control study involving 80,066 persons with an incident diagnosis of pneumonia and 799,881 controls. They found "a strong increase in risk for CAP" with recent initiation of PPI therapy, but not with longer-term current use of PPI therapy [3].

The rationale is that suppression of gastric acid permits upper gastrointestinal tract pathogens to contaminate the oral and respiratory tracts. The fact that acid-suppressive drugs are readily available over the counter should give us pause. Probably we should discuss the risks of use with certain patients, especially high-risk elderly individuals who have previously experienced pneumonia, and perhaps even with other types of respiratory infections.

References

1. Laheij RJF, Sturkenboom MCJM, Hassing RJ. Risk of community-acquired pneumonia and use of gastric acid-suppressive drugs. JAMA. 2004; 292(16):1955–1960.
2. Eurich DT, Sadowski CA, Simpson SH, et al. Recurrent community-acquired pneumonia in patients starting acid-suppressing drugs. Am J Med. 2010; 123(1):47–53.
3. Sarkar M, Hennessy S, Yang YX. Proton-pump inhibitor use and the risk for community-acquired pneumonia. Ann Intern Med. 2008; 149(6):391–398.

###

Metoclopramide (Reglan) Is the Most Common Cause of Drug-Induced Movement Disorders, Such as Tardive Dyskinesia

Metoclopramide is used to treat diabetic gastroparesis and as therapy for gastroesophageal reflux disease resistant to more commonly used therapy. Use of the drug should not exceed three months, but because the diseases treated are chronic in nature, use sometimes exceeds this recommendation, according to a 2009 report from the U.S. Food and Drug Administration (FDA) [1].

The FDA now requires a boxed warning and a risk mitigation strategy for the use of metoclopramide-containing drugs.

Reference

1. FDA requires boxed warning and risk mitigation strategy for metoclopramide-containing drugs. Available at: http://www.fda.gov/bbs/topics/NEWS/2009/NEW01963.html/ Accessed April 8, 2010.

###

Post-Menopausal Women Who Take Estrogen Plus Progestin and Who Develop Lung Cancer Face a Higher Risk of Death

This finding comes from the Women's Health Initiative trial of 16,608 women ages 50–79 assigned to take estrogen + progestin ($n = 8,506$) versus placebo ($n = 8,102$). The study lasted for more than 5 years. There were 109 cases of lung cancer in the hormone-treated group and 85 in the placebo group. The authors found, "Although treatment with estrogen plus progestin in postmenopausal women did not increase incidence of lung cancer, it increased the number of deaths from lung cancer" [1].

This is one more reason to be wary of hormone replacement therapy, especially in women who smoke.

Reference

1. Chlebowski RT, Schwartz AG, Wakelee H. Estrogen plus progestin and lung cancer in post-menopausal women (Women's Heath Initiative trial): a post-hoc analysis of a randomized controlled trial. Lancet. 2009 Oct 10; 374(9697):1243–1251.

###

Long-Term Users of Metformin May Develop a Vitamin B12 Deficiency

Bell describes this deficiency as occurring in 30% of patients who use this drug for type 2 diabetes, and he describes a case presenting as peripheral neuropathy [1].

This fact may be a practice changer. At the very least, I will not make a diagnosis of diabetic neuropathy in chronic metformin user without checking for a vitamin B12 deficiency. I might even begin checking vitamin B12 levels in diabetic patients with a long-term history of metformin therapy.

Reference

1. Bell DSH. Metformin-induced vitamin B12 deficiency presenting as a peripheral neuropathy. Southern Med J. 2010; 103(3):265–267.

###

Quinine Can Cause Thrombocytopenia Accompanied by Bleeding Symptoms

In fact, scores of medications can cause drug-induced thrombocytopenia. Here I choose to focus on quinine. Why? Because you and I just might encounter this adverse effect in a patient next week. For more than a century we have known that quinine can cause acute thrombocytopenia, chiefly encountered in history in connection with the treatment of malaria [1]. Today quinine is seldom used in malaria treatment or prevention; newer, better and safer drugs are now available. The setting in which you and I just might encounter quinine-induced thrombocytopenia is in the patient with nocturnal leg cramps treated with oral quinine tablets, a management strategy actually supported by some published studies and clinical reviews [2, 3, 4]. The problem is that while the published studies allude to the safety issues with quinine, most speak to "short-term treatment" [3]. Despite these warnings, Aster and Bougie opine that therapy of nocturnal leg cramps may be the most common trigger for quinine-induced thrombocytopenia [1].

A curious cause of quinine-induced thrombocytopenia is "cocktail purpura," caused by the ingestion of heroic amounts of tonic water [5]. Tonic water, a quinine-containing beverage, traces its origins to British soldiers stationed in India, who were required to take quinine to ward off malaria. Because quinine is intensely bitter, the enterprising soldiers flavored and diluted the drug solution with lime, lemon and often gin. When a quinine-containing commercial beverage was first introduced in England in the mid 19th century, it was considered to be a tonic – that is, healthful – because of its quinine content.

References

1. Aster RH, Bougie DW. Drug-induced immune thrombocytopenia. N Engl J Med. 2007;357(6):580–587.
2. Man-Son-Hing M, Wells G. Meta-analysis of efficacy of quinine for treatment of nocturnal leg cramps in elderly people. BMJ. 1995;310(6971):13–17.
3. Diener HC, Dethlefsen U, Dethlefsen-Gruber S, Verbeek P. Effectiveness of quinine in treating muscle cramps: a double-blind, placebo-controlled, parallel group, multi-center trial. Int J Clin Pract. 2002;56(4):243–246.
4. Butler JV, Mulkerrin EC, O'Keeffe ST. Nocturnal leg cramps in older people. Postgrad Med J. 2002;78:596–598.
5. Korbitz BC, Eisner E. Cocktail purpura: quinine-dependent thrombocytopenia. Rocky Mt Med J. 1973;70(10):38–41.

###

Mefloquine (Lariam) Can Cause Acute Psychosis

This antimalarial drug is used for prophylaxis and therapy. One possible side effect, however, is the development of acute psychosis, documented in several published reports [1, 2, 3].

This drug should be prescribed with caution for anyone planning to operate a motor vehicle, or perhaps, for that matter, to be in close proximity to wild animals while on safari.

References

1. Sowunmi A, Adio RA, Ouola AM, Ogundahunsi OA, Salako LA. Acute psychosis after mefloquine: report of six cases. Trop Geogr Med. 1995;47(4):179–180.
2. Havaldar PV, Mogale K. Mefloquine-induced psychosis. Ped Inf Dis J. 2000;19(2):166–167.
3. Dietz A, Frölich L. Mefloquine-induced paranoid psychosis and subsequent major depression in a 25-year-old student. Pharmacopsychiatry. 2002;35(5):200–202.

###

Oral Bisphosphonates May Offer Some Protection Against Invasive Breast Cancer

Two studies described at the 32nd Annual San Antonio Breast Cancer Symposium held December 10, 2009, suggest that patients taking oral bisphosphonates for postmenopausal osteoporosis may experience some protection against invasive breast cancer. Dr Rowan Chlebowski of Harbor-UCLA Medical Center in Los Angeles, California analyzed data on 151,592 women in the Womens' Health Initiative trial, of whom 2,216 took oral bisphosphonates. They found 32% less invasive breast cancer in women using bisphosphonates compared with those who did not. There was, however, a higher incidence of ductal carcinoma in situ (DCIS) in bisphosphonate users.

The second paper presented at this conference, by Gar Rennert from Israel, described a case-control study of 2,368 patients with newly diagnosed breast cancer compared with matched control individuals. They found a statistically significant 34% reduction in the incidence of breast cancer. This study found no difference in the incidence of DCIS between the two groups [1].

As of this writing, these reports of these two studies were still not found in the print literature. Although I prefer to present studies readily available for readers to review, I included this new data here because the findings may influence practice decisions.

Reference

1. Presented at the 32nd Annual San Antonio Breast Cancer Symposium, San Antonio, Texas, December 10, 2009. A report can be found at: Oral bisphosphonates may prevent invasive breast cancer. Available at: http://medscape.com/viewarticle/713714?src=mpnews&spon=er&&uac=95007MG/ Accessed April 8, 2010.

Dopaminergic Agents Can Cause Pathologic Gambling

Perhaps this unlikely adverse effect is no longer a secret; I have seen it mentioned in direct-to-consumer television advertisements for these drugs. But what may be noteworthy is that such occurrence is not really rare. A study of 388 Parkinson disease patients conducted in Scotland revealed that 8% of patients taking dopamine antagonists developed problematic gambling [1].

We may remember to monitor our parkinsonian patients using dopaminergic agents for gambling problems, but as in the case of quinine-induced purpura in patients with nocturnal leg cramps, there is another situation in which the drug-induced urge to gamble may occur. Pramipexole (Mirapex) is now a fashionable therapy for the treatment of restless leg syndrome and these patients are not immune from this drug's side effects.

Reference

1. Grosset KA, Macphee G, Pal G. Problematic gambling on dopamine agonists: not such a rarity. Mov Disord. 2006;21(12):2206–2208.

###

Phosphodiesterase Type 5 (PDE5) Inhibitors Can Cause Sudden Hearing Impairment

In April, 2007 Mukherjee and Shivakumar in India reported a single case of sensorineural deafness following use of sildenafil (Viagra) [1]. In response to this single report the FDA, acting with uncharacteristic urgency, searched its adverse event reporting system for similar events. They found 29 instances of sudden hearing loss associated with use of the various PDE5 inhibitors available. The labeling for these drugs now includes a warning about the potential for hearing loss [2].

Kudos to Mukherjee and Shivakumar, whose paper contains the statement, "We could not find any previously reported cases of sildenafil induced hearing loss and to the best of our knowledge, this is the first case report of sildenafil induced sensorineural hearing loss in the world literature" [1]. It seems they were actually the first.

References

1. Mukherjee B, Shivakumar T. A case of sensorineural deafness following ingestion of sildenafil. J Laryngol Otol. 2007;121(4):395–397.
2. FDA Information for Healthcare Professionals: sildenafil (marketed as Viagra and Revatio), vardenafil (marketed as Levitra), tadalafil (marketed as Cialis). Available at: http://www.fda.gov/Drugs/DrugSafety/PostmarketDrugSafetyInformationforPatientsandProviders/ucm124841.htm/ Accessed April 8, 2010.

###

Methylphenidate (Ritalin) Can Cause Complex Visual Hallucinations

A recent report describes a 15 year old boy who received methylphenidate to treat attention-deficit hyperactivity disorder (ADHD). Following the first dose of the drug, he suffered hallucinations of rats running around, and touching and smelling him. The hallucinations ceased when the drug was stopped, but returned when the drug was administered again 7 years later [1].

Long used for children with ADHD, methylphenidate has become a popular treatment for adult ADHD. Thus methylphenidate-induced complex visual hallucinations may be seen in children or adults.

Reference

1. Halevy A, Shuper A. Methylphenidate induction of complex visual hallucinations. J Child Neurol. 2009;24(8):1005–1007.

###

Idiopathic Intracranial Hypertension (ICH), Aka Pseudotumor Cerebri, Has Been Linked to Lithium Therapy

Idiopathic intracranial hypertension presents as a triad of headache, bilateral papilledema and increased intracranial pressure, in the absence of intracranial mass, hydrocephalus or localizing neurologic manifestations. Levine and Puchalski describe two instances in which ICH developed in patients taking lithium as therapy of bipolar disorder [1].

> *The disease is part of the differential diagnosis of chronic headache, although other etiologies, such as migraine, are much more prevalent. ICH can also be related to obesity, steroid therapy, pituitary insufficiency, Vitamin A toxicity, head trauma, Addison disease and Cushing disease.*

Reference

1. Levine SH, Puchalski C. Pseudotumor cerebri associated with lithium therapy in two patients. J Clin Psychiatry. 1991;52(5):239–241.

###

Human Immunodeficiency Virus (HIV)-Infected Patients Are at Greatly Increased Risk of Severe Cutaneous Reactions to Some of the Very Drugs Used to Treat the Disease and Its Complications

The drug-induced effects can include Stevens-Johnson syndrome and toxic epidermal necrolysis, with a potential for severe morbidity and even death. Drug that may precipitate such effects include sulfonamides and antiretroviral medications [1, 2].

Why do HIV-infected patient have such an increased risk of serious cutaneous reactions to drugs? An apparently obvious answer may be repeated exposure to drugs, especially to antibiotics. Other possible contributing factors include abnormalities of the immune system, impaired acetylation of circulating drugs, and the impact of a variety of infections.

References

1. Rotunda A, Hirsch RJ, Scheinfeld N, Weinberg JM. Severe cutaneous reactions associated with the use of human immunodeficiency virus medications. Acta Derm Venereol. 2003;83(1):1–9.
2. Slatore CG, Tilles SA. Sulfonamide hypersensitivity. Immunol Allergy Clin North Am. 2004;24(3):477–490.

###

Gadolinium-Based Contrast Agents Can Cause Nephrogenic Systemic Fibrosis (NSF)

First elucidated in 1997, nephrogenic systemic fibrosis may be one of those diseases we don't think much about, but should. NSF is an iatrogenic, progressive, and potentially fatal multiorgan-system fibrosing disease that occurs when patients with renal impairment are exposed to the gadolinium-based contrast agents used to enhance magnetic resonance (MR) imaging. The link between the disease and MR imaging was not recognized until 2006. We now know that, when gadolinium-based contrast agents are used in patients with severe renal insufficiency, we can expect 4% of these individuals to develop NSF [1].

Mortality following the development of NSF can approach 31%, making this a serious consideration when ordering MR imaging in a patient who may have renal insufficiency.

Reference

1. Schlaudecker JD, Bernheisel CR. Gadolinium-associated nephrogenic systemic fibrosis. Am Fam Phys. 2009;80(7):711–714.

#####

Chapter 11
Drug Interactions and Adventures in Polypharmacy

Every drug we prescribe is an experiment in applied pharmacotherapy.

Taylor RB, Medical Wisdom and Doctoring [1]

The use of two or more drugs simultaneously can be perilous, as shown by the following case:

The patient was an 18-year-old young woman admitted to the hospital with a tentative diagnosis of "viral syndrome with hysterical symptoms." At the time of her admission, she was under treatment with phenelzine (Nardil). About 90 min after entering the hospital, she was given meperidine (Demerol) for agitation. Her agitation increased; she became confused and was thrashing about in the bed, prompting therapy with intramuscular haloperidol (Haldol).

A few hours later she was found to have a high fever, which was followed by respiratory arrest and death.

The patient described above had classic manifestations of the serotonin syndrome, the result of serotonergic stimulation of central nervous system and peripheral receptors. The syndrome is characterized by: (1) mental status changes such as agitation, confusion or hallucinations; (2) somatic effects such as tremor, hyperreflexia, or muscle twitching; and (3) autonomic manifestations such as shivering, tachycardia, hypertension or high fever. Boyer and Shannon points out, "Clinical manifestations of the serotonin syndrome range from barely perceptible to lethal" [2]. The following is a list of just some of the drugs and herbal products that, when used in combination, can be involved in serotonin syndrome:

Monoamine oxidase inhibitors: phenelzine and others
Triptans, such as sumatriptan (Imitrex)
Ergot alkaloids
Meperidine
Dextroamphetamine, found in widely-available cough remedies
Amphetamine derivatives and methylphenidate (Ritalin)
Tricyclic antidepressants: amitriptyline (Elavil) and others
Selective serotonin reuptake derivatives: fluoxetine (Prozac) and others
Serotonin-norepinephrine reuptake inhibitors: trazodone (Desyrel) and others

R.B. Taylor, *Essential Medical Facts Every Clinician Should Know: To Prevent Medical Errors, Pass Board Examinations and Provide Informed Patient Care*, DOI 10.1007/978-1-4419-7874-5_11, © Springer Science+Business Media, LLC 2011

Chlorpheniramine (Chlor-Trimeton)
Lithium (Eskalith)
Oxycodone (OxyContin), hydrocodone, and fentanyl (Actiq)
Valproate (Depakote)
Cocaine
Herbal remedies, including St. John's wort, nutmeg, and Panax ginseng

The astute reader will have recognized the case above as describing the sad tale of Libby Zion, whose death in 1984 at a New York City hospital was the subject of a grand jury investigation, leading to the conclusion that key factors responsible were interns and residents serving for long hours without sleep and without adequate supervision by attending physicians. The outcome was the imposition of an average 80 h workweek with a maximum of 24 consecutive hours for house staff, first in New York State, and later nationally [2, 3].

This chapter presents a selection of drug–drug interactions, as well as the interactions of some drugs with herbal remedies. When we ponder the potential of any patient to take almost any combination of medications, the numbers of possibilities are staggering. Of the literally millions of drug–drug and drug–herb interactions one might encounter, I have tried to present those that are especially clinically relevant.

References

1. Taylor RB. Medical wisdom and doctoring: the art of 21st century medicine. New York: Springer, 2010. Chapter 5.
2. Boyer EW, Shannon M. The serotonin syndrome. N Engl J Med. 2005;352(11):1112–1120.
3. Block AJ. Revisiting the Libby Zion case. Chest. 1994;105(4):977.

###

Our Patients Take a Lot of Drugs and Herbal Remedies, and Hence Have Abundant Opportunities for Drug Interactions

A telephone survey of a random sample of the US population elicited responses from 2,590 adult individuals. Of these, half of all respondents used at least one prescription medication, and 7% took five or more. Who were the leading consumers of prescription medications? Of women age 65 and over, 23% took five or more medications and 12% used at least ten prescription drugs. Of those responding to the survey, 14% reported using herbal/supplement products [1].

And so what about interactions among these drugs? A group of 100 consecutive hospitalized cancer patients were studied for drug interactions. In this study, patients receiving chemotherapy or hormone therapy were excluded. Among these individuals, the average patient was taking eight drugs. Potential interactions were detected in 63 patients, and 18.3% of these potential interactions were considered to be severe [2].

In another study, this one conducted in Brazil, the records of 102 patients in an intensive care setting were reviewed. Of these individuals, 72.5% were exposed to 311 potential drug interactions [3].

Any patient taking five or more drugs lives in a pharmacologic never-land, with the multiple possibilities for advers e effects challenging even the capabilities of today's computer programs.

References

1. Kaufman DW, Kelly JP, Rosenberg L, Anderson TE, Mitchell AA. Recent patterns of medication use in the ambulatory adult population of the United States: the Slone survey. JAMA. 2002;287(3):337–344.
2. Riechelmann RP, Moreira F, Smaletz O, Saad ED. Potential for drug interactions in hospitalized cancer patients. Cancer Chemother Pharmacol. 2005;56(3):286–290.
3. Lima RE, De Bortoli-Cassiani SH. Potential drug interactions in intensive care patients at a teaching hospital. Rev Lat Am Enfermagem. 2009;17(2):222–227.

###

Drugs with a Narrow Therapeutic Range Pose an Extra Risk of Drug–Drug Adverse Effects

Many drug–drug adverse reactions arise when Drug A leads to increased serum levels of Drug B. When Drug B has a narrow therapeutic range, there is a greater risk of toxicity. Here are some drugs that can have a narrow therapeutic range:

Phenytoin
Divalproex
Digitalis
Phenobarbital
Lithium carbonate
Procainamide
Primidone
Quinidine
Theophylline
Procainamide
Tacrolimus

A study by Raebel et al. involving 17,748 patients revealed that many patients taking narrow-therapeutic-range drugs did not receive serum drug concentration monitoring. Specifically they found no monitoring in more than half of all patients taking digoxin, theophylline, procainamide, quinidine, or primidone [1].

Here is an example of what might occur: Two commonly prescribed drugs – ciprofloxacin and cimetidine – can increase serum levels of theophylline. Admittedly, theophylline is not used as commonly as in the past, but neither has it vanished from pharmacy shelves. Both of these drugs are used to treat conditions that might co-exist with asthma or other chronic lung disease treated with theophylline [2, 3]. And in what is probably a historical curiosity, I even found a report of impaired elimination of theophylline after influenza vaccination [4].

References

1. Raebel MA, Carroll NM, Andrade SE, et al. Monitoring of drugs with a narrow therapeutic range in ambulatory care. Am J Manag Care. 2006;12(5):268–274.
2. Raoof S, Wollschlager C, Kahn FA. Ciprofloxacin increases serum levels of theophylline. Am J Med. 1987;82(4A):115–118.
3. Adebayo GI, Coker HAB. Cimetidine inhibition of theophylline elimination: the influence of adult age and the time course. Biopharm Drug Dispos. 2006;8(2):149–158.
4. Renton KW, Gray JD, Hall RI. Decreased elimination of theophylline after influenza vaccination. Can Med Assoc J. 1980;123(4):288–290.

###

Some Adverse Drug–Drug Interactions Involve Decreased Efficacy of One of the Drugs

Such is the case of rifampin and oral contraceptive (OC) drugs. A review of 167 articles revealed at least 30 instances of pregnancies occurring in women taking antibiotics, notably rifampin (Rifadin). Following analysis of data the authors report: "Rifampin impairs the effectiveness of OCs. Pharmacokinetic studies of other antibiotics have not shown any systematic interaction between antibiotics and OC steroids. However, individual patients do show large decreases in the plasma concentrations of ethinyl estradiol when they take certain other antibiotics, notably tetracycline and penicillin derivatives" [1].

Archer and Archer, following a literature review, are more direct, invoking the word "myth." They conclude: "Available scientific and pharmacokinetic data do not support the hypothesis that antibiotics (with the exception of rifampin) lower the contraceptive efficacy of oral contraceptives" [2].

I think two considerations are pertinent here. First of all, many of the reports of oral contraceptive failure associated with antibiotic use are anecdotal, subjective and, in some cases, influenced by litigation. Second, although rifampin is not a drug most of us prescribe every day, tetracycline and penicillin and their cousins are. Strep throat is common in young, fertile women, and penicillin is still a preferred remedy. And, many young women using oral contraceptives have acne, for which a prescription for an oral tetracycline derivative might be considered reasonable.

References

1. Dickinson BD, Altman RD, Nielson NH, Sterling ML, for the Council on Scientific Affairs, American Medical Association. Obstet Gyn. 2001;98(5):853–860.
2. Archer JSM, Archer DF. Oral contraceptives efficacy and antibiotic interaction: a myth debunked. J Am Acad Dermatol. 2002;46(6):917–923.

###

Much of the Risk of Drug–Drug Interactions is Preventable, if Only We Could Reduce the Incidence of Inappropriate Prescribing

Steinman et al. studied 196 outpatients age 65 and older who were taking five or more medications. Of these individuals, 128 (65%) were found to be using one or more inappropriate medications, including 112 (57%) taking a medication that was considered not indicated, ineffective or duplicative. The leading drugs considered to be prescribed inappropriately were: histamine antagonists, digitalis glycosides, loop diuretics, proton pump inhibitors, tricyclic antidepressants, urinary antispasmodics, nasal anti-inflammatory drugs, sedating antihistamines, and non-steroidal antiinflammatory drugs (NSAIDs) [1].

This study also identified some underused drugs, including antihypertensives, anticoagulants, lipid-lowering agents, sublingual nitroglycerin, hypoglycemic agents, and calcium. I found it curious that protein pump inhibitors appeared on both of the lists, the most inappropriate and the most underused medications [1].

In addition to inappropriate prescribing, there are other risk factors for adverse drug interactions. Here are some of them:

- *Age: Infants, young children and the elderly are likely to metabolize drugs less efficiently than those in between these age groups.*
- *Chronic disease: Renal or liver disease may be associated with delayed metabolism or clearance, leading to increased serum levels of drugs.*
- *Acute disease: Severe infection, dehydration, or acute metabolic disturbances, such as diabetic acidosis, may affect drug catabolism or elimination.*
- *Cognitive dysfunction: Persons with diminished mental capacity may not take their medications as advised, and may be prone to overdosage. "If one pill is good, two or three must be better."*
- *Complex dosing regimens: The more confusing the medication plan, the more opportunities there are for error.*

Reference

1. Steinman MA, Landefeld CS, Rosenthal GE, Berthenthal D, Sen S, Kaboli PJ. Polypharmacy and prescribing quality in older people. J Am Geriatr Soc. 2006;54(10):1516–1523.

###

Nonsteroidal Antiinflammatory Drugs Can Blunt the Cardioprotective Effect of Aspirin

Gladding et al. studied the antiplatelet effects of six commonly used NSAIDs in regard to their potential to antagonize the effect of aspirin. The found that four agents – ibuprofen, indomethacin, naproxen, and tiaprofenic acid – block aspirin's antiplatelet action, while sulindac and celecoxib did not [1]. However, a subsequent study by Rimon et al. in dogs found that the administration of celecoxib, a non-steroidal antiinflammatory drug that selectively inhibits cyclooxygenase-2 (COX-2), can interfere with the ability of low dose aspirin to impede platelet aggregation [2].

> In an interview, Dr. William L. Smith of University of Michigan, Ann Arbor, describes a method that might avoid the loss of aspirin's antithrombotic effect. He suggests taking the low-dose aspirin at least 15–30 min before the celecoxib is taken, "because the effect of aspirin on platelets is rather quick." He goes on the state that taking the two drugs simultaneously will make it almost certain that the aspirin "won't be working" [3].
>
> I return to the topic of NSAIDs and the use of low-dose aspirin in Chap. 14, where I tell about a somewhat questionable advertising campaign that seems to contradict the many studies describing the blunting effect on aspirin's antiplatelet activity.

References

1. Gladding PA, Webster MW, Farrell HB, Zeng IS, Park R, Ruijne N. The antiplatelet effect of six non-steroidal anti-inflammatory drugs and their pharmacodynamic interaction with aspirin in healthy volunteers. Am J Cardiol. 2008;101(7):1060–1063.
2. Rimon G, Sidhu RS, Lauver DA, et al. Coxibs interfere with the action of aspirin by binding tightly to one monomer of cyclooxygenase-1. Proc Natl Acad Sci U S A. 2010;107(1):28–33.
3. Nainggolan L. Celecoxib could impede effects of low-dose aspirin. Medscape. Available at http://www.medscape.com/viewarticle/714041?src=mpnews&spon=34&uac=95007MG/. Accessed April 12, 2010.

###

NSAIDs, Including Selective Cyclooxygenase 2 Inhibitors, Can Increase Serum Lithium Concentrations, Leading to Toxicity

A review of the U.S. Food and Drug Administration (FDA) Adverse Event Reporting System and a literature search using PubMed turned up 18 instances of increased lithium serum levels when a COX-2 inhibitor was added to stable lithium therapy [1].

> *Although the study focused on the COX-2 inhibitors, the authors note finding reports of increased lithium levels with aspirin, sulindac and 14 other NSAIDs, making NSAID use a prime suspect when a patient develops lithium toxicity [1].*

Reference

1. Phelan KM, Mosholdler AD, Lu S. Lithium interaction with the cyclooxygenase 2 inhibitors rofecoxib and celecoxib and other nonsteroidal anti-inflammatory agents. J Clin Psychiatry. 2003;64(11):1328–1334.

###

In the Setting of Aspirin and Clopidogrel (Plavix) Used to Prevent Cardiovascular Disease, Doses of Aspirin 100 mg or Greater Taken with Clopidogrel May (Note: *May*) Be Harmful

The data supporting this statement comes from a post hoc observational analysis of data from a double-blind, placebo-controlled, randomized trail involving 15,595 patients with cardiovascular disease or multiple risk factors. Clopidogrel, an anti-platelet drug, is used to prevent blood clots that could cause heart attacks or strokes. In patients taking only aspirin they found no clear benefit for doses of 100 mg or greater. The drug interaction picture is a little murky and did not reach statistical significance. Nevertheless, here is what was found: "In patients also receiving clopidogrel, daily aspirin doses greater than 100 mg seemed to be non-statistically associated with reduced efficacy (adjusted hazard ration, 1.16 [CI, 0.93–1.44]) and increased harm (adjusted hazard ratio, 1.30 [CI, 0.83–2.04])" [1].

> *The increased harm refers to events such as severe or life-threatening bleeding. For me, this study is more evidence supporting the use of low dose versus higher dose aspirin. The issue of dual antiplatelet therapy is yet to be resolved.*

Reference

1. Steinhubl SR, Bhatt DL, Brennan DM. Aspirin to prevent cardiovascular disease: the association of aspirin dose and clopidogrel with thrombosis and bleeding. Ann Intern Med. 2009;150(6):379–386.

###

"Patients at Risk for Heart Attacks or Strokes Who Use Clopidogrel to Prevent Blood Clots Will Not Get the Full Effect of This Medicine if They Are Also Taking Omeprazole." Maybe

The quotation above is from an FDA alert, dated November 17, 2009, regarding clopidogrel (Plavix) and omeprazole (Prilosec) [1]. The "maybe" is added because not all concur with the FDA opinion. Because clopidogrel can cause upper gastrointestinal distress, proton pump inhibitors are often prescribed concomitantly. The cognitive dissonance arises because study results disagree. Gilard reports from France that clopidogrel activity on platelets is diminished in patients receiving proton pump inhibitor (PPI) treatment [2]. Another study of 8,205 patients in U.S. Veterans Affairs hospitals also led to the conclusion: "Concomitant use of clopidogrel and PPI after hospital discharge for acute coronary syndrome (ACS) was associated with an increased risk of adverse outcomes than the use of clopidogrel without PPI, suggesting that the use of PPI may be associated with attenuation of benefits of clopidogrel after ACS" [3].

Other studies, including two randomized trials, have not found that the use of a PPI leads to an impaired response to clopidogrel [4, 5]. In a review of current data, Laine and Henneken conclude: "Thus, current evidence does not justify a conclusion that PPIs are associated with cardiovascular events among clopidogrel users, let alone a judgment of causality" [6].

Of course, there is another issue: the incidence of gastrointestinal bleeding. A cohort study involving 20,596 patients in the Tennessee Medicaid Program involved assessment of prescription records and hospitalizations for gastroduodenal bleeding and serious cardiovascular disease. In this study, the adjusted incidence of hospitalization for gastrointestinal bleeding in concurrent PPI users was 50% lower than in those using clopidogrel alone [7]. Rassen et al., after reviewing the records of 18,565 patients with coronary artery disease treated with clopidogrel with or without PPI use, concluded: "Although point estimates indicated a slightly increased risk of myocardial infarction hospitalization or death in older patients initiating both clopidogrel and a PPI, we did not observe conclusive evidence of a clopidogrel–PPI interaction of major clinical relevance. Our data suggest that if this exists, it is unlikely to exceed a 20% risk increase" [8].

The question of clopidogrel–PPI use continues to linger and further randomized clinical trials will help bring clarity. In the meantime, Laine and Henneken suggest a tactic that may prove useful: "As the presence of PPIs and clopidogrel in plasma is short lived, separation by 12–20 h should in theory prevent competitive inhibition of CYP (cytochrome P450) metabolism and minimize any potential, though unproven, clinical interaction. PPI may be given before breakfast and clopidogrel at bedtime, or PPI may be taken before dinner and clopidogrel at lunchtime" [6].

References

1. Information for Healthcare Professionals: Update to the labeling of clopidogrel bisulfate (marketed as Plavix) to alert healthcare professionals about a drug interaction with omeprazole (marketed as Prilosec and Prilosec OTC). U.S. Food and Drug Administration. Available at: http://www.fda.gov/Drugs/DrugSafety/PostmarketDrugSafetyInformationforPatients andProviders/DrugSafetyInformationforHeathcareProfessionals/ucm190787.htm/. Accessed April 12, 2010.
2. Gilard M, Arnaud B, Cornily JC, et al. Influence of omeprazole on the antiplatelet action of clopidogrel associated with aspirin: the randomized, double-blind OCLA (Omeprazole Clopidogrel Aspirin) study. J Am Coll Cardiol. 2008;51(3):256–260.
3. Ho PM, Maddox TM, Want L, et al. Risk of adverse outcomes associated with concomitant use of clopidogrel and proton pump inhibitors following acute coronary syndrome. JAMA. 2009;301(9):937–944.
4. Siller-Matula JM, Spiel AO, Lang IM, Kreiner G, Christ G, Jilma B. Effects of pantoprazole and esomeprazole on platelet inhibition by clopidogrel. Am Heart J. 2009;157(1):148.e1–e5.
5. O'Donoghue ML, Braunwald E, Antman EM, et al. Pharmacodynamic effect and clinical efficacy of clopidogrel and prasugrel with or without a proton pump inhibitor: an analysis of two randomized trials. Lancet. 2009;374(9694):989–997.
6. Laine L, Henneken C. Proton pump inhibitor and clopidogrel interaction: fact or fiction? Am J Gastroenterol. 2009;105(1):34–41.
7. Ray WA, Murray KT, Griffin MR, et al. Outcomes with concurrent use of clopidogrel and proton-pump inhibitor. Ann Intern Med. 2010;152(6):337–345.
8. Rassen JA, Choudhry NK, Avorn J, Schneeweiss S. Cardiovascular outcomes and mortality in patients using clopidogrel with proton pump inhibitors after percutaneous coronary intervention or acute coronary syndrome. Circulation. 2009;120(23):2322–2329.

###

Carisoprodol (Soma) and Oxycodone (OxyContin) Can Have Additive Depressant Effects on the Central Nervous System (CNS)

Reeves and Mack report the case of a 49 year old woman receiving 40 mg of OxyContin b.i.d. for arthritis of the lumbar spine who developed CNS and respiratory depression following the addition of carisoprodol in a dose increased from one 350 mg tablet q.i.d. to 8–10 tablets daily. She responded promptly to intravenous naloxone.

The authors remind us that Soma is metabolized to meprobamate (Miltown), a controlled substance with CNS depressant activity and abuse potential [1].

A review of Idaho Medicaid pharmacy and medical claims identified long-term users of carisoprodol (n = 340) and other skeletal muscle relaxants (n = 453). The authors of the study found that, when compared to other users of skeletal muscle relaxants, carisoprodol users utilized concomitant opioids more often and had more past diagnoses indicating other drug dependence and abuse [2]. For the record, in our university-based family medicine clinic, we consider a specific patient request for a Soma prescription to be a warning sign that might indicate substance abuse.

References

1. Reeves RR, Mack JE. Possible dangerous interaction of OxyContin and carisoprodol. Am Fam Phys. 2003;67(11):2273.
2. Owens C, Pugmire B, Salness T, et al. Abuse potential of carisoprodol: a retrospective review of Idaho Medicaid pharmacy and medical claims data. Clin Ther. 2007;29(10):2222–2225.

###

Selective Serotonin Reuptake Inhibitors (SSRIs), Notably Paroxetine (Paxil), Can Blunt the Effectiveness of Tamoxifen as Anti-estrogen Adjuvant Treatment of Hormone-Dependent Breast Cancer

In a retrospective, population-based cohort study of 2,430 women with breast cancer treated with tamoxifen and a single SSRI, 374 (15%) died of their disease during follow-up. The chief drug implicated was paroxetine. Patients taking Paxil during more than half of their tamoxifen course of therapy experienced a 54% increase in breast cancer mortality, with the figure rising to a 91% increased risk if paroxetine was used during 75% of the course of tamoxifen therapy. In contrast, the authors report that no such risk was seen with other antidepressants [1].

The effectiveness of tamoxifen as an anti-estrogen depends on its conversion to its metabolite, endoxifen, a conversion that require the action of the hepatic drug-metabolizing enzyme cytochrome P450 2D6 (CYP2D6). A reduction in activity of this enzyme can occur because of the individual's genotype or, more to the point here, by administration of drugs such as paroxetine that inhibit its action [2].

Up to one quarter of women with breast cancer suffer depression in the year following diagnosis, and half of them receive medication. In the setting, an SSRI would seem a logical choice, and so the recent finding of SSRI blunting the effect of tamoxifen is worrisome.

Not all are sanguine that the only culprit is paroxetine; fluoxetine (Prozac) is also as potent inhibitor of CYP2D6 [3]. Lash suggests that citalopram (Celexa) can be safely used in patients taking tamoxifen [4]. Another alternative is to use an aromatase inhibitor instead of tamoxifen in patients requiring SSRI antidepressant therapy; aromatase inhibitors are not affected by CYP2D6 [3].

References

1. Kelly CM, Juurlink DN, Gomes T, et al. Selective serotonin reuptake inhibitors and breast cancer mortality in women receiving tamoxifen: a population based cohort study. BMJ. 2010;340:c693. doi: 10.1136/bmj.c693.
2. Hoskins JM, Carey LA, McLeod HL. CYP2D6 and tamoxifen: DNA matters in breast cancer. Nat Rev Cancer. 2009;9(8):576–586.
3. Tamoxifen, SSRIs, and breast cancer recurrence. Pharmacology Watch. September, 2009; page 1.
4. Lash TL, Cronin-Fentin D, Ahern TP, et al. Breast cancer recurrence risk related to concurrent use of SSRI antidepressants and tamoxifen. Acta Oncol. 2010;49(3):305–312.

###

The Combination of Adderall-XR and Alcohol Can Be Associated with Myocardial Infarction

A brief report describes the death of a young man who suffered a myocardial infarction after taking two 15-mg tablets of Adderall XR with alcohol [1]. A combination of dextroamphetamine and amphetamine, Adderall is used to treat attention deficit/ hyperactivity disorder (ADHD) and narcolepsy. The medication also enjoys some popularity as a "recreational substance."

Rare incidents of sudden death with Adderall, unrelated to alcohol use, have been reported. A review of 20 such deaths, 14 of which occurred in children, prompted Canada to suspend all sales of Adderall-XR in 2005. The U.S. FDA has not taken a similar approach [2].

References

1. Jiao X, Velez S, Ringstad J, Eyma V, Miller D, Bleiberg M. Myocardial infarction associated with Adderall XR and alcohol use in a young man. J Am Board Fam Med. 2009;22(2):197–201.
2. Rosak J. U.S. regulators puzzled by Canada's ruling on safety of ADHD drug. Psychiatric News. 2005;40(5):2.

###

Concomitant Use of an Angiotensin Converting Enzyme (ACE) Inhibitor and an Angiotensin Receptor Blocker (ARB) Brings No Added Benefit when Compared with Adequate Doses of One of the Drugs, but Is Associated with More Adverse Events

Both ACE inhibitors and ARBs are used in patients at risk for vascular events. In a study of patients with vascular disease or high-risk diabetes randomized to receive the ACE inhibitor ramipril (n = 8,576), the ARB telmisartan (n = 8,452) or a combination of both (n = 8,502), researchers looked at a primary composite outcome: death from cardiovascular causes, myocardial infarction, stroke, or hospitalization for heart failure. The telmisartan group had less cough and less angioedema than the ramipril group. As to the primary composite outcome at a median follow-up of 56 months, telmisartan was found to be equivalent to ramipril. However, the authors report, "The combination of the two drugs was associated with more adverse events without an increase in benefit" [1].

Four months after publication of the paper just described there was another paper published by the same group on the same topic of using ACE inhibitors and ARBS. The same participants (a ramipril group of 8,576 subjects, etc.) and same randomization methods are described. The key difference seems to be that here the authors report on renal outcomes, finding telmisartan effects to be similar to those of ramipril, and that combined therapy reduces proteinuria to a greater extent than monotherapy, while overall causing worse major renal outcomes [2].

Paper number 1 was published in the New England Journal of Medicine; paper number 2 was published in Lancet, although with some changes in the authors' names listed. Thus I suspect both papers were under review by different journals at the same time. Was the editor of each prestigious journal aware of the other paper? Would anything have been lost if the renal findings had been included in the first paper? Might some uncharitable reviewer consider these to be Chain Letter Publications in which a research group lets various members be first author by submitting an ongoing series of papers that present just a little more data from an ongoing study? [3] Can we look for future papers to come from the ONTARGET study group?

References

1. ONTARGET Investigators, Yusef S, Teo KK, Pogue J, et al. Telmisartan, ramipril, or both in patients at high risk for vascular events. N Engl J Med. 2008;358(15):1547–1559.
2. Mann JF, Schmieder RE, McQueen M, et al (ONTARGET Investigators). Renal outcomes with telmisartan, ramipril, or both, in people at high vascular risk (the ONTARGET study): a multicentre, randomized, double-blind controlled trial. Lancet. 2008;372(9638): 547–553.
3. Taylor RB. The clinician's guide to medical writing. New York: Springer, 2005; page 217.

###

The Combination of Trimethoprim-Sulfa with Angiotensin-Converting Enzyme Inhibitors or Angiotensin Receptor Blockers Can Result in Hyperkalemia

Antoniou et al. report a study of patients age 66 and older receiving continuous ACE inhibitor or ARB therapy who were prescribed trimethoprim–sulfamethoxazole, amoxicillin, ciprofloxacin, norfloxacin, or nitrofurantoin (the study group). These patients were matched with controls with similar age, sex, and concurrent diseases. At the end of 14 years, during which there were 4,148 admissions involving hyperkalemia, the study group had a nearly sevenfold increased risk (adjusted odds ratio of 6.7) of hyperkalemia-associated hospitalization with the use of trimethoprim–sulfamethoxazole when compared specifically with the use of ampicillin. In fact, increased risk was not found with any of the other comparator antibiotics [1].

*The authors use the phrase "major increase in the risk of hyperkalemia-associated hospitalization relative to other antibiotics" [1]. I think of this in the context of the many instances in which we use trimethoprim–sulfamethoxazole, including urinary tract infections and skin infections suspected of harboring methicillin-resistant Staphylococcus aureus (MRSA). Knowing the drug interaction described here may be a **practice changer** when selecting an antibiotic for use in a patient taking a renin–angiotensin system inhibitor.*

Reference

1. Antoniou T, Gomes T, Juurlink DN, et al. Trimethoprim–sulfamethoxazole-induced hyperkalemia in patients receiving inhibitors of the renin–angiotensin system. Arch Intern Med. 2010;170(12):1045–1049.

###

Combining a Fibrate with a Statin Drug Increases the Risk of Rhabdomyolysis

Chang et al. examined the FDA postmarketing database for reports of rhabdomyolysis in connection with statin or statin-gemfibrozil therapy. They found a total of 866 reported cases. The risk of rhabdomyolysis is more than four times greater with combined therapy than with statin monotherapy: 4.24 cases/100,000 prescriptions for combined therapy versus <1/100,000 for statin use alone [1].

Although rare, statin-induced rhabdomyolysis is serious. Chang et el found that hospitalization for renal failure and dialysis was required in more than 80% of reported cases. The fourfold+ greater risk with combined therapy becomes especially worrisome, since a randomized trial conducted by the ACCORD Study Group of 5,518 patients with type 2 diabetes led to the following conclusion: "The combination of fenofibrate and simvastatin did not reduce the rate of fatal cardiovascular events, nonfatal myocardial infarction, or nonfatal stroke, as compared with simvastatin alone" [2].

References

1. Chang JT, Staffa JA, Parks M, Green L. Rhabdomyolysis with HMG-CoA reductase inhibitors and gemfibrozil combination therapy. Pharmacoepidemiol Drug Saf. 2004;13(7):417–426.
2. ACCORD Study Group. Effects of combination lipid therapy in type 2 diabetes mellitus. N Engl J Med. 2010;362(17):1563–1574.

###

Ketoconazole (Nizoral) Can Increase Plasma Concentrations of Mefloquine (Lariam)

Coadministration of mefloquine and ketoconazole can lead to increased levels of the antimalarial drug, mefloquine, according to an open, randomized two-phase crossover study conducted in eight healthy male volunteers [1].

Mefloquine is frequently used for malaria prophylaxis in travelers to areas where there are susceptible strains of the disease-causing parasite. Mefloquine is also noteworthy for causing an especially troubling side effect, a drug-induced psychosis, as described in Chap. 10, providing an extra incentive for maintaining recommended serum levels of the drug [2].

I include this interaction as potentially relevant to daily practice for this reason: Isn't it just possible that the patient requesting malaria prophylaxis medication just might be taking oral doses of ketoconazole for onychomycosis? Parenthetically, rifampin, used for malaria prophylaxis and tuberculosis therapy, can cause a similar elevation of mefloquine serum levels [3].

References

1. Ridtitid W, Wongnawa M, Mahatthanatrakul W, Raungsri N, Sunbhanich M. Ketoconazole increases plasma concentrations of antimalarial mefloquine in healthy human volunteers. J Clin Pharm Ther. 2005;30:285–290.
2. Sowunmi A, Adio RA, Oduola AM, Ogundahunsi OA, Salako LA. Acute psychosis after mefloquine: report of six cases. Trop Geogr Med. 1995;47(4):179–180.
3. Ridtitid W, Wongnawa M, Mahatthanatrakul W, Chaipol P, Sunbhanich M. Effect of rifampin on plasma concentrations of mefloquine in healthy volunteers. J Pharm Pharmacol. 2000;52(10):1265–1269.

###

Concomitant Use of Clarithromycin and Digitalis Can Lead to Toxic Levels of Digitalis

Several studies have documented this effect. Zapater et al. conducted a prospective observational trial in seven elderly patients taking digitalis, whose digitalis levels were determined before and after the addition of clarithromycin [1]. In another study, Tanaka et el conducted a similar study in eight inpatients with heart failure who received concomitant clarithromycin therapy to treat or prevent pneumonia [2]. In both studies, digitalis/digoxin levels rose following the addition of clarithromycin. In the latter study, researchers found the effect to be dose-dependent on the antibiotic [2].

Here is another familiar clinical picture: a patient taking digoxin for heart failure develops pneumonia and requires an antibiotic. When this happens, remember the potential for a drug–drug interaction.

References

1. Zapater P, Reus S, Tello A, Torrus D, Perez-Mateo M, Horga JF. A prospective study of the clarithromycin–digoxin interaction in elderly patients. J Antimicrob Chemother. 2002;50(4):601–606.
2. Tanaka H, Matsumoto K, Ueno K, Kodama M, Yoneda K, Katayama Y, Miyatake K. Effect of clarithromycin on steady-state digoxin concentrations. Ann Pharmacother. 2003;37(2):178–181.

###

Sildenafil (Viagra) May Relieve Antidepressant-Induced Sexual Dysfunction in Women

The finding described above comes from a study of 49 middle-aged women with depression treated with selective and nonselective serotonin reuptake inhibitors who subsequently reported adverse sexual effects. The subjects, while continuing to take their antidepressant medication, were randomly assigned to take sildenafil or placebo prior to sexual activity. Outcomes were measured using a variety of sexual function scales and also a depression scale. Although the mean Hamilton Depression Scale scores in both cohorts remained consistent with remission, the group taking sildenafil were found to have higher sexual function scores and less adverse sexual effects than the placebo group [1].

I am not sure this can truly be called a drug interaction, since it is really one drug taken to relieve adverse effects of another but, given the powerful effects of placebos in this sort of setting, I find it noteworthy that the researchers found different outcomes in the study and the placebo groups.

Reference

1. Nurnberg HG, Hensley PL, Heiman JR, Croft HA, Debattista C, Paine S. Sildenafil treatment of women with antidepressant-associated sexual dysfunction: a randomized controlled trial. JAMA. 2008;300(4):395–404.

###

The Concomitant Use of Phosphodiesterase-5 Inhibitors and Nitrates Can Cause an Unsafe Drop in Blood Pressure

Guidelines for the American College of Cardiology/American Heart Association recommend that nitrates be withheld for 24 h after taking sildenafil [1]. The concomitant use of tadalafil (Cialis), a commonly prescribed PDE-5 inhibitor, and nitrates is contraindicated [2]. Kloner et al. studied 150 male subjects who received daily doses of tadalafil or placebo, and then were given sublingual doses of nitroglycerin. They found that the hemodynamic interaction (plummeting blood pressure) between tadalafil and sublingual nitroglycerin lasted 24 h, but was not seen at 48 h and beyond [1].

Movies-goers who viewed Something's Gotta Give *were alerted to this drug interaction. In the film, Harry Sanborn, played by Jack Nicholson, is a 63-year old man who dates women in their 20s. During some amorous activity with one of these younger women, Harry suffers a mild heart attack, and his use of Viagra precludes treatment with nitrates.*

References

1. Kloner RA, Hutter AM, Emmick JT, Mitchell ML, Denne J, Jackson G. Time course of the interaction between tadalafil and nitrates. J Am Coll Cardiol. 2003;42(10):1855–1860.
2. Tadalafil(Cialis).EpocratesOnline.Availableat:https://online.epocrates.com/u/10a3560?src=PK/. Accessed March 25, 2010.

###

Smoking Cessation Can Increase Plasma Levels of Clozapine (Clozaril)

In a report on dosing of atypical antipsychotics, de Leon et al. offer a caution regarding smoking cessation and the use of clozapine, and perhaps olanzapine, as well [1].

A warning about the possibility of unanticipated elevations in plasma concentrations in persons who cease smoking is pertinent in a drug that has the potential to cause myocarditis, agranulocytosis and seizures, just to mention a few of the possible adverse reactions.

Reference

1. de Leon J, Armstrong SC, Cozza KL. The dosing of atypical antipsychotics. Psychosomatics. 2005;46(3):262–273.

###

Initiating Treatment with Two Antidepressant Medications May Bring Superior Results

Blier et al. studied 105 patients with major depressive disorder who were randomly assigned to receive one of four treatment regimens: fluoxetine alone, or mirtazapine in combination with fluoxetine, venlafaxine, or bupropion. The primary outcome measure was the score on the Hamilton Depression scale. At the end of the 6-week treatment period the mean scores of subjects showed that those in the three combination groups experienced significantly greater improvement than those in the monotherapy group.

I have sometimes used antidepressants in combination, generally trying to deal with various manifestations of depression such as nighttime insomnia or daytime fatigue, but I have always begun with monotherapy and added the second drug at some later time. Beginning with dual therapy is a new concept, at least to me, and I hope to see more studies with larger numbers of subjects to further assess the merits of this approach.

Reference

1. Blier P, Ward HE, Tremblay P, et al. Combination of antidepressant medications from treatment initiation for major depressive disorder: a double-blind randomized study. Am J Psychiatry. 2010;167(3):281–288.

###

Serum Levels of Warfarin (Coumadin), Whether Increased or Decreased, Can Be Affected by Dozens of Drugs

A useful and well-documented list of drugs that can potentiate or inhibit the action of warfarin is found in a paper by Holbrook et al. [1]. From this paper and other sources, here is a partial list of substances that can interact with warfarin, selected because they are commonly prescribed and thus may unknowingly complicate anticoagulant therapy [1–8].

Selected Drugs, Herbs and Foods That May Increase Warfarin Effect

Acetaminophen
Alcohol
Atorvastatin
Cimetidine
Ciprofloxacin
Cotrimoxazole
Cranberry juice
Diltiazem
Erythromycin and clarithromycin
Fish oil
Mango
Metronidazole
NSAIDs
Omeprazole
Propranolol
Sulfamethoxazole

Selected Drugs, Herbs and Foods That May Decrease Warfarin Effect

Avocado
Barbiturates
Carbamazepine
Chlordiazepoxide
Griseofulvin
Nafcillin
Ribavirin
Rifampin
Sucralfate
Trazodone
Vitamin K supplements

The jury is still out on other substances including: feverfew, garlic, ginkgo, ginseng, green tea, St. John's wort and vitamin K-containing multivitamins [1, 3, 4, 9].

> *The name warfarin comes from WARF- (crediting the University of Wisconsin Alumni Research Foundation), with the added suffix -ARIN, denoting the drug's relationship to its precursor, coumarin, originally found when cattle experienced hemorrhaging after eating feed containing spoiled sweet clover [10].*

References

1. Holbrook AM, Pereira JA, Labiris R, et al. Systematic overview of warfarin and its drug and food interactions. Arch Int Med. 2005;165:1095–1106.
2. Ament PW, Bertolino JG, Liszewski JL. Clinically significant drug interactions. Am Fam Phys. 2000;61:1745–1754.

3. Gardner P, Phillips R, Shaughnessy AF. Herbal and dietary supplements: drug interactions in patients with chronic illnesses. Am Fam Phys. 2008;77(1):73–78.
4. Grant P. Warfarin and cranberry juice: an interaction? J Heart Valve Dis. 2004;13(1):25–26.
5. Suvarna R, Pirmohamed M, Henderson L. Possible interaction between warfarin and cranberry juice. BMJ. 2003;327(7429):1454.
6. Buckley MS, Goff AD, Knapp WE. Fish oil interaction with warfarin. Ann Pharmacother. 2004;38(1):50–52.
7. Schelleman H, Bilker WB, Brensinger CM, et al. Fibrate/statin initiation in warfarin users and gastrointestinal bleeding risk. Am J Med. 2010;123(2);151–157.
8. Fischer HD, Juurlink DN, Mamdani MM, Koop A, Laupacis A. Hemorrhage during warfarin therapy associated with cotrimoxazole and other urinary tract anti-infective agents: a population-based study. Arch Intern Med. 2010;170(7):617–621.
9. Jiang X, Williams KM, Liauw WS, et al. Effect of St John's wort and ginseng on the pharmacokinetics and pharmacodynamics of warfarin in healthy subjects. Br J Clin Pharmacol. 2004;57(5):592–599.
10. Taylor RB. White coat tales – medicine's heroes, heritage and misadventures. New York: Springer, 2008; page 62.

###

Herbal Substances and Dietary Supplements Can Also Interact with Drugs We Prescribe

Warfarin and its many possibilities for drug, herb and food interactions allow me to segue to herbal and dietary supplement interactions. Here I will describe just a few.

A study involving 16 patients with hypercholesterolemia treated with a stable dose of atorvastatin (Lipitor) for 3 months or longer were randomized to also take a commercially available St. John's wort product or to serve as a control. Those taking the St. John's wort product experienced significantly increased levels of total and LDL cholesterol when compared with controls [1].

McRae reports a 74 year old patient whose digoxin levels rose when taking ginseng, fell when ginseng was stopped, and rose again when he resumed ginseng use along with his dose of digoxin [2].

Gardner et al. report a number of suspicious interactions between drugs and herbal and dietary supplements. Among these are case reports of manic-like manifestations, tremulousness, and headache when taking the combination of a monoamine oxidase inhibitor and ginseng, an instance of coma when a patient ingested both gingko and a monoamine oxidase inhibitor, and a report of a patient who experienced drowsiness or serotonin syndrome when using a both an SSRI and St. John's wort.

Experienced physicians know, but sometimes need to be reminded, that patients don't always reveal the herbal and dietary supplements they are taking. They may think the doctor will disapprove or even disparage such use. Nevertheless, the potential for interactions between herbal/dietary supplements and drugs increases each day as the use of unregulated alternative medicine remedies becomes ever more popular.

References

1. Andrén L, Andreasson A, Eggertsen R. Interaction between a commercially available St. John's wort product (Movina) and atorvastatin in patients with hypercholesterolemia. Eur J Clin Pharmacol. 2007;63(10):913–916.
2. McRae S. Elevated serum digoxin levels in a patient taking digoxin and Siberian ginseng. CMAJ. 1996;155(3):293–295.
3. Gardner P, Phillips R, Shaughnessy AF. Herbal and dietary supplements: drug interactions in patients with chronic illnesses. Am Fam Phys. 2008;77(1):73–78.

###

Probiotic Dietary Supplements Help Prevent Antibiotic-Associated Diarrhea (AAD)

Just to show that not all dietary supplement–drug interactions are harmful, I present three studies showing the merits of probiotics, defined as dietary supplements of live bacteria or yeasts, taken with antibiotics to prevent diarrhea. The first is a meta-analysis of ten studies involving 1,862 patients, which led to the following conclusion: "Administration of a *Lactobacillus* single-agent regimen as a prophylactic agent during antibiotic treatment reduced the risk of developing AAD compared with placebo in adults but not in pediatric patients" [1].

In randomized, double-blind placebo-controlled trial of 269 children prescribed antibiotics for acute otitis media and/or respiratory tract infection who also received *S. boulardii* or placebo, the author reported that *S. boulardii* effectively reduced the risk of AAD in children [2].

Probiotic use to prevent AAD also works well in the elderly. A randomized double-blind placebo controlled study of a *Lactobacillus* preparation to prevent diarrhea in a hospital population of patients average age 74 revealed that AAD occurred in 12% of those taking the probiotic compared with a 34% incidence in the control group. The authors found the absolute risk reduction to be 17% (7–27%) and the number needed to treat was six (4–14).

In the last of the three reports described, note the 34% incidence of AAD in hospitalized elderly patients taking antibiotics but not receiving Lactobacillus. That is one third of patients who experienced an unpleasant side effect of antibiotic use that could have been prevented in many by the concomitant use of a safe and inexpensive probiotic supplement.

References

1. Kale-Pradhan PB, Jassai HD, Wilhelm SM. Role of *Lactobacillus* in the prevention of antibiotic-associated diarrhea: a meta-analysis. Pharmacotherapy. 2010;30(2):119–129.
2. Kotowska M, Albrecht P, Szajewska H. *Saccharomyces boulardii* in the prevention of antibiotic-associated diarrhea in children: a randomized double-blind placebo-controlled trial. Aliment Pharmacol Ther. 2005;21(5):583–590.

3. Hickson M, D'Souza AL, Muthu N. Use of probiotic *Lactobacillus* preparation to prevent diarrhea associated the antibiotics: randomized double blind placebo controlled trial. BMJ. 2007;335(7610):80.

Grapefruit Can Increase the Bioavailability of a Number of Medications

Grapefruit juice suppresses the cytochrome P450 enzyme CYP3A4 in the intestinal wall, leading to diminished first-pass metabolism with higher bioavailability, an effect that can persist for 24 h. The following is a list of some medications with known or suspected interactions in which grapefruit juice can increase the drug effect [1–3].

Felodipine
Terfenadine
Verapamil
Nifedipine
Nimodipine
Saquinavir
Cyclosporin
Triazolam
Midazolam
Cisapride
Atorvastatin

This list is certainly incomplete, simply because most other drugs have not been tested.

How did we ever discover that grapefruit juice can have an effect on serum drug levels?
The answer lies in serendipitous observation that occurred during a study of the interaction between the calcium channel antagonist, felodipine, and ethyl alcohol. To mask the taste of alcohol, the investigators added grapefruit juice, more or less making what your local bartender would term a "greyhound." Subsequently they found that those subjects who took both felodipine and the ethanol-in-grapefruit-juice cocktail had greater than expected levels of the drug [3].

References

1. Fuhr U. Drug interactions with grapefruit juice: extent, probable mechanism and clinical relevance. Drug Safety. 1998;18(4):251–272.
2. Arayne MS, Sultana N, Bibi Z. Grapefruit juice–drug interactions. Pak J Pharm Sci. 2005;18(4):45–57.
3. Bailey DG, Malcolm J, Arnold O, Spence JD. Grapefruit juice–drug interactions. Br J Clin Pharmacol. 1998;46(2):101–110.

###

Chapter 12
Alcohol, Nicotine and Caffeine

> *Wine is the most healthful and most hygienic of beverages.*
>
> Louis Pasteur (1822–1895) [1].

> *Tobacco surely was designed*
> *To poison, and destroy mankind.*
>
> American poet and newspaper editor Philip Morin Freneau
> (1752–1832) [2].

> *Caffeine propels both idleness and industry. In the coffee*
> *house, it feeds idleness, whether it is the productive idleness of*
> *talk of politics, art, or social engagement, or the useless and*
> *even inimical idleness of gaming and gossip; in the workplace,*
> *it funnels the mental and physical stimulation that make possi-*
> *ble long hours, punctuality, alertness, and alacrity; and in the*
> *studio, it stirs the artist's imagination and creative energies.*
> *And it does these things with little or no harm to the prudent*
> *user. Of no other drug, nor any agency known to man, can we*
> *say the same.*
>
> Bennett A. Weinberg and Bonnie K. Bealer [3].

The four authors cited above, writing about society's favorite substances, have some interesting back stories. Pasteur, of course, was not a physician and instead was an industrial chemist involved in France's alcohol industry of his time, and the partial heat sterilization technique we call pasteurization and use to make milk safe to drink was originally used to prevent spoilage of beer and wine [4]. Freneau was an American polemicist, nationalist and editor of a newspaper The National Gazette, which published the works of Thomas Jefferson and James Madison; the story of his antipathy to smoking, a socially accepted habit at the time, is unknown, at least by me. After all, it would be a century and a half before we would connect smoking and lung cancer. Bennett A. Weinberg, Ph.D., lead author of the book on caffeine, is a consultant in pharmaceutical communications serving leading industrial companies; he and co-author Bonnie Bealer quickly followed their successful 2001 book with another in 2002 titled *The Caffeine Advantage: How to Sharpen Your Mind, Improve Your Physical Performance, and Achieve Your Goals – The Healthy Way* [5].

R.B. Taylor, *Essential Medical Facts Every Clinician Should Know: To Prevent Medical Errors, Pass Board Examinations and Provide Informed Patient Care*,
DOI 10.1007/978-1-4419-7874-5_12, © Springer Science+Business Media, LLC 2011

Together these authors comment on our most popular drugs – ethanol, nicotine and caffeine – which require no prescription. They share in common that they can affect cognition, that they can have noteworthy adverse effects and – in selected instances – just may even have some health benefits.

Harris J., a successful advertising executive at age 38, came to the hospital emergency department (ED) twice in a month with bouts of atrial fibrillation (AF). In addition, he described episodes of "heart irregularity" occurring at home several times a week, and ending spontaneously after 10 to 30 minutes. The patient was a non-smoker who had no significant past medical history, occasionally drank coffee, and who exercised several times a week. He used no "recreational" or other drugs. He related that he usually had a beer at lunchtime and a martini or two before dinner. In fact, his episodes of "heart irregularity" often seemed to begin after taking a drink. His blood pressure and resting pulse were normal for age, as was his cardiac examination, on both ED visits. Both episodes of AF ceased spontaneously in the ED, and he was referred to his personal physician for management.

Harris' family doctor suspected substance-induced AF. He advised Harris to avoid all use of coffee and alcohol. "Let's try this before we think of using any drugs." Upon ceasing consumption of caffeine and, especially, alcoholic beverages, the episodes of atrial fibrillation virtually ceased – recurring only at rare intervals, and then when under exceptional stress at work.

Harris J. seems to have had substance-induced atrial fibrillation, which can be caused by both illicit drugs and alcohol. Krishnamoorthy et al. describe 88 such patients ages 45 or less admitted to the hospital with electrocardiographically confirmed AF or atrial flutter precipitated by alcohol or illicit drugs. In 19 of these persons (21.5%), alcohol was the precipitating cause of the cardiac abnormality. Upon follow up of 85% of these patients for 12 months, 6 individuals experienced further occurrences of paroxysms, and all 6 reported continued abuse of alcohol or illicit drugs [6].

Because consumption of these three substances – ethanol, nicotine, and caffeine – is so ubiquitous, and because they have so many interactions with drugs clinician prescribe and such diverse effects on health status, I decided to afford our three legal recreational drugs their own chapter in the book.

References

1. Pasteur L. *Études sur le vin*, Pt. I, Ch. 2, Sect B. Quoted in Strauss MB. Familiar medical quotations. Boston: Little, Brown, 1968; page 8.
2. Freneau PM. Poems of Freneau, edited by Clark HH. New York: Harcourt, Brace, 1929.
3. Weinberg BA, Bealer BK. The world of caffeine: the science and culture of the world's most popular drug. New York: Routledge, 2001.
4. Taylor RB. White coat tales: medicine's heroes, heritage and misadventures. New York: Springer, 2008. Page 19.
5. Weinberg BA, Bealer BK. The caffeine advantage: how to sharpen your mind, improve your physical performance, and achieve your goals – the healthy way. New York: Free Press, 2002.
6. Krishnamoorthy S, Lip GYH, Lane DA. Alcohol and illicit drug use as precipitants of atrial fibrillation in young adults: a case series and literature review. Am J Med. 2009;122(9):851–856.

###

Alcohol Leads Both Prescription and Illicit Drugs in Causing Fatal Motor Vehicle Accidents

The finding reported here is from a West Virginia study of fatally injured drivers. The most common culprit, alcohol, was found in 32.5% of decedents tested for both alcohol and drugs [1].

What about drugs? In this study, fatally injured drivers were more likely to have used prescription drugs – notably opioid analgesics and depressants – than illegal drugs [1].

Reference

1. Alcohol and other drug use among victims of motor vehicle crashes – West Virginia, 2004–2005. Morb Mortal Wky Rep. 2006;55:1293–1296.

###

Patients with Breast Cancer and Who Consume 7 or More Alcoholic Beverages Per Week Have an Increased Risk of Developing a Contralateral Breast Cancer

Li et al. studied the effect of lifestyle on 365 patients with estrogen-positive invasive breast cancer and a second primary invasive cancer in the contralateral breast. These individuals were compared to 726 matched controls with an estrogen-positive invasive cancer of one breast only, but without a second tumor in the contralateral breast. Those who drank 7 or more alcoholic beverages per week had a greater risk of a second, contralateral invasive cancer, with an odds ratio (OR) of 1.9. An increased risk of a second cancer was also found for patients who were obese (OR, 1.4) and who smoked cigarettes (OR, 2.2) [1].

Because patients who have cancer in one breast have an increased risk of developing a second cancer, lifestyle changes may be especially important in these persons.

Reference

1. Li C, Daling JR, Porter PL, Tang MT, Malone KE. Relationship between potentially modifiable lifestyle factors and risk of second primary contralateral breast cancer among women diagnosed with estrogen receptor-positive invasive breast cancer. J Clin Oncol. 2009; 27(32):5318–5321.

###

Acute Alcohol Exposure Prior to Trauma Impairs Wound Healing

Acute ethanol exposure inhibits important components of wound healing, including collagen synthesis, blood vessel regrowth, and epithelial regeneration, according to Radek et al. [1].

Note the word "acute." Persons with acute alcohol exposure, a euphemism for inebriated or perhaps even drunk, are especially prone to the very type of traumatic injuries that will necessitate wound healing.

Reference

1. Radek KA, Ranzer MJ, Dipietro LA. Brewing complications: the effect of acute ethanol exposure on wound healing. J Leukoc Biol. 2009;86(5):1125–1134.

###

The Drug Most Often Implicated in Substance-Related Sexual Assault Is Alcohol

Based on a literature review, Madea and Musshoff report that alcohol is involved in approximately 40–60% of cases of drug-facilitated sexual assault. Other substances that may be involved are cannabis and cocaine. They report that "knock-out drugs," such as benzodiazepines and other hypnotics, are involved in very few cases of sexual assault, and that gamma-hydroxybutyric acid (Liquid Ecstasy) is rarely detected with medical certainty [1].

Consider that the literature search described is likely to detect only reportable events, chiefly crimes. The number of unreported instances of drug-facilitated, subsequently-regretted sexual encounters is certainly some multiple of those instances reported.

Reference

1. Madea B, Musshoff F. Knock-out drugs: their prevalence, modes of action, and means of detection. Dtsch Arxtebl Int. 2009;106(20):341–347.

###

African-American Men Seem Especially Prone to Alcohol-Associated Hypertension

That there is a relationship between high consumption of alcohol and the risk of hypertension is widely accepted. But patients are diverse, and not all races/genders may react the same. In a cohort study of 8,334 persons followed for 6 years, there was an increased risk of hypertension in those who consumed 210 g or more of ethanol each week, considered a "large amount" of ethanol, compared with those who did not use alcohol. The research revealed, "Systolic and diastolic blood pressures were higher in black men who consumed low to moderate amounts of alcohol compared with nonconsumers, but not in the other race-gender strata" [1].

This is an important message for all African-American male patients who consume alcohol and who also have a history of elevated blood pressure readings or a family history of hypertension. Simply stated, the African-American male patient has a higher risk of hypertension associated with a low to moderate alcohol consumption.

Reference

1. Fuchs FD, Chambless LE, Whelton PK, Nieto FJ, Heiss G. Alcohol consumption and the incidence of hypertension: the Atherosclerosis Risk in Communities Study. Hypertension. 2001;37(5):1242–1250.

###

Drinking Without Eating May Increase the Risk of Alcohol-Associated Hypertension

In a population-based study of 2,609 white men and women ages 35–80 years, daily drinkers and those consuming alcohol without eating had a significantly greater risk of hypertension than those drinking less than daily and those drinking mostly with food [1].

The study reported also found no consistent association with specific beverage types – wine, beer, or liquor – and the risk of hypertension [1].

Reference

1. Stranges S, Wu T, Dorn JM, et al. Relationship of alcohol drinking pattern to risk of hypertension: a population-based study. Hypertension. 2004;44(6):805–806.

###

Not All Studies Find a Relationship Between Alcohol Consumption and Hypertension

Many studies of alcohol consumption and high blood pressure begin with the premise that there is a link. Common statements include "A close relationship between alcohol consumption and hypertension has been established…" [1] and "Epidemiologic studies have demonstrated a positive relationship between heavy alcohol use and hypertension…" [2].

A recent study, however, suggests a lack of association between alcohol and hypertension.

Halanych et al. followed a diverse group of 4,711 young adults over 20 years. They found the 20-year incidence of hypertension for never, former, light, moderate, and at-risk drinkers was 25.1%, 31.8%, 20.9%, 22.2%, and 18.8%, respectively ($p < 0.001$). Statistical models detected no association between baseline alcohol consumption and incident hypertension, with one exception: There seemed to be a lower risk of hypertension among American women of European ancestry who reported any current alcohol consumption [3].

Although alcohol consumption in any pattern of use seemed not to be related to the development of elevated blood pressure, the study did reveal correlates associated with hypertension risk. These were: age, gender, race, body mass index, education, income, and difficulty paying for basics and medical care [3].

References

1. Fuchs FD, Chambless LE, Whelton PK, Nieto FJ, Heiss G. Alcohol consumption and the incidence of hypertension: the Atherosclerosis Risk in Communities Study. Hypertension. 2001;37(5):1242–1250.
2. Stranges S, Wu T, Dorn JM, et al. Relationship of alcohol drinking pattern to risk of hypertension: a population-based study. Hypertension. 2004;44(6):805–806.
3. Halanych JH, Safford MM, Kertesz SG, et al. Alcohol consumption in young adults and incident hypertension: 20-year follow-up from the Coronary Artery Risk Development in Young Adults Study. Am J Epidem. 2010;171(5):532–539.

###

Weekly Alcohol Consumption May Help Prevent Gallstones

We are easing into the realm of possible beneficial effects of alcohol consumption. The relationship between alcohol use and gallstones was studied in a general population sample of 621 randomly selected persons ages 35–85 years screened for gallstones using ultrasonography at baseline and again 5 years or more later. The researcher found an inverse relationship between gallstones and alcohol consumption [1].

They also found a positive relationship – between gallstones and LDL-cholesterol levels.

Reference

1. Haldestram I, Kullman E, Borch K. Incidence of and potential risk factors for gallstone disease in a general population sample. Br J Surg. 2009;96(11):1315–1322.

###

Beer Drinking Has Been Reported to Increase Bone Mass in Women

From Spain comes a study of 1,697 persons, average age 48.4 years, who were screened for factors that might affect calcium metabolism. The researchers found that beer drinkers have quantitative bone ultrasound values greater than those found in no beer and/or wine drinkers. They speculate that the increased bone density in beer drinkers may be related to the phytoestrogen content of the beverage [1].

> *Beer is not the only alcoholic beverage that may have a claim on improving bone health. The Times of India reports on a paper delivered at the 239th National Meeting of the American Chemical Society, telling how "fructans" from the agave plant enhance the body's absorption of calcium [2]. The agave plant is, of course, the source of the world's agave tequila. Let us all drink our way to stronger bones.*

References

1. Pedrera-Zamorano JD, Lavado-Garcia JM, Roncero-Martin R, Calderon-Garcia JF, Rodriguez-Dominguez T, Canal-Macias ML. Effect of beer drinking on ultrasound bone mass in women. Nutrition. 2009;25(10):1057–1063.
2. Tequila plant may fight osteoporosis. The Times of India. Available at: http://timesofindia.indiatimes.com/articleshow/5718998.cms?prtpage=1/Accessed April 24, 2010.

###

Alcohol Use Is Associated with a Decreased Risk of Benign Prostatic Hyperplasia (BPH)

A meta-analysis of 12 studies relating alcohol use to BPH revealed that an alcohol consumption of 36 g or more daily was associated with a 35% decreased likelihood of BPH, compared to no alcohol use at all [1].

> *In the same report the authors present data from 4 studies looking at alcohol consumption and lower urinary tract symptoms (LUTS). Three of these studies suggest that alcohol is associated with an increased incidence of LUTS [1].*

Reference

1. Parson JK, Im R. Alcohol consumption is associated with a decreased risk of benign prostatic hyperplasia. J Urol. 2009;182(4):1463–1468.

###

The Often-Dramatic Suppression of Essential Tremor Following Alcohol Ingestion Is Related to a Reduction of Cerebellar Synaptic Overactivity

We have long known that the ingestion of even small doses of alcohol can suppress essential tremor, leading to suggestions that this phenomenon can be used to distinguish it from other tremors [1]. Thanks to a more recent study using positron emission tomography (PET) scanning, we now know how the effect occurs. Based on a study of six patients with alcohol-responsive essential tremor and six age-matched normal controls, Boecker et al. found that the response of essential tremor seen following alcohol ingestion is mediated via a reduction of cerebellar synaptic overactivity, and that this effect results in increased afferent input to the inferior olivary nuclei [2].

> It is axiomatic that alcohol is not a routine remedy for any disease [3]. Yet the salutary effect of alcohol on essential tremor, perhaps even a unique phenomenon, can lead older persons with essential tremor to believe that they have found a magic cure. Of course, constant dosing with alcohol can have its own constellation of problems.

References

1. Growdon JH, Shahani BT, Young RR. The effect of alcohol on essential tremor. Neurology. 1975;25(3):259–262.
2. Boecker H, Willis AJ, Ceballos-Baumann A, et al. The effect of ethanol on alcohol-responsive essential tremor: positron emission tomography study. Ann Neurol. 1996;39(5):650–658.
3. Lindsay JA. Medical axioms, aphorisms and clinical memoranda. London: H.K. Lewis Co., 1923. Page 152.

###

Light to Moderate Alcohol Use Seems to Help Protect Against Coronary Heart Disease (CHD)

Of the many epidemiologic studies of this issue, I will present three. Mukamal et al. studied 38,077 male health professionals in regards to alcohol consumption and the incidence of nonfatal myocardial infarction and fatal coronary heart disease over a 12-year period. The found that consumption of alcohol – any type – at least 3–4 days per week was inversely associated with myocardial infarction [1].

A study of 15,630 men and 25,808 women in Spain followed up for a median period of 10 years led researchers to conclude as follows: "In men aged 29–69 years, alcohol intake was associated with a more than 30% lower CHD incidence." For women a negative association was found with p values above 0.05 in all categories of alcohol use [2].

A third study analyzed the National Health Interview Survey between 1987 and 2000, and linked findings to the National Death Index through 2002. The data reveal that in U.S. adults, light and moderate alcohol consumption were inversely associated with cardiovascular disease mortality, even when compared with life-time abstainers [3].

The National Health Interview Survey/National Death Index study highlights an important fact that might be overlooked as we toast alcohol's apparent salutary effect on heart health: This study found that consumption of 3 or more drinks daily increased the risk of cardiovascular mortality compared with taking 2 drinks per drinking day [3]. Simply stated, alcohol use greater than "low to moderate" converts some protective effect to a risk factor for CHD.

References

1. Mukamal KJ, Conigrave KM, Mittleman MA, et al. Roles of drinking pattern and type of alcohol consumed in coronary heart disease. N Engl J Med. 2003;348(2):109–118.
2. Arriola L, Martinez-Camblor P, Larrañaga N, et al. Alcohol intake and the risk of coronary heart disease in the Spanish EPIC (European Prospective Investigation into Cancer) cohort study. Heart. 2010;96(2):124–130.
3. Mukamal KJ, Chen CM, Rao SR, Breslow RA. Alcohol consumption and cardiovascular mortality among U.S. adults, 1987 to 2002. J Am Coll Cardiol. 2010;55(13):1328–1335.

###

Eleven Percent of Women Smoke During Pregnancy

Given that various compounds in tobacco smoke, not just nicotine, are both carcino-gens and can cause fetal harm, it is astounding that more than one in 10 pregnant women smoke cigarettes [1].

Just for starters, women who smoke double their risk of having a preterm or low-birth weight delivery, not to mention other adverse effects on the offspring, a few of which are described next [2].

References

. 1. Carl J, Hill A. Preconception counseling: make it part of the annual exam. J Fam Pract. 2009;58(6):307–311.
2. Oncken C, Dornelas E, Greene J, et al. Nicotine gum for pregnant smokers: a randomized controlled trial. Obstet Gynecol. 2008;112(4):859–867.

###

Newborns Exposed to Maternal Smoking In Utero Can Experience Neurotoxic Effects, Including a Nicotine Withdrawal Syndrome

Pichini and Garcia-Algar characterize the neonatal nicotine withdrawal syndrome as the manifestation of "irritability, tremors and sleep disturbances, most typically observed in newborns of heavy smoking mothers" [1].

A report from Brown Medical School found a dose-response relationship between maternal tobacco use and manifestations of newborn nicotine withdrawal. Their sample was 27 nicotine exposed and 29 control full term infants, all of whose mothers consumed three or less alcoholic drinks per month. Maternal self-reporting and salivary cotinine measured in maternal saliva were used to monitor nicotine exposure. The authors report that finding tobacco-exposed infants to be more excitable and hypertonic. The showed more stress/abstinence signs and required more handling. Excitability, central nervous system and visual stress, and stress/abstinence signs were all found to have a dose-response relationship to maternal salivary cotinine levels [2].

Do we need any more evidence than this that nicotine is an addictive drug?

References

1. Pichini S, Garcia-Algar O. In utero exposure to smoking and newborn neurobehavior: how to assess neonatal withdrawal syndrome. Ther Drug Monit. 2006;28(3):288–290.
2. Law KL, Stroud LR, LaGrasse LL, Niaura R, Liu J, Lester BM. Smoking during pregnancy and newborn neurobehavior. Pediatrics. 2003;111(6):1318–1323.

###

Maternal Smoking Increases the Risk of Attention Deficit Hyperactivity Disorder (ADHD) in Offspring

A study of 1,452 twin pairs ages 5–16 years revealed that, after confounders such as genetic influences were accounted for, maternal smoking during pregnancy was found to have a statistical influence on the risk of developing ADHD [1].

Another effort examined two large case-control family studies of subjects with and without ADHD. Siblings of the probands from these studies (n = 536) were interviewed, including a determination of maternal smoking during pregnancy. The conclusion: "Among all siblings, maternal smoking during pregnancy was significantly associated with ADHD, independent of conduct disorder and other covariates" [2].

What about alcohol? For the record, a review of 21,678 reports of inattention and hyperactivity symptoms in children showed that, when smoking and social adversity were taken into account, low amounts of alcohol consumed during pregnancy were not associated with an increased risk of childhood inattention/hyperactivity symptoms [3].

References

1. Thapar A, Fowler T, Rice F, et al. Maternal smoking during pregnancy and attention deficit hyperactivity disorder symptoms in offspring. Am J Psychiatry. 2003;160(11):1985–1989.
2. Biederman J, Monateaux MC, Faraone SV, Mick E. Parsing the associations between prenatal exposure to nicotine and offspring psychopathology in a nonreferred sample. J Adolesc Health. 2009;45(2):142–148.
3. Rodriguez A, Olsen J, Kotimas AJ, et al. Is prenatal alcohol exposure related to inattention and hyperactivity symptoms in children? Disentangling the effects of social adversity. J Child Psychol Psychiatry. 2009;50(9):1073–1083.

###

The Use of Nicotine Gum by Pregnant Smokers Can Help Increase Birth Weight and Gestational Age

This statement comes from a study of pregnant smokers randomized to take 2 mg of nicotine gum (n = 100) or placebo (n = 94), matched for age, race/ethnicity and smoking history. Nicotine levels were monitored using urine cotinine levels. The birth weight was higher in the nicotine replacement group (7 lb, 3 oz; 3,287 g) versus placebo (6 lb, 8 oz; 2,950 g), with an accompanying increase in gestational age [1].

> What about the safety of nicotine gum in pregnancy? A study of adverse events among smokers in a nicotine replacement therapy (NRT) trial involving records from 157 pregnancies led to this conclusion: "Although race, poor pregnancy history, and use of analgesics were associated with serious adverse events, randomization to NRT during pregnancy was not a significant factor" [2].

References

1. Oncken C, Dornelas E, Greene J, et al. Nicotine gum for pregnant smokers: a randomized controlled trial. Obstet Gynecol. 2008;112(4):859–867.
2. Swamy GK, Roelands JJ, Peterson BL, et al. Predictors of adverse events among pregnant smokers exposed in a nicotine replacement therapy trial. Am J Obstet Gynecol. 2009;201(4):354.e1–e7.

###

Cigarette Smoking Increases the Risk of Colorectal Cancer

From the Department of Epidemiology of the American Cancer Society comes a report of a prospective study of 184,187 persons followed for 13 years. After controlling for other risk factors and screening, the data reveal that long-term cigarette smoking is associated with colorectal cancer, with the greatest relative risk noted among current smokers with 50 or more years of smoking [1].

The paper also reported that the colorectal cancer risk decreased following cessation, varying with the time since cessation and an earlier age at time of cessation [1].

Reference

1. Hannan LM, Jacobs EJ, Thun MJ. The association between cigarette smoking and risk of colorectal cancer in a large prospective cohort from the United States. Cancer Epidemiol Biomarkers. 2009;18(12):3362–3367.

Smokeless Tobacco Can Increase the Risk of Myocardial Infarction and Stroke

Investigators at the International Agency for Research on Cancer in Lyon, France conducted a meta-analysis of 11 observational studies from Sweden and the United States. They concluded, "An association was detected between the use of smokeless tobacco products and risk of fatal myocardial infarction and stroke, which does not seem to be explained by chance" [1].

This risk of myocardial infarction and stroke is in addition to the risk of oral cancer with smokeless tobacco. The National Cancer Institute describes 28 carcinogens in chewing tobacco and snuff [2].

References

1. Boffetta P, Straif K. Use of smokeless tobacco and risk of myocardial infarction and stroke: systematic review with meta-analysis. BMJ 2009;339:b3060. doi: 1136/bmj.b3060.
2. National Cancer Institute Fact Sheet. Available at: http://www.cancer.gov/cancertopics/factsheet/Tobacco/smokeless/Accessed April 25, 2010.

Electronic Cigarettes Are Not Safe, Either

The following is taken directly from an FDA News Release dated July 22, 2009: "The U.S. Food and Drug Administration today announced that a laboratory analysis of electronic cigarette samples has found that they contain carcinogens and toxic chemicals such as diethylene glycol, an ingredient used in antifreeze.

"Electronic cigarettes, also called 'e-cigarettes,' are battery operated devices that generally contain cartridges filled with nicotine, flavor and other chemicals. The electronic cigarette turns nicotine, which is highly addictive, and other chemicals into a vapor that is inhaled by the user.

"These products are marketed and sold to young people and are readily available online and in shopping malls. In addition, these products do not contain any health warnings comparable to FDA-approved nicotine replacement products or conventional cigarettes. They are also available in different flavors, such as chocolate and mint, which may appeal to young people" [1].

The tobacco industry may just have invented a nicotine-delivery device even more efficient than the tobacco-containing cigarette. Like it or not, the e-cigarette may be coming to a middle school near you. This is one more health hazard to discuss with our young patients, who may think that no tobacco means no risk.

Reference

1. FDA and Public Health Experts Warn About Electronic Cigarettes. Available at: http://www.fda. gov/NewsEvents/Newsroom/PressAnnouncements/ucm173222.htm/Accessed April 25, 2010.

###

Asking Two Questions – About Current Smoking and Plans to Quit – Increases the Likelihood that Patients Who Smoke Receive Cessation Counseling

Adding two questions ("Current smoker?" and "Plan to quit?") as vital sign questions in an electronic health record resulted in significantly higher physician-documented counseling rates. In a review of 899 patients, this simple intervention increased the identification of smokers from 18 to 84% and assessment for a plan to quit rose from 25.5 to 51%. The investigators report: "Regression analysis showed that patients who received an assessment for plan to quit were 80% more likely to receive counseling" [1].

Given that 70% of smokers visit a physician annually, the 2-question "vital sign" approach is a low-cost and time-efficient intervention that can have a beneficial health impact.

Reference

1. McCullough A, Fisher M, Goldstein AO, Kramer KD, Ripley-Moffitt C. Smoking as a vital sign: prompts to ask and assess increase cessation counseling. J Am Board Fam Med 2009;22(6):625–632.

###

Smoking Increases the Risk of Type 2 Diabetes

There are, however, some curious findings along the way. First, I will consider the risks. In a study conducted in Sweden involving 3,384 men ages 25–74 years, the age-adjusted risk of prevalent clinically diagnosed diabetes for persons who had ever smoked was 1.88, and for current smokers, 1.74, when compared with never users [1].

A study reported from John Hopkins University involved 10,892 middle-aged adults who did not originally have diabetes who were followed for 9 years. During this time, 1,254 subjects became diabetic and among these, when compared with never users, smokers with the highest pack-year history had an adjusted hazard ratio of incident diabetes of 1.42. Here again, cigarette smoking predicted incident type 2 diabetes [2].

Then there are the quirky findings. In the Sweden study, investigators looked also at the risks associated with using "snus." This is a moist tobacco product, reminiscent of snuff, applied beneath the lip. Used chiefly in Sweden and Norway, snus differs from chewing tobacco in not resulting in the urge to spit, an improvement many smokeless tobacco users and their families would welcome. In this study and in contrast to smoking cigarettes, the use of this nicotine-containing product did not significantly increase the risk of diabetes [1].

The Hopkins study also had an unexpected finding. Although cigarette smoking was clearly linked to type 2 diabetes, stopping smoking led to a higher short-term risk, highest in the first three years after cessation, with a hazard ratio of 1.91 [2].

The last finding is a head-scratcher. A report from the University of Oxford, England involved 1,919 patients followed over 6 years. Of these subjects, 1,216 were initially free of retinopathy and 22% of these developed the pathology over the next 6 years. Of the 703 persons with retinopathy at the onset of the study, 29% progressed by 2 scale steps or more. The authors report: "Development of retinopathy (incidence) was strongly associated with baseline glycemia, glycemic exposure over 6 years, higher blood pressure and not smoking. In those who already had retinopathy, progression was associated with older age, male sex, hyperglycemia (as evidenced by a higher HbA1c) and with not smoking" [3]. In both these subgroups of subjects, note that not smoking had had an unfavorable effect on the development or progression of retinopathy.

References

1. Eliasson M, Asplund K, Nasic S, Rodu B. Influence of smoking and snus on the prevalence and incidence of type 2 diabetes amongst men: the northern Sweden MONICA study. J Intern Med. 2004;256(2):101–110.
2. Yea HC, Ducan BB, Schmidt MI, Wang NY, Brancati FL. Smoking, smoking cessation, and risk for type 2 diabetes. Ann Intern Med. 2010;152(1):10–17.
3. Stratton IM, Kohner EM, Aldington SJ, et al. UKPDS for incidence and progression of retinopathy in Type II diabetes over 6 years from diagnosis. Diabetologia. 2001;44(2):156–163.

###

Tobacco and Also Marijuana Use Can Lead to Reduced Blood Levels of the Human Immunodeficiency Virus (HIV) Drug Atazanavir (Reyataz)

A study presented at the 49th Interscience Conference on Antimicrobial Agents and Chemotherapy in 2009 determined atazanavir trough concentrations, viral loads, and CD4 counts for HIV-positive patients with (n = 32) and without (n = 35) substance abuse disorders. They found, when compared with those with no substance abuse disorder, significantly lower atazanavir trough levels among subjects who used tobacco and marijuana, with subtherapeutic atazanavir levels in 36% of tobacco users and 50% of marijuana users [1].

Of those in the study who reported substance abuse disorders, tobacco was the most popular (49%), followed by alcohol (28%), opioids (19%), marijuana (18%), and cocaine (10%). A quick look at the math makes it clear that many subjects (actually 43%) suffered multiple substance abuse. For the record, alcohol, cocaine and opioid use did not affect atazanavir concentrations [1].

Reference

1. Lennox J. Tobacco, marijuana use decreased blood concentrations. Abstract H-231. Presented September 12, 2009 at the 49th Interscience Conference on Antimicrobial Agents and Chemotherapy, San Francisco, California.

###

Tobacco Smoking May Double the Risk of Active Tuberculosis

Here is the basis for this statement: A study reported from the Harvard School of Public Health involved 17,699 persons in the Taiwan National Health Interview Survey followed for 3 years. The authors of the report found current smoking to be associated with an increased risk of active tuberculosis with an adjusted odds ratio of 1.94. There were significant dose-response relationships for the number of cigarettes smoked per day, total years of smoking, and pack-years [1].

The informed reader may be musing that the incidence of tuberculosis in Taiwan is 74.6 per 100,000 population, and even higher in aborigines (289.8) and persons living in mountainous areas (256.0) [2]. Compare these numbers with the United States, with a tuberculosis incidence of 4.4 per 100,000 population [3]. The first question, then, might be: Can the findings of this study conducted on persons living in Taiwan be generalized to persons living in the United States? The answer involves many issues of culture, race and environment, and may not be known at this time.

Another pertinent consideration might be the relative incidence of tuberculosis among those living within U.S. borders. Tuberculosis rates among Asians living in the United States are 22.9 times higher than among non-Hispanic whites, and foreign-born individuals account for 96.1% of tuberculosis among Asian-Americans [3]. From these data we can identify persons who might benefit from extra efforts directed at smoking cessation and tuberculosis screening.

References

1. Lin HH, Ezzati M, Chang HY, Murray H. Association between tobacco smoking and active tuberculosis in Taiwan: prospective cohort study. Am J Respir Crit Care Med. 2009;180(5):475–480.
2. Hseuh PR, Liu YC, So J, Liu CY, Yang PC, Luh KT. Mycobacterium in Taiwan. J Infection. 2006;52(2):77–85.
3. Trends in tuberculosis – United States, 2007. MMWR Weekly. 2008;57(11):281–285.

###

Tobacco Smoking Seems to Be Inversely Associated with Parkinson Disease (PD)

Tobacco use seems to protect against Parkinson disease, and the effect includes use of cigarettes, cigars, pipes and chewing tobacco, according to a meta-analysis of pooled data by Ritz et al. For cigarette use, the most studied of all variants of tobacco use, the reduction in incidence of Parkinson disease seems to be dose dependent. Education or gender of subjects seemed to play no role [1].

Hancock et al. confirmed the tobacco-related risk reduction and added caffeine to the list, finding that "increasing intensity of coffee drinking was inversely associated with PD" [2]. Another author suggests that, among the otherwise noxious chemicals in tobacco, nicotine may have a protective role related to stimulation of brain dopaminergic systems [3].

When I shared the above with my students, one wisely asked: "Then why not treat Parkinson disease patients with nicotine patches?" Great idea! In searching the literature, I found one report of such a trial, conducted in Lübeck, Germany. In this well-designed study, Vieregge et al. treated 32 non-smoking PD patients with nicotine vs. placebo patches over 12 weeks. The authors conclude that, at least with the doses used and over the time period they were applied, transdermal nicotine was not effective add-on therapy for Parkinson disease [4].

References

1. Ritz B, Ascherio A, Checkoway H. Pooled analysis of tobacco use and risk of Parkinson disease. Arch Neurol. 2007;64(7):990–997.
2. Hancock DB, Martin ER, Stajich JM. Smoking, caffeine, and non-steroidal drugs in families with Parkinson disease. Arch Neurol. 2007;64(4):576–580.

3. Quik M. Smoking, nicotine and Parkinson's disease. Trends Neurosci. 2004;27(9):561–568.
4. Vieregge A, Sieberer M, Jacobs H, Hagenah JM, Vieregge P. Transdermal nicotine in PD: a randomized, double-blind, placebo-controlled study. Neurology. 2001;57(6): 1032–1035.

Nicotine Seems to Improve Some of the Manifestations of ADHD in Adults

An early study compared 6 smokers with 11 non-smokers, all with ADHD diagnosed using DSM-IV criteria. Following overnight smoking deprivation, smokers were given a 21 mg/day nicotine skin patch. Non-smokers were given a 7 mg/day skin patch. The treatment effect of nicotine was measured in various ways, including the Clinical Global Impressions (CGI) scale. The investigators found that nicotine caused a significant overall improvement on the CGI, as well as a significant reduction in reaction time on the Continuous Performance Test and improved accuracy of time estimation. Because nonsmokers, as well as smokers, experienced improvements, the investigators offer the opinion that the favorable effects of nicotine were not simply a relief of withdrawal-induced symptoms [1].

A subsequent report, from the same group at Duke University, presents this conclusion: "This small study (40 participants) provided evidence that nicotine treatment can reduce severity of attentional deficit symptoms and produce improvement on an objective computerized attention task" [2].

There seems to be a peculiar relationship between ADHD and cigarette smoking. To begin, cigarette smokers are overrepresented among adults with ADHD. Then, when compared with adults without ADHD, persons with ADHD are more likely to experience withdrawal symptoms, including irritability and impaired concentration, upon cessation of tobacco use [3].

References

1. Levin ED, Conners CK, Sparrow E, et al. Nicotine effects on adults with attention-deficit/hyperactivity disorder. Psychopharmacology. 1996;123(1):55–63.
2. Levin ED, Conners CK, Silva D, Canu W, March J. Effects of chronic nicotine and methylphenidate in adults with attention deficit/hyperactivity disorder. Exp Clin Psychopharmacol. 2001;9(1):83–89.
3. Pomerleau CS, Downey KK, Snedecor SM, Mehringer AM, Marks JL, Pomerleau OF. Smoking pattern and abstinence effects in smoker with no ADHD, childhood ADHD, and adult ADHD symptomatology. Addict Behav. 2003;28(6):1149–1157.

###

Nicotine Can Enhance Cognitive Function

For this reason, the drug may someday have a role in therapy of dementia and more. Here is some of the background. In 1999, a group at Duke University (Levin and others) used a double-blind, placebo controlled, cross-over study to evaluate the effect of chronic use of nicotine patches in patients with Alzheimer disease. They found an "encouraging" sustained improvement in attention with the nicotine dermal patches, but without a corresponding favorable effect on other cognitive and behavioral domains [1].

In a 2006 overview paper, the Levin/Duke University group went on to describe: "Positive therapeutic effects have been seen in initial studies with a variety of cognitive dysfunctions, including Alzheimer disease, age-associated memory impairment, schizophrenia, and attention deficit hyperactivity disorder" [2].

An interesting study examined the effect of nicotine on cognitive deficits induced by the repeated administration of phencyclidine (PCP), an N-methyl-D-aspartate receptor antagonist that induces cognitive deficits relevant to schizophrenia. Although in this study, at the doses of nicotine and PCP used, the answer was no, the authors do offer the conclusion: "Chronic nicotine had pro-cognitive effects by itself, supporting the hypothesis that cognitive enhancement may contribute to tobacco smoking" [3].

As I summarize these three reports, I have a few random thoughts: The first is a nagging question: Is it a coincidence that a group from Duke, admittedly a premier university despite its tobacco roots, seems to dominate the literature when it comes to nicotine effects? Perhaps this is a moot point, since most of the reports describe research using nicotine dermal patches. Still, I wonder about the source of the nicotine in these patches and about the sources of support for nicotine-related research.

Secondly, although I would never, ever advise a patient to start smoking, and nor would I ever personally light up a cigarette, I wonder what I would do if I were diagnosed with early Alzheimer disease. Might I, like any good physician meddling in self-care, give nicotine dermal patches a try?

Then there is the hypothesis that cognitive enhancement contributes to tobacco smoking. While I respect the opinion of the authors of this paper, I can't help thinking that whatever small role a desire for clearer thinking might play in cigarette smoking, it is overshadowed by the truly addictive properties of the drug nicotine. As evidence I refer you back to the withdrawal symptoms found in newborn offspring of smoking mothers, described on page 246.

References

1. White HK, Levin ED. Four-week nicotine skin patch treatment effects on cognitive performance in Alzheimer disease. Psychopharmacology. 1999;143(2):158–165.
2. Levin ED, McClernon FJ, Rezvani AH. Nicotinic effects on cognitive function: behavioral characterization, pharmacological specification, anatomic localization. Psychopharmacology. 2006;184(3–4):523–539.

3. Amitai N, Markou A. Chronic nicotine improves cognitive performance in a test of attention but does not attenuate cognitive disruption induced by repeated phencyclidine administration. Psychopharmacology. 2009;202(1–3):275–286.

###

The U.S. Food and Drug Administration Now Has the Authority to Regulate Tobacco

Signed into law on June 22, 2009 the Family Smoking Prevention and Tobacco Control Act empowers the FDA to regulate tobacco, including authority to set national standards regarding the manufacture, labeling, advertising and sale of tobacco products [1].

> *Thus the FDA has oversight of tobacco, which has been characterized as the only product under their control which, when used as recommended, may well kill the user. Time will tell what the FDA does with its new power over the leading cause of preventable death in the United States (See Chapter 3).*

Reference

1. Gostin LO. FDA regulation of tobacco: politics, law and the public's health. JAMA. 2009;302(13):1459–1461.

###

Caffeine Is the Most Widely Used of All Drugs

It is also the world's most consumed mood-altering drug. The fact that it is a mood-altering drug is a remarkable statement considering that we add it to beverages – think cola drinks – intended for consumption by children [1].

> *Some persons, a few perhaps even physicians, consume heroic amounts of coffee. As a historical example French author Honoré de Balzac (1799–1850) is reported to have fueled his muse by consuming 50 cups of coffee daily, until his death at age 51 of a "digestive condition, aggravated by caffeine poisoning" [2].*

References

1. Weinberg BA, Bealer BK. The world of caffeine: the science and culture of the world's most popular drug. New York: Routledge, 2001.
2. Conradt S. Writers with strange sources of inspiration. Mental Floss. 2010;9(1):72.

###

Caffeine Can Enhance Cognitive Performance, Even at Quite Low Doses

Smit and Rogers conducted a double-blind, within-subjects study in which 23 subjects abstained from coffee overnight and then completed a test battery before and three times after consuming caffeine or a placebo. Caffeine doses used ranged from 12.5 to 100 mg. Although all doses of caffeine affected cognitive performance, the dose-response relationship was flat. They concluded: "After overnight caffeine abstinence, caffeine can significantly affect cognitive performance, mood and thirst at doses within and even lower than the range of amounts of caffeine contained in a single serving of popular caffeine-containing drinks." They also found that regular caffeine users did not show tolerance to the performance and mood effects of caffeine [1].

Another interesting finding is that the greatest enhancement of performance was seen in individuals with higher levels of habitual caffeine intake [1].

Another study involved subjects (n = 23, and the fact that the study described above also had 23 subjects seems to be a coincidence) who performed a cognitive test and a fatiguing motor task, maximal voluntary contractions of the index finger, singly and simultaneously. Caffeine improved cognitive test performance, both as a single and combined task, but had no effect on the motor performance test [2].

> Isn't consuming caffeine, as with our breakfast coffee, after "overnight caffeine abstinence" just what most of us do? In the Smit and Rogers study, what was interesting is the positive effect on test results of even low doses of caffeine, such as 12.5 or 25 mg, considering that a serving of tea or cola drink may contain 50 mg and a mug of strong coffee may have 100 mg or more of caffeine.

References

1. Smit HJ, Rogers PJ. Effects of low doses of caffeine on cognitive performance, mood and thirst in low and high caffeine consumers. Psychopharmacology. 2000;152(2):167–173.
2. van Duinen H, Lorist MM, Zijdewind I. The effect of caffeine on cognitive task performance and motor fatigue. Psychopharmacology. 2005;180(3):539–547.

###

High Caffeine Consumption Cannot Be Relied Upon to Prevent Age-Related Cognitive Decline

I have tried to craft the previous sentence carefully. Here are two studies that seem pertinent. A study from The Netherlands tested the key hypothesis: that habitual caffeine intake can reduce or postpone age related cognitive decline in healthy adults. A sample of 1,376 adults were studied for 6 years, leading to the conclusion the any "longitudinal effect of habitual caffeine intake is limited and will not promote a substantial reduction in age-related cognitive decline at a population level" [1].

The second study, reported from the United Kingdom, is based on a sample of 923 healthy adults assessed for cognitive function at age 70 in whom results of childhood IQ tests are available. Results seemed to show a positive association between total caffeine consumption and cognitive ability and memory at age 70. That is, until social class and childhood IQ were considered, at which time "most of these associations became nonsignificant" [2].

I am intrigued by two incidental findings from the UK Birth Cohort 1936 study. The first is that investigators noted a "robust" link between drinking ground coffee (e.g. filter and expresso) and scores on cognitive tests. The other is that there seemed to be a trend for coffee drinkers to have higher cognitive scores than tea drinkers [2].

References

1. van Boxtel MPJ, Schmitt JAJ, Bosma H, Jolles J. The effects of habitual caffeine use on cognitive change: a longitudinal perspective. Pharmacol Biochem Behav. 2003:75(4): 921–927.
2. Corley J, Jia X, Kyle JAM, et al. Caffeine consumption and cognitive function at age 70: the Lothian Birth Cohort 1936 study. Psychosom Med. 2010;72(3):206–214.

###

Don't Count on Caffeine to Reverse the Cognitive Impairment Associated with Alcohol Use

Can caffeine counteract the risks of inappropriate or dangerous behavior that can follow drinking? Apparently not. A recent experiment involved mice, which were taught, using an adverse stimulus, to avoid a dead end arm of a maze. When given alcohol, the mice experienced a dose related decrement in both learning and anxiety, while exhibiting increased locomotion. Think of a relaxed but energized person who has had several martinis. When the mice were subsequently given caffeine, there was persistence of the ethanol-induced learning deficits [1].

Consider the currently popular alcohol-energy drink combination. One example is, or was, Spykes, an alcohol-energy drink found in brightly-colored bottles that would seem most attractive to young persons. This beverage is no longer on the market, thanks to the objections of public health experts and parents [2]. A popular cocktail combines vodka (or other alcoholic beverage) with a caffeine-containing beverage such as Red Bull or Rock Star (with the motto: Party Like a Rock Star), a recipe that can result in the ever-popular "wide-awake drunk."

References

1. Gulick D, Gould TJ. Effects of ethanol and caffeine on behavior in C57BL/6 mice in the plus-maze discrimination avoidance task. Behav Neurosci. 2009;123(6):1271–1278.
2. Alcohol, energy drinks, and youth: a dangerous mix. Available at: http://www.marininstitute. org/alcopops/energy_drink_report.htm/Accessed April 30, 2010.

###

Caffeine Can Enhance Athletic Performance, in Some Sports, Sometimes, Maybe

There are many types of sports – from table tennis to skiing to weight lifting. When it comes to athletes, a review by Burke in 2008 points out that although there are an abundance of studies of the effects of caffeine on exercise, the results do not necessarily predict actual athletic performance. Burke cites "a scarcity of field-based studies and investigations involving elite performers." The literature review led to the conclusion that moderate amounts of caffeine (about 3 mg/kg of lean body mass) can yield performance benefits in sports such as endurance events (I think here of marathon races), stop-and-go events (e.g. racquet sports or basketball), or sustained high-intensity events lasting 1–60 min (e.g., swimming or rowing) [1].

Let us review a few studies on cycling, which seems a typical endurance sport. In Scotland, Hunter et al. tested the performance of 8 highly trained cyclists given caffeine tablets or placebo prior to 100-km cycling trials. The caffeine-fueled athletes failed to excel in average power and 100-km time to completion. The article concludes: "Caffeine may be without ergogenic benefit during endurance exercise in which the athlete begins exercise with a defined, predetermined goal measured as speed or distance" [2].

On the other hand, a trial reported by McNaughton et al. in the United Kingdom found a somewhat different result. The subjects were six well-trained cyclists tested after taking caffeine or placebo. Cyclists rode significantly further during the time trail after taking caffeine than after taking the placebo [3].

Slivka et al. studied caffeine and/or carbohydrate use in nine male cyclists in negative energy balance. The conclude: "When co-ingested with carbohydrate, caffeine increased fat use and decreased nonmuscle glycogen carbohydrate use over carbohydrate alone when participants are in negative energy balance; however, caffeine had no effect on the 20 km cycling time trial performance" [4].

Finally, Beedie et al. studied six well-trained male cyclists who were informed that they would receive a placebo, 4.5 mg/kg of caffeine or 9.0 mg/kg caffeine prior to a cycling trial. All received placebos. The response was a "dose-related" effect. Subjects produced 1.4% less power than at baseline when they believed they had received a placebo; 1.3% more power when they believed they had received the moderate dose of caffeine; and 3.1% more power when they believed they had taken the higher dose of caffeine [5]. A logical conclusion seems to be that there are placebo effects of caffeine use that can affect performance [1].

Note that the reports cited above all describe "performance lab" studies. Studies involving actual athletic events/games/contests are complicated by rules, politics, and urgency of actual competition. Furthermore, what occurs in cycling is not the same as what we find in sprints, swimming, or tennis. Hence, the benefit, or lack of benefit, of caffeine on competitive athletic performance remains an area with few solid facts, considerable indirect evidence, and not a little folklore.

References

1. Burke LM. Caffeine and sports performance. Appl Physiol Nutr Metab. 2008;33(6): 1319–1334.
2. Hunter AM, St. Clair Gibson A, Collins M, Lambert M, Noakes TD. Caffeine ingestion does not alter performance during a 100-km cycling time-trial performance. Int J Sport Nutr Exerc Metab. 2002;12(4):438–452.
3. McNaughton LR, Lovell RJ, Siegler J, Midgley AW, Moore L, Bentley DJ. The effects of caffeine ingestion on time trial cycling performance. Int J Sports Physiol Perform. 2008;3(2): 157–163.
4. Slivka D, Hailes W, Cuddy J, Ruby B. Caffeine and carbohydrate supplementation during exercise when in negative energy balance: effects on performance, metabolism, and salivary cortisol. Appl Physiol Nutr Metab. 2008;33(6):1079–1085.
5. Beedie CJ, Stuart EM, Coleman DA, Foad AJ. Placebo effects of caffeine on cycling performance. Med Sci Sports Exerc. 2006;38(12):2159–2164.

###

High Coffee Intake Reduces the Risk of Type 2 Diabetes Mellitus

The consideration of health risks can include reduced risk associated with various actions. A 2004 study from the Harvard School of Public Health and two more recent literature review/meta-analysis reports affirm that something in coffee lowers diabetes risk. Salazar-Martinez in Boston examined the long-term effects of coffee and other carbonated beverages and the incidence of type 2 diabetes mellitus. The subjects were 84,276 women and 41,934 men followed for 12+ years. The investigators found an inverse relationship between habitual coffee use and type 2 diabetes mellitus, with a dose-related pattern; that is, higher levels of coffee consumption seemed to afford a lower risk of diabetes in both women and men [1].

Pimentel, reporting from Brazil, looked at 18 cohort studies, and concluded that moderate coffee intake (4 or more cups daily) is associated with a decreased risk of type 2 diabetes mellitus [2]. From Australia comes a meta-analysis of studies with information on 457,922 participants. This study quantifies the risk reduction: Every additional cup-a-Joe per day was "associated with a 7 percent reduction in excess risk of diabetes relative risk" [3]. This study, by Huxley et al. also found a decreased diabetes risk with decaffeinated coffee and tea consumption.

Interesting. From Brazil and Australia, we have two papers published in the same year, each reviewing exactly 18 studies. Is it possible that there is more than a little overlap in the studies reviewed? No matter, they came to similar conclusions, and each paper found some interesting "asides" to include. The important clinical question is: Will we someday encourage our patients with a family history of diabetes to increase their coffee and tea consumption?

References

1. Salazar-Martinez E, Willett WC, Ascherio A, et al. Coffee consumption and risk for type 2 diabetes mellitus. Ann Intern Med. 2004;140(1):1–8.
2. Pimentel GD, Zemdegs JC, Theodoro JA, Mota JF. Does long-term coffee intake reduce type 2 diabetes mellitus? Diabetol Metab Syndr. 2009;1(1):6.
3. Huxley R, Lee CM, Barzi F. Coffee, decaffeinated coffee, and tea consumption in relation to incident type 2 diabetes mellitus: a systematic review with meta-analysis. Arch Intern Med. 2009;169(22):2053–2063.

#####

Chapter 13
Unforeseen, Counterintuitive and Possibly Prophetic Findings

A discovery is generally an unforeseen relation not included in theory, for otherwise, it would be foreseen.

French Scientist Claude Bernard (1813–1878) [1].

Harriet J. was a 74-year-old woman with complaints of progressive muscle weakness, difficulty walking and impaired thinking, all developing gradually over 6–12 months. Physical examination and laboratory studies revealed skin depigmentation, liver enlargement, a trace of pedal edema, peripheral neuropathy and osteoporosis beyond what might be expected for her age. Extensive testing ruled out pernicious anemia and everything else her physician could bring to mind. What could be the cause of the patient's findings?

One day when Harriet was in the office, the physician was working with a third year medical student, who remarked, "This may sound crazy, but I think I saw something on the web about denture paste causing problems like this."

With that clue, the physician and student searched the web, finding several studies implicating denture adhesives as a cause of copper deficiency, which can result in all the manifestations that Harriet was experiencing. Harriet, a long time user of dentures, anchored them in place each day using generous amounts of denture cream. Focused blood tests confirmed both a copper deficiency and excessively high levels of zinc. The use of zinc-containing dental adhesives was stopped, followed by progressive improvement and eventual disappearance of all symptoms and signs of hypocupremia.

We take our clues where we can get them, even in odd places. In this instance, the key to the puzzle came from an on-line advertisement by some plaintiffs' attorneys, who were trolling the Internet for cases [2]. The physician and medical student reviewed two papers. One was by Nations et al. describing four patients who suffered copper deficiency with profound neurologic disease owing to chronic use of large amounts of denture cream [3]. The second report was by Hedera et al. describing 11 patients with similar findings of progressive myelopolyneuropathy associated with hypocupremia and excessively high blood levels of zinc, all related to inappropriate use of denture creams [4]. The physiologic key to the problem is that zinc and copper are absorbed competitively from the intestine, and thus a high zinc intake can result in a copper deficiency.

R.B. Taylor, *Essential Medical Facts Every Clinician Should Know: To Prevent Medical Errors, Pass Board Examinations and Provide Informed Patient Care*, DOI 10.1007/978-1-4419-7874-5_13, © Springer Science+Business Media, LLC 2011

Serendipity is one of my favorite words. Derived from *Serendip*, the Persian name for Sri Lanka. The word was coined by British author Horace Walpole (1717–1797) to describe the adventures of *The Three Princes of Serendip*, who had the gift of making of accidental, but happy discoveries. I submit that, in the case described above, the medical student viewing and subsequently recalling the legal advertisement describing victims of dental cream toxicity represented an example of serendipity, or accidental sagacity, to use Walpole's phrase. Serendipity also played a role for whoever first connected the dots linking zinc in dental cream and copper deficiency; I feel certain that this unforeseen finding did not start out as a hypothesis.

This chapter is an eclectic collection of serendipitous findings, intriguing facts encountered while meandering through the medical literature as I conducted research for this book. As I read these items, I thought of a quotation by Osler: "… the philosophies of one age have become the absurdities of the next, and the foolishness of yesterday has become the wisdom of tomorrow…" [5]. Some represent "threshold concepts," notions outside the realm of our core knowledge, such as the reduced risk of diabetes in patients with rheumatoid arthritis taking hydroxychloroquine. Sometimes we even encounter "troublesome knowledge," facts that are conceptually truly counter-intuitive to our cherished belief systems [6]. Read on to learn about the long-term effects of minimally invasive radical prostatectomy, and about the worrisome cognitive deficits in patients with "benign" essential tremor. Along the way you will encounter some possibly prophetic concepts, such as the findings of a surgical approach to migraine headache or speculation that antidepressant therapy may have a beneficial effect on the inflammatory processes in patients with heart failure.

References

1. Bernard C. An introduction to the study of experimental medicine, Pt. I, Ch 2, Section iii (Translated by H.C. Green) Quoted in: Strauss MB. Familiar medical quotations. Boston: Little, Brown; 1968. Page 108.
2. Dangers of denture cream causing zinc toxicity. Available at: http://www.zinctoxicitylawyer.com/?gclid=CNCZ4MWluaECFRk7gwodW0E-_Q/ Accessed May 4, 2010.
3. Nations SP, Boyer PJ, Love LA, et al. Denture cream: an unusual source of excess zinc, leading to hypocupremia and neurologic disease. Neurology. 2008;71(9):639–643.
4. Hedera P, Peltier A, Fink JK, Wilcock S, London Z, Brewer GJ. Myelopolyneuropathy and pancytopenia due to copper deficiency and high zinc levels of unknown origin II: the denture cream is a primary source of excessive zinc. Neurotoxicity. 2009;30(6):996–999.
5. Osler W. Aequanimitas with other addresses, 3rd edition. Philadelphia: Blakiston; 1932. Page 266.
6. Meyer JHF, Land R. Threshold concepts and troublesome knowledge: linkages to ways of thinking and practicing within disciplines. In: Improving student learning – ten years on. Rust C, editor. New York: Oxford University Press, 2003.

#

Essential Tremor (ET) Is Often Not "Benign"

Essential tremor (ET), a neurological disease of older persons, is the most commonly encountered movement disorder [1]. Because we are now learning of additional manifestations, essential tremor is no longer considered "benign." A 2001 report comparing 18 ET and 18 Parkinson disease (PD) patients revealed that the ET group had greater impairment in verbal fluency and working memory than those in the PD cohort. Tremor severity did not correlate with cognitive defects [2]. This finding was supported the following year by Lombardi et al. who reported impaired cognitive function in 12 of 13 ET subjects [1]. In 2007, Baerejo-Pareja et al. in Spain found incident dementia in 16 (7.8%) of 206 ET cases, compared with incident dementia in 145 (3.9%) of 3,685 controls, suggesting that ET in the elderly roughly doubles the risk of developing dementia [3].

A more recent study at Columbia University in New York City, describes the use of handwriting samples to identify subjects with ET. The investigators found that ET was associated with increased odds of prevalent dementia (25.0%) and increased risk of incident dementia (18.3%) [4].

Cognitive impairment is not the only risk associated with ET. A study of 250 ET patients compared with 127 PD patients and 127 normal controls revealed worse hearing in the ET group, with the hearing loss tending to be associated with tremor severity [5].

References

1. Lacritz LH, Dewey R Jr, Giller C, Cullum CM. Cognitive functioning in individuals with "benign" essential tremor. J Int Neuropsychol Soc. 2002;8(1):125–129.
2. Lombardi WJ, Woolston DJ, Roberts JW, Gross RE. Cognitive deficits in patients with essential tremor. Neurology. 2001;57(5):785–790.
3. Bermejo-Pareja F, Louis ED, Benikto-León J. Risk of incident dementia in essential tremor: a population-based study. Mov Disord. 2007;22(11):1573–1580.
4. Thawani SP, Schupf N, Louis ED. Essential tremor is associated with dementia: prospective population-based study in New York. Neurology. 2009;73(8):621–625.
5. Ondo WG, Sutton L, Dat Vuong K, Lai D, Jankovic J. Hearing impairment in essential tremor. Neurology. 2003;61(9):1093–1097.

###

Aspirin Rivals Sumatriptan in Providing Relief of Acute Migraine Headache

Since its introduction two decades ago, sumatriptan (Imitrex) has been the gold standard in headache relief, affording hefty profits to its manufacturer, GlaxoSmithKline, and prompting the development of a number of similar "triptans."

Now we find a widely-read 2010 meta-analysis of 13 randomized clinical trials (4,222 subjects) showing that three adult aspirin tablets (900–1,000 mg) yield relief similar to sumatriptan 50 or 100 mg. When the outcome measure was 2-h headache relief and freedom from pain, aspirin alone and sumatriptan showed no difference. When aspirin plus metoclopramide was compared with sumatriptan 100 mg, the "triptan" excelled in providing freedom from pain at 2 h, but not when headache relief was the variable measured. [1]

> This article, as I pointed out in Chapter one is a potential **practice-changer**, especially when we consider the huge cost difference between the two drugs.

Reference

1. Kirthi V, Derry S, Moore RA, McQuay HJ. Aspirin with and without an antiemetic for acute migraine headaches in adults. Cochrane Database Sys Rev. 2010 April 14;4:CD008041.

###

Surgical Deactivation of Migraine Trigger Sites May Prove to Be Useful Therapy for Some

From the Departments of Plastic Surgery and Neurology (an uncommon pairing, to be sure) at Case Western Reserve University in Cleveland, Ohio comes a report of 75 migraineurs randomly assigned to receive actual or sham surgery in their predominant trigger site [1]. Of the 49 patients in the actual surgery group, 41 (83.7%) reported at least 50% reduction in migraine symptoms, when measured by three migraine-specific survey instruments. This compared with 15 (57.7%) of 26 patients in the sham surgery group reporting a 50% relief.

> Given that, as the authors point out, many of America's 30 million migraineurs are not helped by usual therapy, the surgical approach may turn out to have some merit. On a personal note: Because migraine pain has a subjective component, and because many drugs are evaluated as remedies, I have, as described on page 77, told my students that if they wish to evaluate any given drug, fruit or vegetable for its efficacy in treating migraine, they will reach the conclusion that 50% of subjects in the test group experienced 50% improvement.
> Thus, the fact that 83.7% of subjects in the actual surgery group experienced the magic 50% improvement in symptoms means that this approach may be more effective than most other approaches tested.

Reference

1. Guyuron B, Reed D, Kriegler JS, Davis J, Pashmini N, Amini S. A placebo-controlled surgical trial of the treatment of migraine headaches. Plast Reconstr Surg. 2009;124(2):469–470.

###

Women with Migraine Seem to Have a Reduced Risk of Breast Cancer

The statement above is based on a multicenter, population-based case-control study involving nine of the United States' most prestigious research centers (such as the Fred Hutchinson Cancer Research Center in Seattle). Data analyzed involved 4,568 breast cancer cases and 4,678 controls. The result was that women with a history of migraine had a reduced risk of breast cancer, with an odds ratio 0.74, and this finding was independent of exposure to common migraine triggers such as alcohol use. Furthermore the reduced risk of breast cancer was noted with both premenopausal and postmenopausal women [1].

The link here seems to be that breast cancer and migraine are both, to some degree, hormonally mediated diseases [1].

Reference

1. Li CI, Mathes RW, Malone KE, et al. Relationship between migraine history and breast cancer risk among premenopausal and postmenopausal women. Cancer Epidemiol Biomarkers Prev. 2009;18(7):2030–2034.

###

Children with Acute Otitis Media (AOM) Initially Treated with Amoxicillin Have Been Found to Have More Recurrences When Compared with Placebo

A randomized double-blind, placebo-controlled study of 168 children with AOM were treated with amoxicillin or placebo, and studied for recurrence of disease up to 3.5 years.

Of 75 children treated with amoxicillin, 47 (63%) experienced recurrence of AOM, compared with 37 (43%) of 86 subjects in the placebo group. In their conclusion, the authors consider their findings to be "another argument for judicious use of antibiotics in children with acute otitis media" [1].

Although I find the primary outcome of this study to be counterintuitive, I accept the data and their analysis, even though the recurrence reports were based on parental recall evidence.

Also, in this study I find it interesting that of the amoxicillin group, 21% had subsequent ear, nose and throat surgery compared with 30% of the placebo group, which seems more in line with what one might predict.

Reference

1. Bezankova N, Damoiseaux RA, Hoes AW, Schilder AG, Rovers MM. Recurrence up to 3.5 years after antibiotic treatment of otitis media in very young Dutch children: survey of trial participants. BMJ. 2009;338:b2525 doi: 10.1136/bmj2525.

###

Withholding Antibiotic Treatment of Acute Otitis Media Influences the Incidence of Acute Mastoiditis

The incidence of acute mastoiditis is rising. Thorne et al. reviewed the experience at Children's Hospital of Philadelphia from 2000 to 2007. After controlling for case volume, they found an increase in cases of acute mastoiditis with subperiosteal swelling [1].

In 2010, Brook looked at the possible influence of antibiotic therapy of acute otitis media and subsequent suppurative complications. He found that the risk of acute mastoiditis among children whose AOM was treated with antibiotics was 1.8 per 10,000, compared with 3.8 for untreated children [2].

In the early 1940s penicillin was urgently being developed as a tactical weapon in the war effort, and mastoiditis was a dreaded complication of ear infections. Many youngsters bore the scars of surgical mastoidectomies, the treatment of the day.

> *Although it seems clear that antibiotic therapy of AOM lowers the risk of subsequent mastoiditis, how much such therapy is needed? Brook supplies some handy figures. He calculates that to prevent a single instance of acute mastoiditis, 4,831 children with AOM would require antibiotic therapy. The number needed to treat (NNT) drops to about 2,000 + in the older age group. Looking at the United Kingdom as a whole, ceasing all antibiotic treatment of AOM would eliminate 738,775 antibiotic prescriptions per year, at the cost of an additional 255 cases of acute suppurative mastoiditis [2].*
>
> *And, of course, the studies cited do not consider other classic complications of untreated otitis media including meningitis, lateral sinus thrombosis, and chronic suppurative otitis media [3].*

References

1. Thorne MC, Chewaproug L, Elden LM. Suppurative complications of acute otitis media: changes in frequency over time. Arch Otolaryngol Head Neck Surg. 2009;135(7):638–641.
2. Brook I. Antimicrobial therapy of otitis media reduces the incidence of mastoiditis. Curr Infect Dis Rep. 2010;12:1–3.
3. Poole MD. Otitis media complications and treatment failures: implications of pneumococcal resistance. Pediatr Infect Dis J. 1995;14(4 Suppl):S23–S26.

###

Adjuvant Tamoxifen Therapy of Primary Breast Cancer May Increase the Risk of Estrogen Receptor (ER) Negative Contralateral Breast Cancer

The study cited here involved 367 women with both ER-positive invasive breast cancer and a second primary contralateral breast cancer, compared with 728 control women diagnosed with only a first breast cancer. As might be expected, those who used tamoxifen therapy for five or more years had a reduced risk of ER-positive contralateral breast cancer, but had a 4.4-fold increased risk of ER-negative contralateral breast cancer [1].

As the authors point out, although ER-negative contralateral breast cancer is a "relatively uncommon outcome," this subtype has a poorer prognosis than ER-positive tumors [1].

Reference

1. Li CI, Daling JR, Porter PL, Tang MT, Maline KE. Adjuvant hormonal therapy for breast cancer and risk of hormone receptor-specific subtypes of contralateral breast cancer. Cancer Res. 2009;69(17):6865–6870.

###

Breast Cancer in Men, When it Occurs, Is Likely to Be Hormone Receptor Positive

Breast cancer in men accounts for approximately 1% of all breast cancers. Genetic risk factors include BRCA2 mutations, Klinefelter syndrome, and positive family history of breast cancer. Other risks include obesity, cryptorchidism, orchiectomy, radiation exposure, and Jewish ancestry [1, 2].

Giordano et al. reviewed articles concerning male breast cancer published between 1942 and 2000, finding that 81% of breast tumors in men were ER-positive and 74% were progesterone receptor positive [2].

Recognition of the hormone receptor status in male breast cancer is important because, as with women with breast cancer, adjuvant therapy is used to treat male patients who have a substantial risk of recurrence and death from breast cancer [3].

References

1. Weiss JR, Moysich KB, Swede H. Epidemiology of male breast cancer. Cancer Epidemiol Biomarkers Prev. 2005;14(1):20–26.
2. Giordano SH, Buzdar AU, Hortobagyi GN. Breast cancer in men. Ann Intern Med. 2002;137(8):678–687.
3. Giordano SH. A review of diagnosis and management of male breast cancer. Oncologist. 2005;10(7):471–479.

###

Pneumococcal Polysaccharide Vaccination (PPV) May Not Provide Adults the Protection Against Pneumonia We Would Like to Think It Does

Huss et al. review 22 trials involving 101,507 subjects. The investigators note a variety of quality among the trials examined, and report that in studies with the best methodologic quality, there was little evidence of vaccine protection against presumptive pneumonia (relative risk [RR] 1.20) and against all-cause pneumonia (RR 1.19). When vaccine protection was studied in the setting of the most vulnerable populations, elderly persons and chronically ill adults, there was also scant evidence of protection against presumptive pneumococcal pneumonia (RR 0.89) and all-cause pneumonia (RR 1.00) [1].

These findings generally support the conclusion of a 2003 Cochrane Database review of randomized studies that concluded: "While polysaccharide pneumococcal vaccines do not appear to reduce the incidence of pneumonia or death in adults with or without chronic illness, or in the elderly (55 years and above), the evidence from the non-randomized studies suggests that the vaccines are effective in reducing the incidence of the more specific outcome, invasive pneumococcal disease among adults and the immunocompetent elderly (age 55 years and above)." The authors of this study offer a handy estimate of the number-needed-to-treat: 20,000 vaccinations per infection avoided and perhaps 50,000 per death avoided [2].

A 2008 Cochrane Database review, actually an update of the 2003 review cited above, examined 22 studies involving 62,294 subjects. The review found evidence to support the use of pneumococcal vaccine to prevent invasive pneumococcal disease in adults, but did not "provide compelling evidence to support the routine use of PPV to prevent all-cause pneumonia or mortality" [3].

Just to add another wrinkle to this issue, a study of 3,415 patients with community-acquired pneumonia (CAP) revealed that those with prior PPV immunization had a 40% lower rate of death or intensive care unit admission compared with those not previously vaccinated [4].

> *Here is another personal reflection. Although I know the difference between an antibiotic prescription and an immunization, I am struck by the NNT when it comes to treating acute otitis media with antibiotics (about 2,000, see above) to prevent acute mastoiditis in older children with AOM and the NNT with pneumococcal vaccine (about 20,000) to prevent a case of pneumococcal pneumonia.*

References

1. Huss A, Scott P, Stuck AE, et al. Efficacy of pneumococcal vaccination in adults: a meta-analysis. CMAJ. 2009;180(1):48–58.
2. Dear K, Holden J, Andrews R, Tatham D. Vaccines for preventing pneumococcal infection in adults. Cochrane Database Sys Rev. 2003;(4):CD000422.

3. Moberley SA, Holden J, Tatham DP, Andrews RM. Vaccines for preventing pneumococcal infection in adults. Cochrane Database Sys Rev. 2008;(1):CD000422.
4. Johnstone J, Marrie TJ, Eurich DT, Majumdar SR. Effect of pneumococcal vaccination in hospitalized adults with community-acquired pneumonia. Arch Intern Med. 2007; 167(18):1938–1943.

###

Pneumococcal Vaccine Does Seem to Offer Protection to Human Immunodeficiency Virus (HIV)-Infected Adults Against Recurrent Pneumococcal Infection

A study was conducted in Malawi of the efficacy of 7-valent conjugate pneumococcal vaccine in 496 predominately HIV-infected subjects who had recovered from documented invasive pneumococcal disease. The authors concluded, "The 7-valent pneumococcal conjugate vaccine protected HIV-infected adults from recurrent pneumococcal infection by vaccine serotypes or serotype 6A" [1].

It seems to me that, whatever decision might be made about the use of pneumococcal vaccine in the elderly, patients with HIV should be afforded protection.

Reference

1. French N, Gordon SB, Mwalukomo T, et al. A trial of 7-valent pneumococcal conjugate vaccine in HIV-infected adults. N Engl J Med. 2010;362(9):812–822.

###

Statins May Play a Beneficial Role in Patients with Chronic Obstructive Lung Disease (COPD)

Two studies support this theory. The first, from the University of British Columbia in Vancouver, Canada was a systematic review of nine studies, all of which showed benefits involving various outcome measures for COPD patients. These favorable outcome measures included exercise capacity, pulmonary function, the number of COPD exacerbations, the number and the time to intubation, COPD mortality, and all-cause mortality [1].

In the second study, reported from The Netherlands, investigators studied 3,371 patients undergoing vascular surgery for peripheral vascular disease. Of these subjects, 1,310 (39%) had COPD. All were followed for a median of 5 years for lung or extrapulmonary mortality. Investigators found COPD linked to a doubling of the risk of lung cancer (hazard ratio [HR] 2.06) and an increased risk of extrapulmonary cancer death (HR 1.43). Study results showed a lower risk of cancer mortality in COPD patients using statins when compared with COPD patients not using statins (HR 0.57). The also found a lower risk of extrapulmonary cancer mortality among statin users with COPD (HR 0.49) [2].

These papers suggest that we should have a low threshold for prescribing statins in COPD patients with high cholesterol levels. One might wonder if we will someday prescribe statins for all our COPD patients, as we recommend angiotensin converting enzyme (ACE) inhibitors for persons found to have non-diabetic, non-nephrotic proteinuria [3].

References

1. Janda S, Park K, FitzGerald JM, Etminan M, Swiston J. Statins in COPD: a systematic review. Chest. 2009;136(3):734–743.
2. van Gestel YR, Hoeks SE, Sin DD, et al. COPD and cancer mortality: the influence of statins. Thorax. 2009;64(11):963–967.
3. Ruggenenti P, Perna A, Gherardi G, et al. Renoprotective properties of ACE-inhibition in non-diabetic nephropathies with non-nephrotic proteinuria. Lancet. 1999;354(9176): 359–364.

Statins May Reduce Proteinuria and Slow the Rate of Kidney Function Loss, Especially in Patients with Cardiovascular Disease

I came across this paper while checking my facts on statins, COPD, and proteinuria. Sandhu et al. performed a meta-analysis of 27 studies involving 39,704 subjects to assess the effect of statins on urinary protein excretion and changes in renal function. They found that "the standardized mean difference for the reduction in albuminuria or proteinuria as a result of statin therapy was statistically significant." Patients with cardiovascular problems seemed to benefit most.

This is one more benefit of statin use to keep in mind when making treatment decisions in our patients with cardiovascular disease.

Reference

1. Sandhu S, Wiebe N, Fried LF, Tonelli. Statins for improving renal outcomes: a meta-analysis. Oncologist. 2005;10(7):471–479.

###

In Patients with Worsening Heart Failure (HF), Statin Use May Improve Left Ventricular Ejection Fraction (LVEF) and Decrease the Risk of Hospitalization

A meta-analysis of 10 studies involving 10,192 patients taking one of three statin drugs followed for 3–47 months revealed a 4.2% increase in LVEF and a significant decrease in hospitalization for worsening HF upon follow-up [1].

This chapter is beginning to seem like an "Ode to Statins." In fact, my research has even led me to a study whose authors wonder if "universal statin therapy for older U.S. adults warrants investigation" [2]. In the meta-analysis cited above, just to show that no drug does everything, the investigators did not find that statins improve cardiovascular or all- cause mortality in the heart failure patients studied. Nor did statins make these outcomes worse [1]. Also, a meta-analysis by Ray et al. "did not find evidence for the benefit of statin therapy on all-cause mortality in a high-risk primary prevention set-up" [3].

References

1. Lipinski MJ, Cauthen CA, Biondi-Zoccai GG, et al. Meta-analysis of randomized controlled trials of statins versus placebo in patients with heart failure. Am J Cardiol. 2009;104(12): 1708–1716.
2. Muntner P, Mann D, Razzouk L, et al. Is measuring C-reactive protein useful for guiding treatment in women ≥60 years and men ≥50 years of age? Am J Cardiol. 2009;104(3): 354–358.
3. Ray KK, Seshasai SR, Erquo S, et al. Statins and all-cause mortality in high-risk primary prevention: a meta-analysis of 11 randomized controlled trials involving 65,229 participants. Arch Intern Med. 2010;170(12):1024–1031.

Appendicitis and Mesenteric Lymphadenitis When Young Reduces the Risk of Adult Ulcerative Colitis

Frisch et al. in Copenhagen conducted a study that covered a heroic 11.1 million years of follow-up of patients who had undergone appendectomy for appendicitis in childhood or adolescence. They found that no matter whether or not persons had a family history of inflammatory bowel disease (IBD), the risk of developing ulcerative colitis during adulthood was significantly reduced following appendectomy for appendicitis. Furthermore, in those with a family history of IBD, a cohort who notoriously have an increased risk of developing ulcerative colitis, the risk after appendectomy for appendicitis was halved [1].

In this study and in another reported in 2010, appendectomy in the absence of appendicitis offered no protection against the development of ulcerative colitis [1].

Reference

1. Frisch M, Pedersen BV, Andersson RE. Appendicitis, mesenteric lymphadenitis, and subsequent risk of ulcerative colitis: cohort studies in Sweden and Denmark. BMJ. 2009;338:b716. Doi. 10.1136/bmj.b716.

###

A Family History of Colorectal Cancer May Offer a Reduced Risk of Cancer Recurrence and Death in Patients with Stage III Colon Cancer

Chan et al. at the Dana-Farber Cancer Institute in Boston conducted a prospective study of 1,087 patients with stage III colon cancer who were receiving adjuvant chemotherapy. Of those who had a family history of colorectal cancer, the incidence of cancer recurrence or death was 29%, compared with a 38% incidence of cancer recurrence or death in those with no family history of colorectal cancer.

This finding seems paradoxical, given that a family history of colorectal cancer in a first-degree relative increases the risk of developing colorectal cancer, but will be some comfort to stage III colon cancer patients with positive family histories.

Reference

1. Chan JA, Meyerhardt JA, Niedzwieki D et al. Association of family history with cancer recurrence and survival among patients with Stage III colon cancer. JAMA. 2008; 299:2515–2523.

###

Screening Colonoscopy Reduces the Prevalence of Colorectal Cancer, But Chiefly in Regard to Neoplasms in the Left Colon

A trial by Brenner et al. in Germany studied 3,287 persons undergoing screening colonoscopy. Of those undergoing previous colonoscopy within the prior 10 years 6.1% were found to have advanced neoplasms, compared to 11.4% of those who had received no prior screening. What is arguably unforeseen was the finding of a 67% risk reduction with prior colonoscopy that was limited to left-sided neoplasms and did not extend to right-sided tumors [1].

Why was the reduction in neoplasms with screening colonoscopy within 10 years of colonoscopy limited to left-sided lesions? Yes, most colorectal neoplasms occur on the left, but this does not truly answer the question? The reason must be the technical difficulties related to examining the right colon compared to the left.

Reference

1. Brenner H, Hoffmeister M, Arndt V, Stegmaier C, Altenhofen L, Haug U. Protection from right- and left-sided colorectal neoplasms after colonoscopy: population-based study. J Natl Cancer Inst. 2010;102(2):89–95.

###

The Venerated Digital Rectal Examination (DRE) May Be as Harmful as Helpful in Diagnosis, at Least in Patients with Undifferentiated Abdominal Pain

Quass et al. studied the merits of the digital rectal examination in the evaluation of undifferentiated abdominal pain, a setting in which a rectal exam would seem a reasonable part of the physical examination. Of 893 patients with undifferentiated abdominal pain, 538 (60%) had a DRE performed. In only 44 of these subjects did the examining physicians consider the DRE as influential in formulating their differential diagnosis. Of the 538 patients, 17 (3%) were diagnostically helped and 12 (2%) were diagnostically harmed. The statisticians on the study calculate that unless all 11 of the subjects lost to follow-up were "helped," the help-harm balance was a dead heat [1].

> *William J. Mayo (1861–1939) once wrote, "The examining physician often hesitates to make the necessary examination because it involves soiling the finger" [2]. Even now, woe to the medical intern who fails to perform a digital rectal examination on every hospital patient, a comment that highlights the finding by Yeong et al. that the digital rectal examination is often performed by the most inexperienced physician and frequently not verified by a more senior colleague [3]. Perhaps there is a better way. The authors of the cited study advise: "Given the discomfort and minimal predictive value of the DRE in this setting (undifferentiated abdominal pain), highly selective use seems reasonable" [1].*

References

1. Quass J, Lanigan M, Newman D, McOsker J, Babayev R, Mason C. Utility of the digital rectal examination in the evolution of undifferentiated abdominal pain. Am J Emerg Med. 2009;27(9):1125–1129.
2. Mayo WJ. In: Journal-Lancet 1915;35:339. Quoted in: Strauss MB. Familiar medical quotations. Boston: Little, Brown; 1968. Pages 164–165.
3. Yeung JM, Yeeles H, Tang SW, Hong LL, Amin S. How good are newly qualified doctors at digital rectal examination? Colorectal Dis. DOI: 10.1111/j.1463-1318.2009.02116.x. Published online Nov. 6, 2009.

###

Diabetic Self-Monitoring May Risk Depression with No Gain in Glycemic Control

O'Kane et al. in Northern Ireland conducted a study of newly diagnosed type 2 diabetic men. Of these, 96 were randomized to self-monitoring and 88 to serve as controls. HbA1c values determined monthly for 1 year showed no significant differences at any time. However, patients engaged in self-monitoring scored 6% higher on a depression scale [1].

Should every patient with type 2 diabetes know the technique of self-monitoring? I say, yes. Should every patient with type 2 diabetes monitor their blood glucose levels regularly – several times daily or weekly? The cited study suggests that the answer is, no.

Reference

1. O'Kane MJ, Bunting B, Copeland M, Coates VE: the ESMON Study Group. Efficacy of self-monitoring of blood glucose in patients with newly diagnosed type 2 diabetes (ESMON Study): randomized controlled trial. BMJ. 2008;336(7654):1174–1177.

###

Bariatric Surgery May Yield a Dividend Beyond Weight Loss: Remission of Type 2 Diabetes

A 2002 paper, from a surgery institute in France, reviewed the literature pertaining to weight loss surgery and glucose metabolism, coming to the conclusion: "Gastric bypass and biliopancreatic diversion seem to achieve control of diabetes as a primary and independent effect, not secondary to the treatment of overweight" [1].

In 2009, Dixon reported a remission of type 2 diabetes in 50–85% of persons following bariatric surgery [2]. This was followed in 2010 by a report by Hauser et al. describing the results of laparoscopic Roux-en-Y gastric bypass in 70 patients with a mean age 52 years. Of the 35 patients (50%) in this group with type 2 diabetes, 91% experienced a normalization of their glycosylated hemoglobin levels, while another 6% showed improvement [3].

Of course, we really should not use the word "cure" in connection with diabetes [1]. Nevertheless there seems to be solid evidence that bariatric surgery can be followed by remission. Will we soon be recommending surgery chiefly for management of difficult-to-control diabetes in individuals who happen to be obese?

References

1. Rubino F, Gagner M. Potential of surgery for curing type 2 diabetes mellitus. Ann Surg. 2002;236(5):544–549.
2. Dixon JB. Obesity and diabetes: the impact of bariatric surgery on type-2 diabetes. World J Surg. 2009;33(10):2014–2021.
3. Hauser DL, Titchner RL, Wilson MA, Eid GM. Long-term outcomes of laparoscopic Roux-en-Y gastric bypass in US veterans. Obes Surg. 2010;20(3):283–289.

###

Persons Taking Hydroxychloroquine for Rheumatoid Arthritis Seem to Have a Reduced Risk of Developing Diabetes

An 18 month study of 4,905 adults with rheumatoid arthritis – 1808 taking hydroxychloroquine and 3,097 who had never taken the drug – followed for a truly impressive 21.5 years showed a lower incidence of diabetes in the hydroxychloroquine group – 5.2 versus 8.9 cases of diabetes per 1,000 patient-years of observation – with the risk of diabetes significantly reduced with increased duration of use [1].

This is an interesting study, but I am still pondering how to use the observation in practice.

Reference

1. Wasko MCM, Hubert HB, Lingala VB. Hydroxychloroquine and risk of diabetes in patients with rheumatoid arthritis. JAMA. 2007; 298(2): 187–193.

###

In Patients with Both Heart Failure and Diabetes Mellitus, There Is a "Sweet Spot" in the Middle Range of Glycosylated Hemoglobin Values When Risk of Death Is Considered

Aguilar et al. studied 5,815 veterans with both HF and diabetes, and divided their HbA1c values into five quintiles. In the 2 years of the trial, the highest death rates occurred the top and bottom quintiles, that is, in the quintiles with the highest and lowest glycosylated hemoglobin levels. The middle quintile, with HbA1c values of 7.1–7.8%, fared the best [1].

In this study, the same "sweet spot" phenomenon was not found in regard to hospitalization rates for HF. The investigators did report a non-statistically-significant linear relationship among HbA1c quintiles and hospitalization rates for HF; that is, higher hospitalization rates with higher HbA1c levels [1].

Reference

1. Aguilar D, Bozkurt B, Ramasubbu K, Deswal A. Relationship of hemoglobin A1c and mortality in heart failure patients with diabetes. J Am Coll Cardiol. 2009;54:422–428.

###

Type 2 Diabetics at High Risk for Cardiovascular Events May Not Benefit from Rigorous Blood Pressure Control

This was a nicely designed study in which 4,733 subjects with type 2 diabetes mellitus were randomly assigned to intensive antihypertensive therapy with a target of 120 mmHg systolic pressure, or to receive usual therapy. Patients were followed for a mean of 4.7 years, with primary outcomes of major cardiovascular events: nonfatal myocardial infarction, nonfatal stroke, or cardiovascular death. At the end of this time, data revealed the following: "In patients with type 2 diabetes at high risk for cardiovascular events, targeting a systolic blood pressure of less than 120 mmHg, as compared with less than 140 mmHg, did not reduce the rate of a composite of fatal and nonfatal major cardiovascular events" [1].

*For those who have advocated for especially intensive antihypertensive therapy in type 2 diabetic patients, this report may be a **practice changer.***

Reference

1. ACCORD Study Group, Cushman WC, Evans GW, Byington RP, et al. Effects of intensive blood-pressure control in type 2 diabetes mellitus. N Engl J Med. 2010;362(17):1575–1585.

###

In Patients with Diabetic Neuropathy, High Dose B-Vitamins Can Adversely Affect Renal Function and Increase the Risk of Vascular Events

This study was a multicenter, randomized, double blind, placebo-controlled trial involving 238 subjects with type 1 or type 2 diabetes complicated by diabetic neuropathy. Patients were given a single daily tablet of B vitamins containing folic acid (2.5 mg), vitamin B6 (25 mg), and vitamin B12 (1 mg) or matching placebo. At 36 months patients taking high-dose B vitamins had a greater decrement in glomerular filtration rate and a higher rate of myocardial infarction and stroke [1].

> *Given that the stated objective of the study was "To determine whether B-vitamin therapy can slow progression of diabetic neuropathy and prevent vascular events," the outcome – reduced renal function and more heart attacks and strokes in the B-vitamin cohort – must have been a truly unforeseen result.*

Reference

1. House AA, Eliasziw M, Cattran DC, et al. Effect of B-vitamin therapy on progression of diabetic neuropathy: a randomized controlled trial. JAMA. 2010;303(16):1603–1609.

###

In One Study, Placebo Therapy Both Helped and Harmed Patients with Benign Prostatic Hyperplasia (BPH)

The study examined what happened to 303 patients enrolled in the placebo cohort of a trial evaluating the use of the antiandrogen finasteride (Proscar) in the management of BPH. Just to emphasize, this involved a "placebo-only" group of subjects. Over the 25 months of follow-up, there was a rapid and significant improvement in symptom scores and in maximum urinary flow rate (Qmax), all in the face of an 8.4% average progressive increase in prostate volume. But there were some problems with this otherwise promising *placebo* therapy: Some patients (6.3%) reported decreased libido and another 6.3% told of impotence. Adverse side effects prompted 13.2% of patients to discontinue the placebo therapy [1].

> *This strikes me as an amazing example of the power of placebo therapy. Note that the Qmax is an objective measurement of urinary flow rate. It also seems an enviable example of "data mining," which I define as searching mountains of data, data collected for some other reason, hunting for a nugget of clinical value.*

Reference

1. Nickel JC. Placebo therapy of benign prostatic hyperplasia: a 25-month study. Canadian PROSPECT Study Group. Br J Urol. 1998;81(3):383–387.

###

Minimally Invasive Radical Prostatectomy (MIRP) Offers Short Term Advantages, But a Greater Risk of Long Term Problems When Compared with Open Retropubic Radical Prostatectomy (RRP)

Hu et al. studied men with prostatic cancer treated with robotic-assisted MIRP (n = 1938) or RRP (n = 6,899). How did they compare? Compared with the RRP patients, MIRP patients had a shorter length of hospital stay (median stay, 2.0 vs. 3.0 days), fewer postoperative respiratory complications (4.3% vs. 6.6%); fewer miscellaneous surgical complications (4.3% vs. 5.6%); and lower transfusion rates (2.7% vs. 20.8%). On the other hand, compared with RRP, patients undergoing MIRP had a greater incidence of genitourinary complications (4.7% vs. 2.1%); incontinence (15.9 vs. 12.2 per 100 person-years); and erectile dysfunction (26.8 vs. 19.2 per 100 person-years) [1].

> As of the time of this writing, this is the latest and best series to have been reported. Robot-assisted radical prostatectomy is a relatively new and rapidly evolving technique, involving nerve-sparing maneuvers and other advances, and so we look for future changes in comparative outcomes. As for this study, it seems an example of the "troublesome knowledge" described by Meyer and Land [2]. I enjoyed reading the authors' reflection: "In light of the mixed outcomes associated with MIRP, our finding that men of higher socioeconomic status opted for a high-technology alternative despite insufficient data demonstrating superiority over an established gold standard may be a reflection of a society and health care system enamored with new technology that increased direct and indirect health care costs but had yet to uniformly realize marketed or potential benefits during early adoption" [1].
>
> Of course, all of this begs the question of when, if ever, to operate on men with prostate cancer. And in the data above, note the 20.8% transfusion rate with RRP, a figure I would consider worrisome were I a patient.

References

1. Hu JC, Xiangmei G, Lipsitz SR, et al. Comparative effectiveness of minimally invasive vs. open radical prostatectomy. JAMA. 2009;302(14);1557–1564.
2. Meyer JHF, Land R. Threshold concepts and troublesome knowledge: linkages to ways of thinking and practicing within disciplines. In: Improving student learning – ten years on. Rust C, editor. New York: Oxford University Press, 2003.

###

Vertebroplasty Seems to Offer "No Beneficial Effect" in the Treatment of Painful Osteoporotic Vertebral Fractures

From Australia comes a report of a multicenter, randomized, double-blind, placebo-controlled trial to assess the merits of vertebroplasty in relieving the pain of osteoporotic vertebral fractures. Of an original 78 subjects with painful osteoporotic vertebral fractures randomized to receive vertebroplasty or a sham procedure, 35 of 38 who underwent vertebroplasty and 36 of 40 who had placebo surgery completed the 6-month follow-up. Although both groups showed gradual improvement in pain, physical functioning, and quality of life, the investigators did not find vertebroplasty to "result in a significant advantage in any measured outcome at any point in time" [1].

Vertebroplasty as a treatment of painful osteoporotic fractures has a relatively short history; a 2002 paper describes it as a "new treatment strategy for osteoporotic compression fractures" [2]. I might even compare its rise to popularity as similar to that of robot-assisted radical prostatectomy. Now we have a paper that seems to show no benefit. Of course there are the risks and inevitable misadventures associated with a surgical procedure, whether needed or not. I am reminded of a favorite quote by American biochemist Lawrence Henderson (1878–1942): "Somewhere between 1910 and 1912 in this country, a random patient, with a random disease, consulting a doctor chosen at random had, for the first time in the history of mankind, a better than fifty-fifty chance of profiting from the encounter" [3]. (Henderson was probably alluding to the discovery at that time by Paul Ehrlich of the organoarsenic compound arsphenamine, aka Salvarsan, as a treatment for syphilis). I wonder today if we do not still face the same risk:benefit ratio when considering some of our currently popular surgical procedures and medical therapy recommendations.

The apparent lack of effectiveness of vertebroplasty, with the attendant operative risks, is especially ironic, given that a well-designed systematic review in 2005 of 5 trials involving 246 subjects with painful osteoporotic compression fractures revealed that "calcitonin significantly reduced the severity of pain using a visual analogue scale following diagnosis," and shortened the time to mobilization [4]. In this study, not a single surgical complication occurred.

References

1. Buchbinder R, Osborne RH, Ebeling PR, et al. A randomized trial of vertebroplasty for painful osteoporotic vertebral fractures. N Engl J Med. 2009;361(6):557–568.
2. Eck JC, Hodges SD, Humphrews SC. Vertebroplasty: a new treatment strategy for osteoporotic compression fractures. Am J Orthop. 2002;31(3):123–127.
3. Henderson LJ. Quoted in: Aring CD. A random patient consulting a physician at random. JAMA. 1974;229(7):785–786.
4. Knopp JA, Diner BM, Blitz M, Lytitis GP, Rowe BH. Calcitonin for treating acute pain of osteoporotic vertebral compression fractures: a systematic review of randomized, controlled trials. Osteoporosis Int. 2005;16(10):1281–1290.

Conventional Non-steroidal Antiinflammatory Drugs (NSAIDs) May Harm Knee Cartilage, While Cyclooxygenase (COX)-2 Inhibitors May Have Beneficial Effects on Knee Cartilage

In JAMA there is a report of a trial of 395 randomly selected adults, ages 51–80 years, who had magnetic resonance imaging (MRI) of the knee at baseline and 2.9 years later. Findings were correlated with NSAID use, as recorded by questionnaire.

Most (n = 334) used no NSAIDs at all. Those who used conventional NSAIDS (n = 21) had more knee cartilage defect development and greater knee cartilage volume loss than those subjects (n = 40) using COX-2 inhibitors, who had decreased knee cartilage defect development and less knee cartilage volume loss [1].

This study is limited by the relatively small numbers of subjects in the two cohorts. However, if the findings are confirmed by subsequent research, this might herald a change in the management of symptomatic osteoarthritis of the knees. Of course, such a change would be tempered by reports, 3 of them in one 2005 issue of the New England Journal of Medicine, documenting unforeseen cardiovascular events associated with COX-2 inhibitor use [2–4].

References

1. Ding C, Cicuttini F, Jones G. Do NSAIDs affect longitudinal changes in knee cartilage volume and knee cartilage defects in older adult? JAMA. 2009;122(9):836–842.
2. Solomon SD, McMurray JJV, Pfeffer MA, et al. Cardiovascular risk associated with celecoxib in a clinical trial for colorectal adenoma prevention. N Engl J Med. 2005;352(11): 1071–1080.
3. Nussmeier NA, Whelton AA, Brown MT, et al. Complications of the COX-2 inhibitors parecoxib and valdecoxib after cardiac surgery. N Engl J Med. 2005;352(11):1081–1091.
4. Bresalier RS, Sandler RS, Quan H, et al. Cardiovascular events associated with rofecoxib in a colorectal adenoma chemoprevention trial. N Engl J Med. 2005;352:1092–1102.

###

Men with Restless Leg Syndrome (RSL) Are at Increased Risk of Having Erectile Dysfunction (ED)

A sample of 23,119 men, all free of diabetes and arthritis, were evaluated regarding the incidence of RSL and ED, including noting the frequency of RSL symptoms. The authors report: "Men with RSL had a higher likelihood of concurrent ED, and the magnitude of the observed association was increased with a higher frequency of RSL symptoms" [1]. The authors postulate shared common determinants, notably dopaminergic hypofunction in the central nervous system.

RLS and ED seem to have a shared origin in dopamine dysfunction, and dopamine agonists are now routinely used to treat RLS [2]. What about dopamine agonists in ED? In fact, there are studies describing the use of apomorphine, with one study by Dula et al. describing sublingual apomorphine as "an effective and safe treatment for ED, with 2 and 4 mg providing the most acceptable therapeutic index" [3]. Will we ever see the day when a new dopamine agonist challenges the phosphodiesterase-5 inhibitors for the huge ED therapy market?

References

1. Gao X, Schwarzschild MA, O'Reilly EJ, Wang H, Ascheroi A. Restless legs syndrome and erectile dysfunction. Sleep. 2010;33(1):75–79.
2. Ekbom K, Ulfberg J. Restless legs syndrome. J Int Med. 266(5):419–431.
3. Dula E, Keating W, Siami PF, Edmonds A, O'Neil J, Buttler S. Efficacy and safety of fixed-dose and dose-optimization regimens of sublingual apomorphine versus placebo in men with erectile dysfunction. The Apomorphine Study Group. Urology. 2000;56(1):130–135.

###

Depression Is an Inflammatory State with Implications for Cardiac Disease

In healthy individuals, depression is associated with a 1.5 to 2.0 relative risk of developing coronary artery disease (CAD), and depressed patients with existing CAD have a relative risk of mortality between 1.5 and 2.5 [1]. Coexistent depression also increases the risk of mortality in coronary heart disease [2]. The most likely link is described by Dinan as a proinflammatory response, manifested as elevated levels of C-reactive protein (CRP) and cytokines such as tumor necrosis factor (TNF)-alpha [3].

In 2008 Tousoulis et al. helped to clarify the underlying inflammatory link. They studied 250 HF patients, 154 of whom suffered from major depression. These major depression patients were taking selective serotonin reuptake inhibitors (SSRIs) (n = 120), or tricyclic antidepressants (TCAs) and/or serotonin/norepinephrine reuptake inhibitors (SNRIs) (n = 34). The investigators report: "TNF-alpha and CRP levels were significantly lower in patients receiving TCA/SNRI compared to patients receiving SSRIs or those without depression." They conclude that treatment of patients with both HF and major depression with TCAs/SNRIs is associated with lower levels of TNF-alpha and CRP, and furthermore that the choice of antidepressant medication may have a significant effect on the underlying inflammatory process [4].

The link between depression and heart disease is not unexpected. What I did not anticipate was finding the difference between classes of antidepressants described by Tousoulis et al. Their comment regarding the "choice of antidepressant medication" having a significant effect on the inflammatory process seems to say that, in the setting of known or suspected heart disease, TCA and/or SNRI therapy may be better than SSRI use.

References

1. Lett HS, Blumenthal JA, Babyak MA, Sherwood A, Strauman T, Robins C, Newman MF. Depression as a risk factor for coronary artery disease: evidence, mechanisms, and treatment. Psychosom Med. 2004;66(3):305–315.
2. Barth J, Schumacher M, Herrmann-Lingen C. Depression as a risk factor for mortality in patients with coronary heart disease: a meta-analysis. Psychosom Med. 2004;66(6):820–823.
3. Dinan TG. Inflammatory markers in depression. Curr Opin Psychiatry. 2009;22(1):32–36.
4. Tousoulis D, Drolias A, Antoniades C, et al. Antidepressive treatment of inflammatory process in patients with heart failure: effects of proinflammatory cytokines and acute phase protein levels. Int J Cardiol. 2009;134(2):238–243.

###

Overweight Older Children and Adolescents Consume Fewer Calories than Their Healthy Weight Peers

In this book, I have presented very few facts based on posters and similar reports that have not been subject to peer review and publication, but I believe that this unanticipated finding merits a mention. Skinner of the University of North Carolina reviewed the dietary self-reports of 12,316 children and adolescents enrolled in the National Health and Nutrition Examination Study (NHANES). In the younger age group – 2 years of age and younger – the caloric intake of overweight/obese children exceeded that of healthy weight children. But about age 7, things changed, and by age 9 and older, healthy weight children consumed more calories than overweight/obese children. For example, in children ages 9–11, overweight/obese children consumed 1,988 kcal daily compared with 2,069 kcal for healthy weight children. Although boys consumed more calories than girls, the differences in caloric intake in the two cohorts extended to both sexes [1].

> The obvious explanation might seem to be a difference in physical activity in the two groups. Nevertheless, finding that the healthy weight cohort consumed less calories than those who were obese of is a bit counterintuitive, especially to anyone who has taken a good look lately at what overweight (and sometimes even healthy weight children) eat at a MacDonald's restaurant.

Reference

1. Skinner AC. Poster presentation 2863.511. Presented May 4, 2010 at the Pediatric Academic Societies 2010 Annual Meeting, Vancouver, BC.

###

Women Who Have Menopausal Night Sweats May Enjoy a Reduced Risk of Death Over the Following 20 Years

A study by Svartberg et al. involved 867 postmenopausal women with an average follow-up of 11.5 years. The found that women who, in addition to hot flashes, also had night sweats had an almost 30% lower all-cause mortality risk compared with women without this symptom, independent of the various risk factors possible, including estrogen use [1].

I cannot think of a clinical intervention that will come from this study, but it may be some comfort to our menopausal patients experiencing hot flashes with night sweats.

Reference

1. Svartberg J, von Mühlen D, Kritz-Silverstein D, Barrett-Connor E. Vasomotor symptoms and mortality. Menopause. 2009;16(5):888–891.

###

Marijuana Use May Be Associated with a Reduced Risk of Head and Neck Squamous Cell Carcinoma (HNSCC)

A sample 434 patients were matched with 547 controls, and all were surveyed for lifetime marijuana use. After adjusting for potential confounders such as tobacco and alcohol use, investigators found that subjects with a 10–20 year history of marijuana use had a significantly reduced risk (odds ratio 0.38) compared with those who had never used marijuana [1].

The astute reader will note that I am wandering into the land of esoterica, odd and unlikely findings that lack clinical application, as least for today. Certainly I am not going to recommend that anyone begin marijuana use just to reduce the risk of head and neck cancer. But in the future, who knows what might evolve from this and other observations? Read on to learn about some other fascinating findings.

Reference

1. Liang C, McClean MD, Marsit C, et al. A population-based case-control study of marijuana use and head and neck squamous cell cancer. Cancer Prev Res. 2009;2(8):759–768.

###

Eating Egg Yolks – 4 a Day, and Maybe Even Just 2 a Day – Reduces the Risk of Dry, Age-Related Macular Degeneration

The study involved 37 subjects with low macular pigment optical density, who were taking cholesterol-lowering statins and ate 2 or 4 egg yolks a day for 5 weeks, with determination of macular pigment optical density at baseline and at the end of the trial. The biochemical basis of the trial was that egg yolks contain lutein and zeaxanthin, postulated to augment macular pigment concentrations. The authors conclude: "Consumption of 4 egg yolks/d, and possibly of 2 egg yolks/d, for 5 wk benefited macular health in older adults" [1].

An interesting side note on this study is that of the subjects involved, HDL cholesterol increased by 5%, while LDL cholesterol did not change. Perhaps we will see different outcomes in studies lasting longer than 5 weeks, but perhaps not. Whatever the outcome, I would like to see the next study supported by some agency other than the American Egg Board.

Reference

1. Vishwanathan R, Goodrow-Kotyla EF, Wooten BR, Wilson TA, Nicolosi RJ. Consumption of 2 and 4 egg yolks/d for 5 wk increases macular pigment concentrations in older adults with low macular pigment taking cholesterol-lowering statins. Am J Clin Nutr. 2009;90(5):1271–1279.

###

Metformin Inhibits Endometrial Cancer Cell Proliferation In Vitro

Cantrell et al. studied the impact of metformin on endometrial cancer cell lines, finding potent inhibition of cell proliferation [1].

Given that diabetes and obesity both increase the risk of endometrial cancer, this fact has some implications in medication choice, especially in women who are at increased risk for endometrial cancer. And, looking to the future, might there be some cancer treatment possibilities here?

Reference

1. Cantrell LA, Zhou C, Mendivil A, Malloy KM, Gehrig PA, Bae-Jump VL. Metformin is a potent inhibitor of endometrial cancer cell proliferation – implications for a novel treatment strategy. Gynecol Oncol. 2010;116(1):92–98.

###

Transmission of Rabies Virus from an Organ Donor to Transplant Recipients Has Been Reported

Four persons received transplanted organs – kidneys, liver, and an arterial segment – from one donor, and within 30 days, all four developed encephalitis and died within 13 days of the onset of neurologic manifestations. A diagnosis of rabies was confirmed in all. The donor had died of a subarachnoid hemorrhage; he also had told of being bitten by a bat [1].

This unfortunate case highlights the importance of an exhaustive donor history in any organ transplantation setting.

Reference

1. Kusne S, Smilack J. Transmission of rabies virus from an organ donor to four transplant recipients. Liver Transpl. 2005;11(10):1295–1297.

Massive Cola Ingestion Can Cause Hypokalemic Myopathy

Tsimihodimos et al. describe a literature search that turned up six reports of muscle signs and symptoms, ranging from mild weakness to paralysis, in patients who consumed large amounts of cola drinks and who were found to have low serum potassium levels. One mechanism postulated is a fructose-induced chronic osmotic diarrhea, leading to potassium depletion.

I have visited areas of the United States where colas are the beverages of choice, and "water is for washing." Into this culture of widespread cola use, we have added the "supersize" containers. Hence we now need to worry about hypokalemia (albeit rare) as well as excessive caloric intake and obesity.

Reference

1. Tsimihodimos V, Kakaidi V, Elisaf M. Cola-induced hypokalemia: pathophysiologic mechanisms and clinical implications. Int J Clin Pract. 2009;63(6):900–902.

###

Electromagnetic Field (EMF) Exposure Has Shown Benefit in Both Normal Mice and Transgenic Mice Destined to Develop Alzheimer-Like Cognitive Impairment

The study cited used long-term high-frequency electromagnetic field exposure in the range found in cell phones. Alzheimer-prone mice subjected to this treatment showed reduced brain amyloid-beta deposition. The mice also showed increased neuronal activity and increased cerebral blood flow. As the authors state in the title to their paper: "Electromagnetic field treatment protects against and reverses cognitive impairment in Alzheimer disease mice" [1].

Yes, the subjects were mice and not humans, it being difficult to persuade human subjects to volunteer for brain biopsies during research studies. Still, wouldn't be ironic if EMF exposure turned out to be beneficial?

This study adds to the body of literature – and controversy – regarding the impact of electromagnetic waves on the human brain. Another recent study, this one in humans, involved interviewing 2,708 persons with glioma and 2,409 with meningioma with matched controls in regard to mobile telephone use. Subjects were recruited from 13 countries. In conclusion, the authors report that "no increase in risk of glioma or meningioma was observed with use of mobile phones." However, the article conclusion goes on to muddy the water just a little: "There were suggestions of an increased risk of glioma at the highest exposure levels, but biases and error prevent a causal interpretation" [2].

References

1. Arendash GW, Sanchez-Ramos J, Mori T, et al. Electromagnetic field treatment protects against and reverses cognitive impairment in Alzheimer disease mice. J Alzheimer Dis. 2010;19(1):191–210.
2. The INTERPHONE Study Group. Brain tumor risk in relation to mobile telephone use: results of the INTERPHONE International case-control study. Int J Epidemiol. 2010;39(3):675–694.

A Study Has Reported Finding No Evidence to Support the Contention that Resident Fatigue Leads to Increased Medical Errors

Mitchell et al. studied sentinel events (major medical mistakes) in a Dallas health system from 2004 to 2008, searching for the reasons these events happened. Concerning the 110 events identified, they report, "Root cause analysis showed no evidence of resident fatigue involvement" [1]. This finding seems to be supported by a review of the Joint Commission national databank, described by the authors, of 4,817 sentinel events from 1995 to 2007. (Note that this paper includes an era prior to 2003, when the 80-h workweek was implemented.) This review showed "no documented evidence of resident fatigue was found" [1].

Above I have presented some unforeseen and counter-intuitive findings. I end the chapter with this report, published in a surgery journal. As one who has struggled (as we physicians all have) with decision-making during times of sleep deprivation, I find that the conclusion contradicts one of my cherished belief systems. It also contradicts the story ascribed to a surgeon who served on the front lines in World War I, who reported that following long hours of surgery he would be aware that while his technical skills were intact, his judgment was impaired. Forced by circumstances of the battle to continue to operate, he would ask a less fatigued surgical colleague to examine that patient and confirm his diagnosis and surgical plan [2]. Still, data are data, and I suspect that we will see more studies of this issue in the future.

References

1. Mitchell CD, Mooty CR, Dunn EL, Ramberger KC, Mangram AJ. Resident fatigue: is there a patient safety issue? Am J Surg. 2009;198(6):811–816.
2. L'Etang HL. Ill health in senior officers, 1939–45: an unexplored influence on command decisions. In: The pathology of leadership. New York: Hawthorn Press; 1970. Chapter 9.

#####

Chapter 14
Some Timeless Truths About Medical Practice

*Truth is a constant variable. We seek it, we find it, our view-
point changes, and the truth changes to meet it.*

U.S. Surgeon William J. Mayo (1861–1939) [1]

*Caring for the patient encompasses both the science and the art
of medicine. The science of medicine embraces the entire stock-
pile of knowledge accumulated about man as a biologic entity.
The art of medicine consists of the skillful application of this
knowledge to a particular person for the maintenance of health
or amelioration of disease. Thus the meeting place of the science of medicine and the art of medicine is in the patient.*

U.S. Physician Hermann L. Blumgart (1895–1977) [2]

This final chapter of the book is to remind us that medicine is not just about
epidemiologic data, clinical correlates, diagnostic pearls, physical findings, drug
effects and intriguing reports in the medical literature. It is intended to put the prior
287 pages in perspective, emphasizing that essential medical facts really matter
only when we use them to help improve the health of our patients.

Sometimes we use these essential facts to lead us to the difficult diagnosis, or to
make the insightful therapeutic recommendation. And other times we somehow
process the information presented and then draw upon our reservoir of past lessons
learned – the triumphs, the near-misses, and the care gone wrong we wish we could
forget, but cannot – and we make what turns out to be the right, albeit not exactly
evidence-based, medical decision, based on our clinical intuition. The following
describes one such instance [3].

The setting is 2001, the time of the anthrax postal scare when letters containing anthrax
spores were mailed to two U.S. senators and to several news media offices. All suspicious
envelopes passed through the facilities of the U.S. Postal Service. In this case, or actually
series of cases, dubbed *Amerithrax* by the Federal Bureau of Investigation, at least 22
persons, perhaps more, were infected, and 5 of these individuals died. This true story
involves two of these victims of bioterrorism.

Patient A was a postal employee who consulted his physician, reported the finding of
anthrax at his workplace and described vague, flu-like symptoms. Public health experts
were consulted, advising Patient A's physician that, given the clinical facts presented,

R.B. Taylor, *Essential Medical Facts Every Clinician Should Know: To Prevent Medical
Errors, Pass Board Examinations and Provide Informed Patient Care*,
DOI 10.1007/978-1-4419-7874-5_14, © Springer Science+Business Media, LLC 2011

anthrax was a highly unlikely diagnosis. They advised against the use of antibiotics. Within days, the patient was dead of anthrax.

Patient B, also a worker at a postal facility where there had been an anthrax scare, presented a similar history of vague symptoms. In this instance, the doctor – unaware of Patient A – followed a different course. The doctor listened carefully as the patient described, "I know my body and something's just not right." Call it a hunch, but this physician started the patient on ciprofloxacin and admitted him to the hospital where, before long, a diagnosis of anthrax was confirmed, validating the empiric use of antibiotics and hospitalization.

Patient B survived, thanks largely to decisions made by the physician of first contact. This doctor listened to what the patient had to say, related this history to the known facts about the anthrax scare, probably considered the risks of anthrax as a must-not-miss diagnosis, and acted on sound clinical intuition.

> Now here I am, in a book about medical facts, extolling the virtues of intuition – or listening to your gut. But intuition is not anti-facts. Actually, in a sense, it is perhaps the loftiest application of knowing essential facts, when you have reached a point where, when faced with a complex clinical problem, your instincts point you in the right direction without apparent conscious thought.
> This brings me to the first of 9 process-oriented medical facts described in this chapter.

The Best Physicians Often Employ Fact-Based, Intuition-Guided Decision-Making

When I think of the phenomenon of clinical intuition, I think of Sherlock Holmes, the brainchild of physician-turned-writer Sir Arthur Conan Doyle. Holmes once told someone who sought his help, "Never mind, it is my business to know things. Perhaps I have trained myself to see what others overlook. If not, why should you come to consult me" [4]. I concur that training certainly plays a role, but training is clearly not the whole story. All of us have gone to professional school and received postgraduate training. The physicians for Patients A and B described above surely did, and yet only one followed the intuitive, and eventually life-saving, course.

Perhaps the secret is experience. Unfortunately, there is a common misconception that years of practice confer wisdom and that the more a doctor sees, the more he or she knows. This is certainly true up to a point, and the recent residency graduate has seen many fewer instances of aortic dissection, spinal osteomyelitis, and meningococcemia, just to name a few of the sometimes-difficult-to-diagnosis, but must-not-miss clinical entities. Yet some physicians seem immune to learning from experience, and some even seem determined to provide proof for the adage offered by American Surgeon J Chambers DaCosta (1863–1993): "What we call experience is often a series of ghastly mistakes" [5].

As we consider the relationship of experience to clinical intuition, and indeed to quality of care, and also to provide some evidence from the literature, I offer the report by Choudhry et al. in which the authors report their systematic review of 62 articles relating years in practice to various quality outcomes. They found that in 52% of the studies reviewed, there was evidence of decreasing performance with increasing years in practice for all outcomes assessed. Their conclusion: "Physicians who have been in practice longer may be at risk for providing lower quality care" [6].

If a long history of experience is not the key to intuitive practice, what about evidence-based medicine? Here we come to what Greenhalgh describes as "Intuition and evidence – uneasy bedfellows" [7]. From its emergence in the early 1990s, evidence based medicine (EBM) has become the *summum bonum* of academicians and house officers, alike. Protocols, ideally but not always, based on randomized clinical trials guide the actions of inexperienced physicians. Many of these protocols are guideline based, an apparently safe haven until one comes to recognize that some organizations promulgating guidelines have special interests to protect. For example, the American Urologic Association recommends that "prostate-specific antigen (PSA) should be offered to well-informed men aged 40 years or older who have a life expectancy of at least 10 years" [8]. This contrasts with recommendations by other major groups, such as the U.S. Preventive Services Task Force, a group that has no professional investment in performing prostate surgery.

In some other guidelines, evidence has been considered, and then guidelines have been promulgated, without actually using the results of the randomized clinical studies available, and instead incorporating the experience of the experts present. Such guidelines are called GOBSAT guidelines – "good old boys sat around a table" guidelines.

The conclusion must be that properly evaluated evidence, based on randomized clinical trials, can be highly useful in clinical practice, even if some of the guidelines derived are slightly suspect. Furthermore, we must also be wary of guideline-based protocols that limit our thinking. We should practice evidence-based, but not "evidence-burdened" medicine [7]. EBM is not really a radical change in how we think (The results of properly designed clinical trials have always been part of our decisions) and it has not changed the nature of medical practice. Rather, in the words of Djulbegovic, "We should consider EBM as a continually evolving heuristic structure for optimizing medical practice" [9].

The synthesis of all this, in my opinion, is as follows: Wise physicians who have actually learned from their clinical experience have better clinical outcomes than those who are rigidly protocol-driven in their approach to patients [7]. Why do some doctors learn from instances when things go wrong, and others make the same errors time after time? The difference may be a sense of curiosity, or the quality of humility, or maybe it is some inherited ability to see how things can be better. Whatever the reason, some gifted physicians achieve better outcomes by following a subtle, contextual decision-making pathway that, although it requires some degree of experience, is based on the creative integration of current facts and past lessons learned. In other words these physicians are willing to listen to their hunches – their intuition. Of course, these same physicians also probably have developed the skill of listening attentively to patients and families.

References

1. Mayo WJ. Writing the Annals of Surgery (1931;94:799). Quoted in Strauss MB. Familiar medical quotations. Boston: Little, Brown; 1968.
2. Blumgart HL. Caring for the patient. N Engl J Med. 1964;270(9):449–456.

3. Pink DH. A whole new mind: why right-brainers will rule the world. New York: Riverhead Books, 2005. Page 169.
4. Doyle AC. A case of identity. London: Strand (magazine), 1888.
5. DaCosta JC. The trials and triumphs of the surgeon. Philadelphia: Dorrance & Co, 1944.
6. Choudhry NK, Fletcher RH, Soumerai SB. Systematic review: the relationship between clinical experience and quality of health care. Ann Intern Med. 2005;141(4):260–273.
7. Greenhalgh T. Intuition and evidence – uneasy bedfellows. Br J Gen Pract. 2002; 52(478):395–400.
8. American Urological Association. AUA counters mainstream recommendations with the new best practice statement on prostate-specific antigen testing. Available at: http://www.auanet.org/content/press/press_releases/article.cfm?articleNo=129/ Accessed May 23, 2010.
9. Djulbegovic B, Guyatt GH, Ashcroft RE. Epistemologic inquiries in evidence-based medicine. Cancer Control. 2009;16(2):158–168.

###

Only Rarely Does a Patient Have Just One Disease

You have a patient newly diagnosed with Crohn disease, episodic cluster headache, or one of the more uncommon rheumatic diseases. It is time to think about management. As a careful and conscientious physician who doesn't encounter uncommon diseases every day (That is why we call them "uncommon."), you consult the panoply of current clinical practice guidelines (CPGs). Here is where we encounter a small problem with most published CPGs: They are promulgated by experts on the entity in question, and they assume the patient has only that single disease. They fail to account for co-morbidity.

What is the likelihood of any adult patient having multiple health problems? In fact, the probability is quite high, especially as the age of the patient increases. Among house staff, there is a humorous aphorism: "Good health means you haven't fully evaluated the patient." Consider the following data, all having to do with adult individuals living in the United States:

- The overall prevalence of episodic tension-type headache is 38.3% [1]. Frankly, I believe this to be a low figure but, of course, data trumps personal experience.
- The age-adjusted prevalence of obesity is 30.5% [2].
- In persons ages 40–59 the prevalence of hypertension is 32.6%, and is 66.3% in persons age 60 and above [3].
- Diabetes occurs in 13.7% of men and 11.7% of women age 30 and over [4].
- The American Heart Association estimates that 17,600,000 of us have some form of coronary heart disease [5].
- Heart failure is found in 17.4% of persons age 85 and older [6].
- Up to 4% of men and 8% of women have a clinically significant depressive disorder. Depressed mood, without the modifier "clinically significant" is so common that depression can be considered the common cold of mental illness [7].

Add to these possibilities the widespread prevalence of food allergy, drug intolerance, chronic anxiety states, irritable bowel syndrome, backache, and various types of chronic dermatitis, and you can see the potential for any given adult person to have a fairly long medical problem list. In a study of medical students logging problems per patient they encountered, the average patient had 2.4 health problems and one patient had as many as 14 problems [8]. I have personally seen longer lists than this.

Next, consider what happens when your patient has a list of 3–5 preexisting problems and then develops one of the uncommon problems mentioned as examples above: Crohn disease, episodic cluster headache, or one of the more uncommon rheumatic diseases. Guidelines may prompt you, sooner or later, to prescribe non-steroidal anti-inflammatory drugs (NSAIDs), lithium, sulfasalazine, methotrexate, steroids, or other medications that may affect other diseases the patient may have. What happens then?

Boyd et al. reviewed currently available guidelines for the 15 most common chronic diseases, including atrial fibrillation, hypercholesterolemia, osteoarthritis, and chronic obstructive pulmonary disease. Reviewers assessed each guideline in the setting of older patients with multiple comorbid diseases, differing patient preferences, various life expectancies and more. They found that "most CPGs did not modify or discuss the applicability of their recommendations for older patients with multiple comorbidities." They concluded that, when treating an older person with multiple comorbidities, following current CPGs could have undesirable effects [9].

In a 2009 editorial published in the Journal of the American Medical Association, Shaneyfelt and Centor discuss bias in clinical guidelines: "The most widely recognized bias is financial. Guidelines often have become marketing tools for device and pharmaceutical manufacturers... Financial ties between guideline panel members and industry are common. So-called experts on guideline panels are more likely to receive industry funding for research, consulting fees, and speakers' honoraria" [10]. Caveat emptor!

References

1. Schwartz BS, Stewart WF, Simon D, Lipton RB. Epidemiology of tension-type headache. JAMA. 1998;279(5):381–383.
2. Flegal KM, Carroll MD, Ogden CL, Johnson CL. Prevalence and trends in obesity among US adults, 1999–2000. JAMA. 2002;288(14):1723–1727.
3. Ong KL, Cheung BMY, Man YB, Lau CP, Lam KSL. Prevalence, awareness, treatment, and control of hypertension among United States adults 1999–2004. Hypertension. 2007;49(1):69–75.
4. Danaei G, Friedman AB, Oza S, Murray CJ, Ezzati M. Diabetes prevalence and diagnosis in the US states: analysis of health surveys. Popul Health Metr. 2009;25(9):7–16.
5. American Heart Association: Heart attack and angina statistics. Available at: http://www.americanheart.org/presenter.jhtml?identifier=4591/ Accessed May 24, 2010.
6. Bleumink GS, Knetsch AM, Sturkenboom MC, et al. Quantifying the heart failure epidemic: prevalence, incidence rate, lifetime risk and prognosis of heart failure: the Rotterdam Study. Eur Heart J. 2004;25(18):1614–1619.
7. Lehtinen V, Joukamaa M. Epidemiology of depression: prevalence, risk factors and treatment situation. Acta Psychiatr Scand. 2007;89(s377):7–10.
8. Sumner W 2nd. Student documentation of multiple diagnoses in family practice patients using a handheld student encounter log. Proc AMIA Symp. 2001:687–690.

9. Boyd CM, Darer J, Boult C, Fried LP, Boult L, Wu AW. Clinical practice guidelines and quality of care for older patients with multiple comorbid diseases: implications for pay for performance. JAMA. 2005;294(6):716–724.
10. Shaneyfelt TM, Centor RM. Reassessment of clinical practice guidelines: go gently into that good night. JAMA. 2009;301(8):868–869.

###

No Drug Has Only One Action

Occasionally you will encounter the patient with only one disease. You will never find the drug with only one action. Never. Even the placebo has potent side effects. Consider the action of placebo therapy on patients with benign prostatic hypertrophy, including improvement in the maximum urinary flow rate (Qmax) at the expense of an increased incidence of erectile dysfunction, described in Chap. 13.

When we prescribe a drug, we hope for a desired action, such as relief of arthritis pain. With the use of a nonsteroidal antiinflammatory drug (NSAID), the patient may also experience dizziness, tinnitus, gastrointestinal bleeding or exacerbation of heart failure. The protein pump inhibitor omeprazole (Prilosec) illustrates the wide spectrum of drug effects. Available in the United States without prescription, omeprazole is widely used for the symptoms of gastroesophageal reflux disease (GERD) and peptic ulcer disease. Yet, as beneficial and as seemingly safe (sold over-the-counter, after all) as the drug may be, there is a spectrum of problems. For example, direct side effects of omeprazole include diverse manifestations, including anaphylaxis, urticaria, pancreatitis, gynecomastia, myalgia, photosensitivity, and vertigo. There are also drug-drug reactions, with the most notorious being the interaction with clopidogrel, in which omeprazole seems to reduce the antiplatelet effect of clopidogrel [1]. Also consider an adverse outcome of the desired action of the drug, the suppression of gastric acid; Dial et all report the increased incidence of community-acquired *C. difficile* disease in persons using proton pump inhibitors [2]. Omeprazole can even interact with herbal remedies, as shown by Yin et al. whose study suggests a decreased effect of omeprazole when used concomitantly with ginkgo biloba [3].

Undesirable drug reactions can be much more than a mild heartburn or transient rash. A prospective observational study in England of 18,820 hospitalized adult patients revealed that 1,225 (6.5%) of these admissions were related to adverse drug reactions (ARDs) with the ADR being the direct cause of admission in 80% of cases. These authors report that the drugs most commonly implicated were: aspirin (low dose), diuretics, warfarin, and non-aspirin NSAIDs [4]. In another report, describing a review of 39 prospective studies from U.S. hospitals, the investigators found an overall 6.7% incidence of serious ADRs and 0.32% fatal ADRs in hospitalized patients [5].

The significance of no drug having only one effect is as follows: Adverse drug effects and associated risks have been mentioned often in this book. As new drugs are developed and new drug-drug interactions discovered, keeping up with the actions of medications will test the limits of our memories and our computers. Certainly we should be responsible for knowing the hazards of the drugs we prescribe often, and have a healthy suspicion of those we encounter seldom. Groopman has written, "Every clinical event has a core of uncertainty; no outcome is ever completely predictable" [6]. In no setting is this thought more pertinent than in prescribing for patients.

References

1. Norgard NB, Mathews KD, Wall GC. Drug-drug interaction between clopidogrel and the proton pump inhibitors. Ann Pharmacother. 2009;43(7):1266–1274.
2. Dial S, Delaney JAC, Barkun AN, Suissa S. Use of gastric acid-suppressive agents and the risk of community-acquired Clostridium difficile-associated disease. JAMA. 2005;294(23):2989–2995.
3. Yin OQ, Tomlinson B, Waye MM, Chow AH, Chow MS. Pharmacogenetics and herb-drug interactions: experience with ginkgo biloba and omeprazole. Pharmacogenetics. 2004;14(12):841–850.
4. Pirmohamed M, James S, Meakin S, et al. Adverse drug reactions as a cause of admission to hospital: prospective analysis of 18,820 patients. BMJ. 2004;329:15–19.
5. Lazarou J, Pomeranz BH, Corey PN. Incidence of adverse drug reactions in hospitalized patients: a meta-analysis of prospective studies. JAMA. 1998;279(15):1200–1205.
6. Groopman J. How doctors think. Boston: Houghton Mifflin, 2007. Page 113.

###

Just Being in a Medical Journal Doesn't Make it True

"It's not the things you don't know that get you, but the things you know that ain't so," according to Mark Twain. You are nearing the end of a book about medical facts, most of them coming from articles in medical journals. The best of them are reports of randomized clinical trials, published in widely-read peer-reviewed publications. I have also included a number of meta-analyses, a handy method of accumulating data regarding a huge number of subjects. In a few instances, I have cited review articles, internet sites, and even anecdotal case reports, while recognizing that the plural of "anecdote" is not data. Still, most of the facts presented are backed up by what seem to be credible studies. So is there an issue?

The issue is that what is found in medical journals must always be read critically. There are many ways misleading information finds its way into print, yes, even in our most prestigious journals. How does this happen? Just some of the ways include: the scientific hoax, the influence of study sponsors, faulty research design and statistical shading of analysis, publication bias including the impact of studies never published as all, and even the content of pharmaceutical advertisements.

Scientific hoaxes enjoy a rich history. Here is an early and amusing example: It concerns *penis captivus* – the medical condition in which a man and woman become inseparably connected during sexual intercourse. The story begins with an editorial by Theophilus Parvin printed in *Medical News* in 1884, describing *penis captivus* [1]. It was a pedantic and largely theoretical article, unlikely to be helpful to physicians of the day. Not long thereafter the same journal published a vividly described case report, involving "an uncommon form of vaginismus." The article relates that after a number of methods were tried, chloroform, administered to the woman, allowed separation of the couple [2]. The author of the case description, listed as Dr. Egerton Yorrick Davis, was none other than Sir William Osler. The piece was written to poke fun at the pomposity of Dr. Parvin, and was just one manifestation of Osler's mischievous side. In fact, Silverman et al. tell how Osler at one time, afflicted with renal colic, added small quartz stones to his urine specimen, and how he once, while traveling with his wife, signed the hotel register with his alias: Dr. Egerton Yorrick Davis. We can assume that Mrs. Osler was not amused [3].

The paper by Davis, aka Osler, was intended as a humorous prank. Not all spurious reports are published with similar impish intent. Some hoaxes seem to arise in the quest for grants, professional credibility, and perhaps even academic tenure. Here are a few examples: In the now famous "painted mouse" caper, a respected researcher at the Sloan-Kettering Institute for Cancer Research claimed to have achieved successful skin grafts between different stain of mice, presenting as evidence two mice whose skin had been painted with a felt-tip pen [4]. A researcher involved in a Harvard University study on sleep apnea in morbidly obese patients has been disciplined by the U.S. Department of Health and Human Services for falsifying data included in a published report [5].

In 2005, Lancet published a report by Sudbø and 13 co-authors that involved 9,241 subjects, and concluded, "Long-term use of NSAIDs is associated with a reduced incidence of oral cancer (including in active smokers), but also with an increased risk of death due to cardiovascular disease" [6]. Now, the "fact" that NSAIDs can reduce the incidence of oral cancer, even in smokers, might logically have appeared in one of the earlier chapters of this book, except for one small problem. The data in this study are false, concocted from "thin air" [7] One must wonder about the role of the 13 co-authors.

The "most-harm-caused" award for bogus studies goes to Dr. Andrew J. Wakefield who, with 12 co-authors, published a report linking the measles-mump-rubella (MMR) vaccine to autism, a report I described in Chap. 3 under the heading: "Childhood vaccines do not cause autism" [8]. Upon review of the paper and the methods used in the study, questions arose having to do with the small number of subjects (n = 12), the selection of subjects (not "consecutively referred," as claimed), and a sizeable contribution to Wakefield's research from attorneys representing families of children believed to have been harmed by the MMR vaccine. Lancet has fully retracted the paper from the published record [9].

I am not sure that many therapeutic recommendations were based on the "painted mice" caper, but reports concerning sleep apnea in morbidly obese patients and also of NSAIDs reducing the risk of oral cancer could influence clinical decisions. Consider the hypothetical smoker who begins using daily NSAIDs to prevent oral cancer and subsequently develops gastrointestinal bleeding. However, the prize goes to Wakefield et al. whose misleading report has undermined public confidence in childhood immunization practices and deterred tens of thousands of children from receiving the MMR vaccine.

The following few sections offer more reasons to question what we read in the medical literature.

References

1. An uncommon form of vaginismus (Editorial). Med News. 1884;45:602.
2. Davis EY. Vaginismus. Med News. 1884;45:673.
3. Silverman ME, Murray TJ, Bryan CS. The quotable Osler. Philadelphia: American College of Physicians; 2003. Page xxix.
4. Ariyan S. Of mice and men: honesty and integrity in medicine. Ann Surg. 1994;220(6):745–750.
5. Mirviss LG. Erstwhile medical school professor falsified sleep study data. The Harvard Crimson. Available at: http://www.thecrimson.com/article.aspx?ref=527563/ Accessed May 27, 2010.
6. Sudbø J, Lee JJ, Lippman SM, et al. Non-steroidal anti-inflammatory drugs and the risk of oral cancer: a nested case-control study. Lancet. 2005;366(9494):1359–1366.
7. Marris E. Doctor admits Lancet study is fiction. Nature. 2006;439(7074):248–249.
8. Wakefield AJ, Murch SH, Anthony A, et al. Ileal-lymphoid-nodular hyperplasia, non-specific colitis, and pervasive developmental disorder in children. Lancet. 1998;351(9103):637–641.
9. The editors of The Lancet. Retraction-Ileal-lymphoid-nodular hyperplasia, non-specific colitis, and pervasive developmental disorder in children. Lancet. 2010; 375(9713):445.

###

Statistical Analysis Can Be Misleading

We may not, as individual clinicians, always spot scientific fraud, but fortunately we can count on statistics and peer review to assure that what we are reading is true. But can we? After all, we clinicians – who are chiefly concerned with a patient's history, physical findings, diagnosis and response to therapy – generally have long since forgotten how to calculate analysis of variance or a Cox regression analysis. We rely on experts – the statisticians.

A researcher friend once quipped, "I can prove that the amount of damage in a fire is directly related to the number of fire trucks on the scene." This seems to suggest that the fire trucks cause the damage but, of course, they don't. The fire truck story seems to support the thesis of the book *How to Lie with Statistics* [1]. I went back to read the paper by Sudbø et al. the one with the fabricated data [2]. Here the authors offered readers statistical niceties such as standard deviations, hazard ratios, confidence intervals, and p values. Even Wakefield and his 12 co-authors found a p value somewhere in their study of 12 children [3].

Creative statistical analysis of questionable data is not the only problem. We must acknowledge the extreme pressure to have one's paper published in a well-regarded, high-impact journal, considering that the best journals accept only a small fraction of submitted manuscripts. Sadly, in an effort to publish the ground-breaking, career-making paper, some researchers yield to the temptation to manipulate data [4].

Other authors in search of a publisher sometimes resort to "spin" in their reports. Boutron et al. reviewed 72 published reports in which a parallel-group randomized clinical trial with a clearly identified clinical outcome yielded a statistically nonsignificant result (that is, $P \geq 0.5$), looking for reporting and interpretation of findings that were inconsistent with results. They found spin in 18.0% of titles. When maintext

Results, Discussion, and Conclusions sections were reviewed they found that spin in at least two of these sections in more than 40% of reports [5].

The extent of self-serving statistical legerdemain and inventive reporting has led one critic to offer the opinion, "There is increasing concern that most current published research findings are false... Simulations show that for most study designs and settings, it is more likely for a research claim to be false than true" [6]. Although the viewpoint that so much of what we read is false seems a little extreme to me, it does remind me of the description of some hapless author, attributed to Scots anthropologist Andrew Lang (1844–1912): "He uses statistics as a drunken man uses lamp posts, for support rather than illumination."

A special form of statistical shenanigans can occur in the selection of papers for a meta-analysis. Cleland offers an example: the long-term use of aspirin for coronary artery disease. He asked if we are being deceived by a biased presentation of the evidence. Here is what he writes: "A recent meta-analysis concluded that considerable uncertainty exists regarding the wisdom of giving aspirin for the prevention of a first vascular event in populations who are at a low or intermediate cardiovascular risk. This meta-analysis did not include three recent primary prevention trials – these were resoundingly neutral or showed evidence of harm" [7]. Had these three papers been included in the not-quite-systematic review, might the conclusion have been different?

References

1. Huff D, Geis I. How to lie with statistics, edition 12. New York: Norton, 1993.
2. Sudbø J, Lee JJ, Lippman SM, et al. Non-steroidal anti-inflammatory drugs and the risk of oral cancer: a nested case-control study. Lancet. 2005;366(9494):1359–1366.
3. Wakefield AJ, Murch SH, Anthony A, et al. Ileal-lymphoid-nodular hyperplasia, non-specific colitis, and pervasive developmental disorder in children. Lancet. 1998;351(9103):637–641.
4. Ncayiyana DJ. "Truth" in medical journal publishing. South African Med J. 2010; 100(2):71–72.
5. Boutron I, Dutton S, Ravaud P, Altman DG. Reporting and interpretation of randomized controlled trials with statistically nonsignificant results for primary outcomes. JAMA. 2010; 303(20):2058–2064.
6. Ioannidis JPA. Why most published research findings are false. PLoS Med. 2005;2(8):e124. Doi:10.1371/journal.pmed.0020124. Accessed May 28, 2010.
7. Cleland JGF. Long-term aspirin for coronary artery disease: are we being deceived by a biased presentation of the evidence? Future Cardiol. 2010;6(2):141–146.

Publication Bias Can Influence What We Read

Publication bias takes many forms. One type of bias arises in what happens to reports submitted for publication. As a hypothetical example, a study showing that a new antibiotic, tigercillin, is no more effective than peanut butter does not sound very exciting, even if the authors present a huge cohort of subjects and brilliant statistical analysis of data. Peer reviewers may well conclude that no one cares about a "wonder drug" that isn't very wonderful. Hopewell et al. studied publication bias by searching a number of databases of published studies and, very importantly, contacting researchers to identify additional studies. They concluded that clinical trials that show a "positive" outcome are more likely to be published and to be published more quickly than studies with "negative" outcomes [1].

Of course, the paper describing the woeful efficacy of tigercillin may well never be submitted for publication at all. This is especially likely to occur when a study is supported by a pharmaceutical company. Let us imagine that were 10 trials of the effectiveness of tigercillin sponsored by its pharmaceutical manufacturer parent, and that five studies showed some efficacy and five did not. Consider further that perhaps the five that showed "negative" results were never submitted for publication and merely languished in someone's desk drawer. In this scenario, however unlikely it may seem, clinicians would read only about the merits of the drug.

Can this sort of situation occur? The following is an example, described by Lurie and Wolfe; here I use the author's words to be sure the facts are stated correctly. "In 1996, due to reports of paradoxical bronchospasm associated with the use of GlaxoSmithKline's (GSK's) newly approved, long-acting inhaled β agonist salmeterol, and previous epidemics of asthma-related deaths in patients taking other long-acting β agonists, the company initiated a randomized trial comparing salmeterol (Serevent, known as Advair when combined with the steroid fluticasone) to placebo. The results have never been published. We only know the detailed results of this crucial study because the drug came before the U.S. Food and Drug Administration (FDA) Pulmonary-Allergy Drugs Advisory Committee on July 13, 2005. These documents provide insight into the manner in which the company manipulated the data it submitted to the FDA in an apparent attempt to convince the agency that the risks were smaller" [2].

I detect two transgressions here. The first is failure to submit the data for peer review and publication after finding some troubling asthma-related deaths. The second is apparent statistical slight-of-hand, which is described by Lurie and Wolfe [2]. The outcome was that a few months later, in November 2005, the FDA issued an advisory regarding the risk that use of long acting β agonists could lead to aggravation of bronchospasm and even asthma-related deaths.

In 1997 the British Medical Journal and more than 100 other medical journals worldwide offered an "amnesty" for unpublished trials, inviting readers to send information on unpublished studies [3]. I am not aware that there was a robust response to this invitation.

References

1. Hopewell S, Loudon K, Clarke MJ, Oxman AD, Dickerson K. Publication bias in clinical trials due to statistical significance or direction of trial results. Cochrane Database Sys Rev. 2009;(1):MR000006.
2. Lurie P, Wolfe SM, Misleading data analyses in salmeterol (SMART) study – GlaxoSmithKline's reply. Lancet. 2005;366(9493):1262–1265.
3. Smith R, Roberts I. An amnesty for unpublished trials. BMJ. 1997;315:622.

###

Pharmaceutical Advertisements, Even Those Appearing in Esteemed Medical Journals, Must Be Read with Great Care

Like it or not, some of the knowledge we use about drugs comes from pharmaceutical advertising, and here we must be careful about what we accept as "fact." In April, 2010, while working on this book and searching for pertinent facts, I came across an advertisement for Aleve brand of naproxen that appeared in a leading US medical journal [1]. One of the claims made in the ad was this: "Ibuprofen may decrease the antiplatelet benefit of aspirin. ALEVE doesn't impact the antiplatelet benefit in patients taking low-dose aspirin, according to a pharmacodynamic study." If true, this could influence a lot of prescribing decisions. The reference cited for ibuprofen is Advil Labeling by Wyeth Consumer Healthcare, 2006. Well and good, and this assertion is supported by a peer-reviewed study published in the *New England Journal of Medicine* that concludes: "Treatment with ibuprofen in patients with increased cardiovascular risk may limit the cardioprotective effects of aspirin" [2]. No disagreement here.

However my curiosity was aroused by the claim that naproxen was somehow exempt from this interaction. To support its superiority, the ad offers one study, described as Abstract 858, Arthritis Rheum. 2007;56(9 suppl):s359. I sought to read this publication, and I hunted in my usual handy sites: PubMed, Google Scholar, and our university's library website. No luck.

I did however, come across an editorial about coxibs written by the lead author, and here I learned of consultancies with Bayer, Merck, Novartis, Pfizer, and Sanofi [3]. Hmmm.

Not to be deterred, I went to the web site listed on the ad: the Naproxen Clinical Data Center [4].

Here I found a list of 12 publications relevant to naproxen. Among them was an article by Capone et al. which concludes: "Naproxen interfered with the inhibitory effect of aspirin on platelet COX-1 activity and function. This pharmacodynamic interaction might undermine the sustained inhibition of platelet COX-1 that is necessary for aspirin's cardioprotective effects" [5]. But doesn't this conclusion contradict the claim in the ad?

Not listed on the Naproxen Clinical Data Center is a 2008 paper by Gladding et al. that states: "In conclusion, ibuprofen, indomethacin, naproxen, and tiaprofenic acid all block the antiplatelet effect of aspirin" [6].

Finally, near the end of the list of 12 citations, I found the elusive "Abstract 858." Actually it was a poster, presented at a 2007 meeting of the American College of Rheumatology [7]. The authors of the poster reveal consultant and research support by Bayer (Guess what company makes Aleve.) and others. I was able to print out and study the poster, which concluded: "In the present study OTC doses of naproxen sodium 220 mg tid as well as acetaminophen 1,000 mg qid did not interfere with the antiplatelet effect of EC-ASA." Is a broad generalization being made from a study involving only 37 subjects and using only low doses of naproxen? I wondered why a full report of this study did not seem to have been published. Can we really trust the assertion made in the advertisement that Aleve doesn't impact the antiplatelet benefit in patients taking low-dose aspirin?

I don't want to join the current pummeling of the companies that make the drugs we use each day. But shouldn't "ethical" drug manufacturers be presenting ads with validity that stands up to a quick citation check? And what about the responsibility of medical journals that carry these ads, and thereby lend some legitimacy to the stated claims?

Here is an update to this story. In June, 2010 the report described above was – finally – published [8]. In the report, the authors note the small sample size and open-label design as study limitations. Despite the fact that this modest study has found its way into print, I wonder about the decision to use it as the basis for a major advertising campaign in the face of similar studies that report contradictory results [5, 6].

References

1. Pharmaceutical advertisement of Aleve. JAMA. 2010;303(14):1338.
2. Catella-Lawson F, Reilly MP, Kapoor SC, et al. Cyclooxygenase inhibitors and the antiplatelet effects of aspirin. N Engl J Med. 2001;345(25):1809–1817.
3. Brune K. Do case control studies on coxibs tell us anything new? Rheumatology 2007;46(3):435–438.
4. Naproxen Clinical Data Center. Available at: http://www.naproxenclinicals.com/ Accessed May 2, 2010.
5. Capone ML, Sciulli MG, Tacconelli S, et al. Pharmacodynamic interaction of naproxen with low-dose aspirin in healthy subjects. J Am Coll Cardiol. 2005;45(8):1295–1301.
6. Gladding PA, Webster MW, Farrell HB, Zent IS, Park R, Ruijne N. The antiplatelet effect of six non-steroidal anti-inflammatory drugs and their pharmacodynamic interaction with aspirin in healthy volunteers. Am J Cardiol. 2008;101(7):1060–1063.
7. Brune K, Hochberg MC, Schiff M, Oldenhof J, Zlotnick S. The platelet inhibitory effects of the combination of naproxen sodium or acetaminophen with low-dose aspirin. Poster 858. Presented at the American College of Rheumatology (ACR) 71st Annual Meeting, November 6–11, 2007. Boston, MA.
8. Oldenhof J, Hochberg M, Schiff M, Brune K. Effect of maximum OTC doses of naproxen sodium or acetaminophen on low-dose aspirin inhibition of serum thromboxane B2. Curr Med Res Opin. 2010;26(6):1497–1504.

The section above is adapted from a previously published paper: Taylor RB. Pharmaceutical advertisements, citations and trust. Fam Med. 2010;42(10):744–745. Used with permission.

###

Some of Today's Great Ideas – and the "Facts" We Cherish – Will Prove to Be Wrong

Richard Smith, editor of the British Medical Journal (BMJ), has been quoted as saying, "The BMJ is not in the business of publishing 'the truth'" [1]. Facts describe what we believe today, forming the basis of current decisions. Truth changes over time, as today's facts fall by the wayside and more are discovered.

The sections above illustrate just some of the ways in which our current beliefs may be careless, misguided, spurious, and possibly even the result of some statistical manipulation.

If anyone doubts the fate of medical facts, consider the following: Phenacetin was known to be a safe analgesic and was combined with aspirin and caffeine to make the popular over-the-counter painkiller APC, containing aspirin, phenacetin and caffeine. Then in 1953 we began to recognize chronic kidney disease in those who used large amounts of the drug, giving rise to the clinical epithet: phenacetin kidney. First marketed in 1956 as a remarkably safe and mild sedative, thalidomide was sold without prescription in Europe, safe even for use in children, and became so popular it was dubbed "the West German baby sitter." It was also considered safe for use in pregnancy. Then in 1961 physicians began to connect the dots between thalidomide and the rising number of children born with phocomelia [2]. Diethylstilbestrol, a synthetic estrogen synthesized in 1938 was considered a safe and effective remedy for premature labor, until it was found in 1971 to cause defects in the offspring of these pregnancies [3].

Today we all recognize the dangers of using large doses of phenacetin, and administering thalidomide or diethylstilbestrol to pregnant women. But these are "highlight films" of evolving medical facts. Other so-called facts, generally involving correlations instead of fatal nephritis or deformed children, have tended to linger. In 2007 Tatsioni et al. reported an intriguing study, looking at how findings based on observational studies tend to endure even after refutation by randomized controlled trials (RCTs). Among their examples, the authors cite "articles published in 2006 that referenced highly cited articles proposing benefits associated with beta-carotene for cancer (published in 1981 and contradicted long ago by RCTs in 1994–1996) and estrogen for Alzheimer disease (published in 1996 and contradicted recently by RCTs in 2004)" [4].

Whenever I think of the sometimes transitory nature of medical knowledge, I think of venerated American cardiologist Paul Dudley White, who believed that hypertension just might be needed – that is, "essential" – to push blood through the hardened arteries of older persons. In his 1931 book *Heart Disease*, White theorized that "hypertension may be an important compensatory mechanism which should not be tampered with..." [5]. Even the wisest of us are sometimes eventually proven wrong, and I can accept that some of the facts presented in these pages will not stand the test of time. New studies will be published, and some of our beliefs will change. If only you and I could predict which ones will fall by the wayside our lives would be much simpler, but we can't, and so, for the time being and based on the studies cited, the facts you will encounter here are the best I can offer today.

> *The message here, and throughout this chapter is this: Truth in medicine is a goal that will always be a little beyond our reach. Perhaps the word is not relevant to medicine. This is because knowledge evolves and today's facts can change. We clinicians must read constantly, question dogma and avoid the myth of certainty.*

References

1. Ncayiyana DJ. "Truth" in medical journal publishing. South African Med J. 2010;100(2):71–72.
2. Cartwright FF. Disease and history: the influence of disease in shaping the great events of history. New York: Crowell; 1972. Page 215–216.
3. Taylor RB. White coat tales: medicine' heroes, heritage and misadventures. New York: Springer; 2008. Pages 209–210.
4. Tatsioni A, Bonitsis NG, Ioannidis JP. Persistence of contradicted claims in the literature. JAMA. 2007;298(21):2517–2526.
5. White PD. Heart disease. New York: Macmillan; 1931. Page 326.

###

In the End, the Best Physicians, Like the Best Generals, Make the Fewest Errors

Since this book is about the using our knowledge of facts to help avoid medical errors, it seems reasonable to pause here to consider the problem of clinical missteps. I have tracked this "fewest errors" maxim back to English surgeon and anatomist Sir Astley Paston Cooper (1768–1841) who practiced eye surgery at Guy's Hospital in London. Dr. Cooper's exact words were: "I have made many mistakes myself; in learning the anatomy of the eye I dare say I have spoiled a hatful; the best surgeon, like the best general, is he who makes the fewest mistakes" [1]. (Parenthetically, the same quote – doctor, general and fewest mistakes – is also attributed to Sir William Osler [2].)

The most spectacular medical errors – most often occurring in the operating room – are the stuff of headlines. We have all heard of accidentally ligated ureters, various instruments left in surgical sites, and even one instance in which a 78 year old woman admitted for knee surgery instead was the recipient of a new prosthetic anal sphincter [3]. Then there is the series of three incidents in a single hospital in which surgeons operated on the wrong sides of patients' heads [4]. Most medical errors occur outside the operating room and, fortunately, most are not quite as egregious as, for example, enucleation of the wrong eye.

Non-operative medical errors fall into two broad categories: diagnostic and therapeutic, the latter chiefly related to medications. A retrospective study of 307 closed malpractice claims revealed that 181 (59%) of claims involved diagnostic errors resulting in harm to patients. Key factors contributing to these errors were failures in judgment in 79% of cases, vigilance or memory in 59%, and knowledge in 48% of cases [5]. Here I highlight the failure of *knowledge* in almost half of all cases. If the doctor does not know the significance of a right-sided varicocele, an intra-abdominal tumor may be missed (see Chap. 6). The physician unaware of the significance of the sudden onset of labored, rapid breathing in an otherwise healthy person may overlook a diagnosis of pulmonary embolism (see Chap. 8). Even failing to recognize harmful drug effects constitutes diagnostic error. Lacking the knowledge that sumatriptan can cause ischemic colitis or that metoclopramide is the most common cause of drug-induced movement disorders such as tardive dyskinesia can yield devastating results if the physician fails to act appropriately when a patient begun on one of these drugs calls to report abdominal pain or strange neurologic manifestations (see Chap. 10).

Medication errors are common in the hospital and in the doctor's office. Ridley et al. examined prescriptions written in 24 critical care units for 4 weeks. They found that 15% of these prescriptions had one or more errors, with failure to adhere to recommended drug use and ambiguous orders being common causes [6]. A study of medication errors by primary care physicians showed that 70% were prescribing errors. Somehow, the physician in each instance didn't know or didn't bring to mind some important fact about the drug [7]. Facts matter.

> *Any poker player will tell you that the key to coming out ahead at the end of the game is simple: Don't lose! Playing wisely, staying in when it makes sense and throwing in your hand when it doesn't is what makes a good player. Losing big hands is what hurts you most.*
>
> *I think there is an analogy here. To return to Dr. Cooper's aphorism: The best doctors make the fewest errors. They especially make the fewest BIG errors. And this brings me to an important point: They are not good doctors just because they make the fewest errors and especially the fewest big errors. Instead they make the fewest errors because they are good doctors. In my last book I called such a healer a Wise Physician [8]. This term describes a physician who is compassionate, thorough, vigilant, resourceful, and who knows the essential medical facts that can help avoid medical errors and provide informed patient care.*

References

1. Cooper Sir AP. Quoted in: Fraser's Magazine. 1862;66:574.
2. Osler Sir W. Valedictory address to graduates in Medicine and Surgery, McGill University. Can Med Surg J. 1875;3:433–442.
3. Pescovitz D. Surgeons perform erroneous anal surgery. Available at: http://boingboing.net/2008/03/21/surgeons-perform-err.html/ Accessed May 30, 2010.
4. Catalano K. Have you heard? The saga of wrong site surgery continues. Plas Surg Nurs. 2008;28(1):41–44.
5. Gandhi TK, Kachalia A, Thomas EJ, et al. Missed and delayed diagnosis in the ambulatory setting: a study of closed malpractice claims. Ann Intern Med. 2006;145(7):488–496.
6. Ridley SA, Booth SA, Thompson CM, et al. Prescription errors in UK critical care units. Anesthesia. 2004;59(12):1193–1200.
7. Kuo GM, Phillips RL, Graham D, Hickner JM. Medication errors by US family physicians and their office staff. Qual Saf Health Care. 2008;17(4):286–290.
8. Taylor RB. Medical wisdom and doctoring: the art of 21st century practice. New York: Springer, 2010.

#####

A Clinician's Glossary of Statistical Terms

Here is an admittedly incomplete and over-simplified glossary of statistical terms, intended to help patient care clinicians better understand published reports of clinical studies.

Absolute risk reduction (ARR)   Typically referring to adverse events, absolute risk describes the probability of an event in the population under study, and ARR is the arithmetic difference in the rates of events between study and control groups. Relative risk reduction (RRR) is the percentage difference in outcomes between the study and control groups. Here is an example: If a treatment, such as use of an antiplatelet agent, decreases the risk of a stroke from 2/1,000 to 1/1,000, than the absolute risk reduction is 1/1,000. And in this scenario, the relative risk reduction (described below) is 50%.

Bias   Also called systematic error, bias describes something that might confound the validity of a study. Examples include selection bias, recall bias and referral bias (see below).

Case–control study   A retrospective comparison of a group of subjects with a disease or outcome of interest with a group without the disease or outcome of interest, seeking a probable cause for the disease or outcome in the study (case) group that is absent in the control group. In other words, this study design starts with the disease or outcome and looks back to identify antecedent events, exposures or risk factors.

Cochrane collaboration   A network of physicians and scholars who perform systematic reviews and meta-analyses of randomized clinical trials and other research studies. The results of their efforts are found in *The Cochrane Database of Systematic Reviews*. The Cochrane database can be accessed at: http://www.cochrane.org/. The name commemorates the British physician and epidemiologist Archie Cochrane (1909–1988), who advocated for systematic summaries of best evidence to improve the effectiveness and efficiency of care.

Cohort   A defined group of people (subjects). A study group and a control group might each be called a cohort. A study cohort may share one of many types of attributes: year of birth, race, exposure to a disease, presence of a disease, use of a

R.B. Taylor, *Essential Medical Facts Every Clinician Should Know: To Prevent Medical Errors, Pass Board Examinations and Provide Informed Patient Care*,
DOI 10.1007/978-1-4419-7874-5, © Springer Science+Business Media, LLC 2011

drug, or something else. In contrast to a case–control study, a cohort study starts with the exposure and follows subjects to determine the outcome.

Cohort study   Research which involves examination of a study group (who received an intervention or were exposed to a risk) versus a control group. A long term follow-up of a group of persons accidentally exposed to radiation in an industrial accident versus a control group of unexposed persons would be a cohort study.

Hazard ratio (HR)   According to the National Cancer Institute, the hazard ratio describes how often a particular event happens in one group compared to how often it happens in another group, over time. In cancer research, hazard ratios are often used in clinical trials to measure survival at any point in time in a group of patients who have been given a specific treatment compared to a control group given another treatment or a placebo, generating the familiar "survival curves." In this setting, a hazard ratio of 1 means that there is no difference in survival between the two groups. A hazard ratio of greater than one or less than one means that survival was better in one of the groups.

Incidence   A measurement of the number of previously unaffected persons who develop a condition during a particular period of time, such as a year, 5 years or even a lifetime. Knowing the incidence of a disease helps us understand the likelihood that a disease will occur in a given person over a given time frame. For example, think of a cruise ship carrying 1,000 passengers on a week long voyage. If, during that voyage, 95 persons develop acute gastroenteritis, then the incidence of that disease in that population of passengers for that 7-day time interval is 95/1,000 or 9.5%.

Likelihood ratio (LR)   The likelihood that a given test result would be expected in a patient with the specific disease compared to the likelihood that that same result would be expected in a patient without the target disorder. The LR is helpful in assessing the probability that a specific diagnostic test will be useful. It does so by providing a direct estimate of how much a test result will change the odds of having a disease, and incorporates both the sensitivity and specificity of the test. The likelihood ratio for a positive test result is: sensitivity/1 – specificity. The likelihood ratio for a negative test result is: 1 – sensitivity/specificity. A LR less than 1 indicates a lower likelihood of disease, while a LR greater than 1 indicates a higher likelihood of disease. Tests with LRs less than 0.2 or greater than 5.0 tend to be the most useful clinically.

Meta-analysis   A type of systematic review (see below) that involves quantitative methods and rigorous pooling of data from applicable clinical trials. Perhaps the best known of the meta-analyses are the reports from the Cochrane Collaboration.

Number needed to treat (NNT)   The number of persons who must receive an intervention in order for one additional person to benefit. It can be calculated as the inverse of absolute risk reduction (1/ARR). In a report described in Chap. 13, the author calculates that to prevent a single instance of acute mastoiditis, 4,831 children (the NNT) with acute otitis media would require antibiotic therapy. The other side of the coin would be the **number needed to harm (NTH)**.

p-Value   See Statistical significance, below.

Post-test probability   The proportion of patients with a particular test result who have the target disorder. In deciding whether or not to invest in a specific test – for example, a magnetic resonance scan in a patient with headache – the post-test probability will help the clinician decide if the test result is likely to make a difference in the treatment of the patient.

Predictive value   A ratio, stated as a percentage, of the patients with a positive tests for a disease who actually have the disease. Chapter 9 describes a report of chest radiography to assess 58 bedridden patients for pneumonia; in this study the sensitivity was found to be 65%, the specificity 93%, and the positive and negative predictive values were 83 and 65%, respectively. Predictive value is strongly affected by the prevalence of a disease, even if the sensitivity and specificity of the test remain constant.

Pre-test probability   A measurement of the likelihood of a positive test result determined before the result of a test is known. For example, if we know, hypothetically, that in a large population of 50 year old asymptomatic women, the vitamin D level will be low in 9% of subjects, this figure represents the pre-test probability of finding a low serum level in the next asymptomatic 50-year-old woman tested.

Prevalence   A measurement of the total number of cases of the disease in the population at a given time. It may be stated as a percentage: the total number of cases in the population (the numerator) divided by the number of individuals in the population (the denominator). Hypertension, for example is often stated as having a 28–30% prevalence in the U.S. population. Prevalence tells us how common a disease is. In contrast, incidence tells us how many new cases occur in a given time frame.

Prospective study   A "looking-forward" study in which the outcome event has not yet occurred. An example might be a study of what happens when a group of overweight persons are treated with a new appetite suppressant versus the outcome in a similar group of persons who do not receive the drug. Randomized trials are all prospective studies, as are some cohort studies.

Randomized controlled trail (RCT)   The gold standard of clinical therapeutic research, the RCT is a study design that involves random allocation of subjects and interventions. With successful randomization of subjects, study and control group have comparable characteristics (even if we don't know what the relevant characteristics are!) and selection bias is absent.

Recall bias   A systematic error in a research study that occurs when evidence is collected by relying on the patient's memory. Think of a study that involves use of a new vaccine evaluated by an interview a few weeks later, asking about possible side effects.

Referral bias A type of systematic error related to who is assigned to the study versus the control group, typically seen when patients are referred from the community to a study in a tertiary care center, and decisions are made based on patient characteristics as to who should be in which cohort. The result is a non-randomized study.

Relative risk (RR) Also sometimes called the risk ratio. The probability of an adverse outcome occurring during a specified time interval in a study group exposed to some sort of event versus the outcome without the exposure. For example, we might be concerned with the relative risk of stroke among persons with and without hypertension.

Relative risk reduction (RRR) An expression of the degree to which an intervention decreases the probability of developing a disease, complication or other adverse outcome. An example presented in Chap. 9 is a meta-analysis of the relative risk reduction by age in regard to major cardiovascular events afforded by various categories of antihypertensive agents.

Reliability The consistency of an assessment method. If the speedometer on my car happens to be set to read 50 miles per hour (mph) when the actual speed is 60 mph, it will reflect this error every time, and thus be reliable even though it is not accurate. This will make scant difference to the traffic officer who writes the summons for speeding.

Retrospective cohort study An examination of what has already happened to a group of individuals who experienced an exposure or intervention compared with an otherwise similar group who did not experience the exposure or intervention. An example of such a study might be the record review to determine the uterine cancer risk that has already occurred in women exposed to hormone replacement therapy (HRT) compared to a similar group with no HRT exposure. A prospective cohort study, in contrast, would follow exposed and unexposed women into the future.

Selection bias In a cohort or case control study, selection bias occurs when, for one reason or another, study groups and control groups differ from the start. Suppose, for instance, that in a cohort study to determine the outcome of treating hypertension with a specific drug, the intervention group had far more diabetic patients than the control group.

Sensitivity (Sn) A measurement of the portion of items correctly detected as present. This usually has to do with tests used to detect disease. Thus a test with 100% (also stated as 1.0) sensitivity for tuberculosis, for example, would identify all persons with the disease, and a test with a 0.5 sensitivity would detect half of those infected. Compare this term with Specificity, described below. A test with a high sensitivity will have few false negatives.

Specificity (Sp) A measurement of the proportions of items correctly identified as not present, often represented as the percentage of healthy people who are correctly identified as not having a particular disease. Thus a test with 100%

(or alternatively, 1.0) specificity for tuberculosis, for example, would not identify (incorrectly) anyone from the healthy group as sick. A test with a high specificity will have few false positives. In Chap. 2, I describe a report of nitroglycerine used to identify a cardiac origin of chest pain; In the subjects studied, the diagnostic sensitivity of sublingual nitroglycerine was 72%, and the specificity was 37%. Thus using nitroglycerine to make decisions about the origin of chest pain will detect some, but not all, patients with coronary artery disease, but will yield a lot of false positives.

Statistical significance   Used often in this book, the term refers the likelihood that a result could occur by chance, usually expressed as a **p-value**. The smaller the p-value the less likely it is that the findings reported are the result of chance. If the level is 0.05, then there is only a 5% chance that the findings occurred by chance. In research terminology, a setting in which a so-called null hypothesis is often employed, the *smaller* the p-value, the *less* likely the null hypothesis is true, and consequently the more statistically significant the reported result is considered. Thus a p-value of 0.01 represents a higher level of statistical significance than a p-value of 0.05. Chapter 12 presents an example of the use of the p-value and statistical significance: A study of 15,630 men and 25,808 women in Spain followed up for a median period of 10 years led researchers to conclude that in men aged 29–69 years, alcohol intake was associated with a more than 30% lower coronary heart disease incidence. However, for women a similar benefit could not be demonstrated, with p values above 0.05 in all categories of alcohol use.

Stratification   A polysyllabic word that describes separating research subjects into clinically relevant subgroups for analysis. For example, we might stratify the analysis of a drug for treating hypertension by separately examining patients with and without elevated creatinine levels. This is one strategy for reducing confounding; another strategy would be to simply exclude patients with high creatinine levels from a study.

Systematic review   A general term describing a look-back at multiple published reports on a single topic in an attempt to answer one or more focused questions relevant to the topic. Using a reproducible search strategy in bibliographic data bases, and selecting all articles that meet specified criteria (e.g., sample size, randomization, or other design features) are the characteristics that make a review "systematic," in contrast to "what's in my file drawer."

Validity   A description of the extent to which a study accurately measures what the researcher set out to measure. There are various types of validity: **Face validity** is the research "sniff test:" Do the study design and results reported seem to make sense? **Internal validity** has to do with the integrity of the research design. **External validity** is a description of the extent to which the study conclusions are generalizable to other populations. These all differ from **reliability** – the reproducibility of the actual measuring instrument or procedure.

Index